Practical Emergency Resuscitation and Critical Care

D1388572

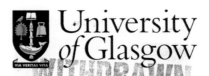

Practical Emergency Resuscitation and Critical Care

Edited by

Kaushal Shah, MD

Residency Director for the Emergency Medicine residency at Mount Sinai in New York City,
Chair of the SAEM Trauma Interest Group,
and Chair of the Education Committee for the New York chapter of ACEP

Jarone Lee, MD, MPH

Critical Care Attending
Quality Director, Surgical Critical Care
Division of Trauma, Emergency Surgery, Surgical Critical Care,
Massachusetts General Hospital
Harvard Medical School
Boston, MA, USA

Kamal Medlej, MD

Assistant Professor of Clinical Emergency Medicine,
Department of Emergency Medicine,
American University of Beirut Medical Center, Beirut, Lebanon

Scott D. Weingart, MD

Department of Emergency Medicine at the
Elmhurst Hospital Center; and Associate Professor and the
Director of ED Critical Care at the Mount Sinai School of Medicine, NY, USA

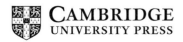
CAMBRIDGE
UNIVERSITY PRESS

CAMBRIDGE
UNIVERSITY PRESS

University Printing House, Cambridge CB2 8BS, United Kingdom

Published in the United States of America by Cambridge University Press, New York

Cambridge University Press is part of the University of Cambridge.

It furthers the University's mission by disseminating knowledge in the pursuit of
education, learning and research at the highest international levels of excellence.

www.cambridge.org
Information on this title: www.cambridge.org/9781107626850

First published 2013

Printed in the United Kingdom by TJ International Ltd. Padstow Cornwall

A catalogue record for this publication is available from the British Library

Library of Congress Cataloguing in Publication data
Practical emergency resuscitation and critical care / [edited by] Kaushal Shah,
Jarone Lee, Kamal Medlej, Scott D. Weingart.
   p. ; cm.
Includes bibliographical references and index.
ISBN 978-1-107-62685-0 (pbk.)
I. Shah, Kaushal, editor of compilation.   II. Lee, Jarone, editor of compilation.
III. Medlej, Kamal, editor of compilation.   IV. Weingart, Scott, editor of compilation.
[DNLM: 1. Critical Care–Handbooks.   2. Emergency Medical Services–Handbooks.
3. Resuscitation–Handbooks. WX 39]
RC86.7
616.02′5–dc23
2013022964

ISBN 978-1-107-62685-0 Paperback

Contents

Section 3: Neurological emergencies

Section editor: Michael N. Cocchi

Section 4: Cardiovascular emergencies

Section editor: Todd A. Seigel

Section 5: Respiratory emergencies

Section editor: Susan Wilcox

Section 6: Gastrointestinal emergencies

Section editor: Ruth Lamm

Section 7: Renal emergencies

Section editor: John E. Arbo

Section 8: Hematology–oncology emergencies

Section editor: Graham Walker

Section 9: Infectious disease emergencies

Section editor: Syed S. Ali

Section 10: Endocrine emergencies

Section editor: Brandon Godbout

Contributors

Syed S. Ali, MD
Assistant Professor of Medicine, Section of Emergency Medicine, Department of Medicine, and Director of Emergency Critical Care, Ben Taub General Hospital, Baylor College of Medicine, Houston, TX, USA

Nathan Allen, MD, FAAEM
Assistant Professor of Medicine and Medical Ethics, Assistant Residency Program Director, Section of Emergency Medicine, Department of Medicine, Baylor College of Medicine, Houston, TX, USA

John E. Arbo, MD
Assistant Professor of Medicine, Division of Emergency Medicine and Pulmonary Critical Care Medicine, Weill Cornell Medical College, New York Presbyterian Hospital, New York, NY, USA

Elizabeth Arrington, MD
Emergency Medicine Resident, Baylor College of Medicine, Houston, TX, USA

Ani Aydin, MD
Clinical Instructor, Department of Emergency Medicine, Yale-New Haven School of Medicine, New Haven, CT, USA

Kenneth R. L. Bernard, MD, MBA
Emergency Medicine Resident, Massachusetts General Hospital & Brigham and Women's Hospital, Boston, MA, USA

Amy Caggiula, MD
Resident Physician, Department of Emergency Medicine, St Luke's-Roosevelt Hospital Center, New York, NY, USA

Nolan Caldwell, MD
Chief Resident, Stanford/Kaiser Emergency Medicine Residency, Stanford, CA, USA

Jennifer L. Carey, MD
Toxicology Fellow, Department of Emergency Medicine, University of Massachusetts Medical School, Worcester, MA, USA

Jennifer Carnell, MD
Ultrasound Director, Section of Emergency Medicine, Department of Medicine, Baylor College of Medicine, Houston, TX, USA

Jayaram Chelluri, MD
Resident Physician, Department of Emergency Medicine, Icahn School of Medicine at Mount Sinai, New York, NY, USA

Michael N. Cocchi, MD
Director of Critical Care Quality, Assistant Professor of Medicine, Harvard Medical School, Beth Israel Deaconess Medical Center, Boston, MA, USA

Cristal Cristia, MD
Attending Physician, Department of Emergency Medicine, Beth Israel Deaconess Hospital-Milton, Milton, MA, USA

Vishal Demla, MD
Department of Emergency Medicine, Mount Sinai Medical Center, New York, NY, USA

Bram Dolcourt, MD
Assistant Professor of Emergency Medicine, Wayne State University School of Medicine, Detroit, MI, USA

Andrew Eyre, MD
Resident, Harvard Affiliated Emergency Medicine Residency, Brigham and Women's Hospital & Massachusetts General Hospital, Boston, MA, USA

Shawn Fagan, MD
Medical Director, Division of Burns, Massachusetts General Hospital, Harvard Medical School, Boston, MA, USA

Brandy Ferguson, MD
Resident Physician, Department of Emergency Medicine, Icahn School of Medicine at Mount Sinai, New York, NY, USA

Sarah Fisher, MD
Resident, Department of General Surgery, Emory University, Atlanta, GA, USA

Jonathan Friedstat, MD
Resident Physician, Plastic and Reconstructive Surgery, University of North Carolina, Chapel Hill, NC, USA

Brian C. Geyer, MD, PhD, MPH
Emergency Medicine Resident, Harvard Affiliated Emergency Medicine Residency, Massachusetts General Hospital & Brigham and Women's Hospital, Boston, MA, USA

Brandon Godbout, MD
Attending Physician, Department of Emergency Medicine, Director of Simulation Medicine, Lenox Hill Hospital, New York, NY, USA

Jeremy Gonda, MD
Critical Care Fellow, Department of Critical Care Medicine, Stanford University School of Medicine, Stanford, CA, USA

Jeremy Goverman, MD
Attending Surgeon, Division of Burns, Massachusetts General Hospital, Harvard Medical School, Boston, MA, USA

Ashley L. Greiner, MD, MPH
Resident Physician, Beth Isreal Deaconness Medical Center, Boston, MA, USA

Casey Grover, MD
Chief Resident, Stanford/Kaiser Emergency Medicine Residency, Stanford, CA, USA

Carla Haack, MD
Assistant Professor of General and GI Surgery, Emory University, Atlanta, GA, USA

Abigail Hankin, MD
Clinical Instructor of Emergency Medicine, Tufts University School of Medicine, Attending Physician, Maine Medical Center, Portland, ME, USA

John W. Hardin, MD
Resident Physician, Harvard Affiliated Emergency Medicine Residency, Beth Israel Deaconess Medical Center, Boston, MA, USA

Katrina L. Harper, MD
Mount Sinai School of Medicine, New York, NY, USA

Gregory Hayward, MD
Department of Emergency Medicine, Rhode Island Hospital, Providence, RI, USA

Stephen Hendriksen, MD
Resident Physician, Department of Emergency Medicine, Alpert Medical School of Brown University, Providence, RI, USA

Daniel Herbert-Cohen, MD
Resident Physician, Department of Emergency Medicine, St Luke's-Roosevelt Hospital Center, New York, NY, USA

Nadine Himelfarb, MD
Memorial Hospital of Rhode Island, Pawtucket, RI, USA

Calvin E. Hwang, MD
Resident Physician, Stanford/Kaiser Emergency Medicine Residency, Stanford, CA, USA

Jacob D. Isserman, MD
Department of Emergency Medicine, Icahn School of Medicine at Mount Sinai, New York, NY, USA

Joshua Jauregui, MD
University of Washington School of Medicine, Division of Emergency Medicine, Seattle, WA, USA

Joshua W. Joseph, MD
Resident in Emergency Medicine, Beth-Israel Deaconess – Harvard Affiliated Emergency Medicine Residency, Boston, MA, USA

Elena Kapilevich, MD
Resident Physician, Department of Emergency Medicine, Alpert Medical School of Brown University, Providence, RI, USA

Feras H. Khan, MD
Assistant Professor, Department of Internal Medicine, Division of Pulmonary and Critical Care Medicine, Department of Emergency Medicine, University of Maryland, Baltimore, MD, USA

Sarvotham Kini, MD, FACEP, FACS
Staff Physician, Atlanta VA Medical Center, Decatur, GA, USA

Karen A. Kinnaman, MD
Resident, Harvard Affiliated Emergency Medicine Program, Partners Healthcare, Boston, MA, USA

Ruth Lamm, MD, FACEP
Assistant Professor of Emergency Medicine, Assistant Professor of Surgery, Emory University School of Medicine, Department of Emergency Medicine, Atlanta, GA, USA

Calvin Lee, MD
Resident Physician, Harvard Affiliated Emergency Medicine Residency, Massachusetts General Hospital & Brigham and Women's Hospital, Boston, MA, USA

Jarone Lee, MD, MPH
Critical Care Attending, Quality Director, Surgical Critical Care, Division of Trauma, Emergency Surgery, Surgical Critical Care, Massachusetts General Hospital, Harvard Medical School, Boston, MA, USA

Charles Lei, MD
Chief Resident, Stanford/Kaiser Emergency Medicine Residency, Stanford, CA, USA

John Lemos, MD
Attending Physician, Department of Emergency Medicine, Emory University, Atlanta, GA, USA

Daniel J. Lepp, MD
Resident in Emergency Medicine, St. Luke's-Roosevelt Hospital Center, New York, NY, USA

Elisabeth Lessenich, MD, MPH
Emergency Medicine Resident, Massachusetts General Hospital & Brigham and Women's Hospital, Boston, MA, USA

Brandon Maughan, MD, MHS
Emergency Medicine Resident, Alpert Medical School of Brown University, Providence, RI, USA

Julie Mayglothling, MD, FACEP
Associate Professor, Department of Emergency Medicine, Department of Surgery, Division of Trauma/Critical Care, Virginia Commonwealth University, Richmond, VA, USA

Kevin McConnell, MD
Assistant Professor of Surgery, Acute and Critical Care Surgery, Emory University School of Medicine, Atlanta, GA, USA

Laura Medford-Davis, MD
Emergency Medicine Resident, Baylor College of Medicine, Houston, TX, USA

Kamal Medlej, MD
Assistant Professor of Clinical Emergency Medicine, Department of Emergency Medicine, American University of Beirut Medical Center, Beirut, Lebanon

Heather Meissen, ACNP-BC
Director of NP/PA Critical Care Residency, Surgical Intensive Care Unit, Emory University Hospital, Emory Healthcare, Atlanta, GA, USA

Payal Modi, MD
Resident Physician, Department of Emergency Medicine, Alpert Medical School of Brown University, Providence, RI, USA

Joel Moll, MD, FACEP
Assistant Professor of Emergency Medicine, Director of Emergency Medicine Administration Fellowship, Director of Academic and Clinical Integration and Assistant Residency Director, Department of Emergency Medicine, Emory University School of Medicine, Atlanta, GA, USA

Jolene H. Nakao, MD, MPH
Resident Physician, Department of Emergency Medicine, St. Luke's-Roosevelt Hospital Center, New York, NY, USA

Matthew Nicholls, ACNP
Surgical Intensive Care Unit, Emory University Hospital, Atlanta, GA, USA

Lindsay Oelze, MD
Resident Physician, Baylor College of Medicine, Section of Emergency Medicine, Department of Medicine, Houston, TX, USA

Carolyn Maher Overman, MD
Emergency Medicine Resident, Emory University School of Medicine, Atlanta, GA, USA

Viral Patel, MD
Emergency Medicine Resident, St. Luke's-Roosevelt Hospital Center, New York, NY, USA

Timothy C. Peck, MD
Chief Resident, Harvard Affiliated Emergency Medicine Residency, Beth Israel Deaconess Medical Center, Boston, MA, USA

Jeffrey Pepin, MD
Resident Director of Medical Student/Intern Academic Affairs, Department of Emergency Medicine, Lincoln Medical and Mental Health Medical Center, Bronx, NY, USA

Candace Pettigrew, MD
Resident Physician, Baylor College of Medicine, Section of Emergency Medicine, Department of Medicine, Houston, TX, USA

Byron Pitts, MD
Resident Physician, Department of Emergency Medicine, Emory University, Atlanta, GA, USA

Zubaid Rafique, MD
Assistant Professor of Medicine, Section of Emergency Medicine, Department of Medicine, Baylor College of Medicine, Houston, TX, USA

Chanu Rhee, MD
Infectious Disease Fellow, Massachusetts General Hospital & Brigham and Women's Hospital, Boston, MA, USA

Jonathan C. Roberts, MD
Attending Physician, Department of Emergency Medicine, Beth Israel Deaconess Hospital-Milton, Milton, MA, USA

Daniel Rolston, MD, MS
Chief Resident, St. Luke's-Roosevelt Hospital Center, New York, NY, USA

Steven C. Rougas, MD
Department of Emergency Medicine, Warren Alpert Medical School of Brown University, Providence, RI, USA

Benjamin Schnapp, MD
Resident Physician, Department of Emergency Medicine, Mount Sinai Medical Center, New York, NY, USA

Kathryn A. Seal, MD
Resident Physician, Emory University, Atlanta, GA, USA

Raghu Seethala, MD
Emergency Medicine and Critical Care Attending, Brigham and Women's Hospital, Harvard Medical School, Boston, MA, USA

Todd A. Seigel, MD
Assistant Professor of Emergency Medicine, Warren Alpert Medical School of Brown University, Providence, RI, USA

Navdeep Sekhon, MD
Assistant Professor, Baylor College of Medicine, Houston, TX, USA

Kaushal Shah, MD
Residency Program Director, Department of Emergency Medicine, Icahn School of Medicine at Mount Sinai, New York, NY, USA

Robert L. Sherwin, MD
Assistant Professor of Emergency Medicine, Wayne State University School of Medicine, Detroit, MI, USA

Kirill Shishlov, MD, MPH
Resident Physician, Department of Emergency Medicine, St Luke's-Roosevelt Hospital Center, New York, NY, USA

Ashley Shreves, MD
Assistant Professor, Department of Emergency Medicine, Brookdale Department of Geriatrics and Palliative Medicine, Mount Sinai School of Medicine, New York, NY, USA

Sebastian Siadecki, MD
Resident Physician, Department of Emergency Medicine, St Luke's-Roosevelt Hospital Center, New York, NY, USA

Jeffrey N. Siegelman, MD
Assistant Professor of Emergency Medicine, Emory University, Atlanta, GA, USA

Liza Gonen Smith, MD
Assistant Professor of Emergency Medicine, Tufts University School of Medicine, Attending Physician, Baystate Medical Center, Springfield, MA, USA

Ted Stettner, MD
Assistant Professor of Emergency Medicine, Emory University, Atlanta, GA, USA

Marie Carmelle Tabuteau, DO, MBA
Emergency Medicine Resident, Emory University, Atlanta, GA, USA

Joseph E. Tonna, MD
Resident Physician, Stanford/Kaiser Emergency Medicine Residency, Stanford, CA, USA

N. Seth Trueger, MD
Health Policy Fellow and Adjunct Instructor in Emergency Medicine, George Washington University Hospital, Washington, DC, USA

Chad Van Ginkel, MD, MPH
Resident Physician, Department of Emergency Medicine, Alpert Medical School of Brown University, Providence, RI, USA

Bina Vasantharam, MD
Resident Physician, Emergency Medicine, Emory University, Atlanta, GA, USA

Graham Walker, MD
Staff Physician, Stanford/Kaiser Emergency Medicine Residency, Massachusetts General Hospital & Brigham and Women's Hosptial, Boston, MA, USA

Susan Wilcox, MD
Attending Physician, Department of Emergency Medicine, Department of Anesthesia, Critical Care, and Pain Medicine, Massachusetts General Hospital, Harvard Medical School, Boston, MA, USA

Sandra J. Williams, DO, MPH
Assistant Professor of Emergency Medicine, Baylor College of Medicine, Houston, TX, USA

Matthew L. Wong, MD, MPH
Resident, Beth Israel Deaconess Medical Center, Boston, MA, USA

Nelson Wong, MD
Resident Physician, Department of Emergency Medicine, Mount Sinai Medical Center, New York, NY, USA

Samantha Wood, MD
Assistant Professor of Emergency Medicine, Tufts University School of Medicine and Attending Physician, Maine Medical Center, Portland, ME, USA

John Woodruff, MD
Resident Physician, Department of Emergency Medicine, Emory University, Atlanta, GA, USA

Benjamin Zabar, MD
Resident Physician, Department of Emergency Medicine, St Luke's-Roosevelt Hospital Center, New York, NY, USA

Preface

Every day more and more critically ill patients arrive at the emergency department (ED) requiring both rapid stabilization and the full spectrum of treatments that are normally delivered in intensive care units (ICU). This book's content is unique in that it was written, researched, and edited by physicians with training in both emergency medicine and critical care from leading medical institutions throughout the world. It describes the initial steps in the stabilization of acutely ill patients, and also details the management if they continue to further decompensate. This book fills an important niche by providing concise, evidence-based summaries of key material and concepts. Although it was designed with the medical student and junior resident in mind, it will surely help practitioners at all levels of experience better manage their critically ill patients. Not only does it provide key points and details of well-established and evidence-based interventions in bullet point format, it is easy to read and portable – ideal for the busy clinician at the bedside.

Abbreviations

AA	aortic stenosis
AAA	abdominal aortic aneurysm
ABG	arterial blood gases
ABI	ankle-brachial index
AC	assist control (assist volume control)
ACE	angiotensin-converting enzyme
ACLS	advanced cardiac life support
ACS	abdominal compartment syndrome
ACS	acute coronary syndrome
ACTH	corticotropin (adrenocorticotropic hormone)
ADH	antidiuretic hormone
ADHF	acute decompensated heart failure
AEF	aortoenteric fistula
AG	anion gap
AGA	American Gastroenterological Association
AIP	intra-abdominal pressure
AKI	acute kidney injury
ALI	acute lung injury
ALT	alanine aminotransferase
AMI	acute myocardial infarction
AMS	altered mental status
ANC	absolute neutrophil count
ANT	acute tubular necrosis
AP	anteroposterior
APRV	airway pressure release ventilation
AR	aortic regurgitation
ARDS	acute respiratory distress syndrome
AST	aspartate aminotransferase (same as SGOT)
ATLS	advanced trauma life support
ATP	adenosine triphosphate
AV	atrioventricular
AVM	arteriovenous malformation
AVNRT	atrioventricular nodal reentrant tachycardia

Bi-PAP	bi-level positive airway pressure
BISAP	bedside index of severity in acute pancreatitis
BMV	bag-mask ventilation
BNP	brain (or B-type) natriuretic peptide
BP	blood pressure
bpm	beats per minute
BRBPR	bright red blood per rectum
CAP	community-acquired pneumonia
CBC	complete blood count
CDC	Centers for Disease Control
CHF	congestive heart failure
CI	cardiac index
CMV	controlled mandatory ventilation
CMV	cytomegalovirus
CNS	central nervous system
CO	cardiac output
COPD	chronic obstructive pulmonary disease
CPAP	constant positive airway pressure
CPK	creatine phosphokinase
CPP	cerebral perfusion pressure
CPR	cardiopulmonary resuscitation
CRP	C-reactive protein
CRT	cardiac resynchronization therapy
CSF	cerebral spinal fluid (CSF)
c-spine	cervical spine
CT	computed tomography
CTA	CT-angiography
CVA	cerebrovascular accident
CVC	central venous catheter
CVP	central venous pressure
CVVH	continuous veno-venous hemofiltration
CVVHD	continuous venous-venous hemodiafiltration
CXR	chest radiograph/chest radiography
DI	diabetes insipidus
DIC	disseminated intravascular coagulation
DKA	diabetic ketoacidosis
DNI	do not intubate
DNR	do not resuscitate
DO_2	oxygen delivery
DOL	diagnostic peritoneal lavage
DSI	delayed sequence intubation
DVT	deep vein thrombosis
EAST	Eastern Association for the Surgery of Trauma
ECG	electrocardiogram

ECMO	extracorporeal membrane oxygenation
ED	emergency department
EDT	emergency department thoracotomy
EEG	electroencephalogram/electroencephalography
EGA	extraglottic airways
EGDT	early goal-directed therapy
ELM	external laryngeal manipulation
EMG	electromyography
EMS	emergency medical services
EOR	endpoint of resuscitation
ERCP	endoscopic retrograde cholangiopancreatography
ESR	erythrocyte sedimentation rate
ET	endotracheal tube
$EtCO_2$	end-tidal carbon dioxide
ETT	endotracheal tube
EUS	emergency ultrasonography
EVD	external ventricular drain
FAST	Focused Assessment with Sonography in Trauma
FEV_1	forced expiratory volume in 1 second
FFP	fresh frozen plasma
FiO_2	fraction of inspired oxygen
FSP	fibrin split products
FVC	forced vital capacity
FVCA	four-vessel cerebrovascular angiography
GCS	Glasgow Coma Score
GCSE	generalized convulsive status epilepticus
GFR	glomerular filtration rate
GI	gastrointestinal
GOLD	Global Initiative for Chronic Obstructive Lung Disease
GSW	gunshot wounds
HbA	hemoglobin A
HBO	hyperbaric oxygen
HCAP	healthcare-associated pneumonia
hCG	human chorionic gonadotropin
Hct	hematocrit
HELLP	hemolysis, elevated liver enzymes, and low platelet count
HFOV	high-frequency oscillatory ventilation
Hgb	hemoglobin
HSV	herpes simplex virus
I/E ratio	ratio of inspiratory time to expiratory time
ICH	intracerebral hemorrhage
ICP	intracranial pressure
ICU	intensive care unit
IFR	inspiratory flow rate

iHD	intermittent hemodialysis
INR	international normalized ratio
IRIS	immune reconstitution inflammatory syndrome
IV	intravenous
IVC	inferior vena cava
IVDA	intravenous drug abuse
IVDU	intravenous drug use
IVF	intravenous fluid
IVIg	intravenous immunoglobulin
IVP	intravenous push
JVD	jugular venous distension
KDIGO	Kidney Disease Improving Global Outcomes
L	liter
LAD	left anterior descending artery
LCX	left circumflex artery
LDH	lactate dehydrogenase
LFT	liver function tests
LOS	length of stay
lpm	liters per minute
LRINEC	laboratory risk indicator for necrotizing fasciitis
LVAD	left ventricular assist device
LVEDV	LV end-diastolic volume
MAE	mesenteric arterial embolism
MAHA	microangiopathic hemolytic anemia
MAP	mean arterial pressure
MASCC	Multinational Association for Supportive Care in Cancer
MAST	military anti-shock trousers
MAT	mesenteric arterial thrombosis
MDI	metered-dose inhaler
MEN-2	multiple endocrine endpoint neoplasia type 2
MESS	mangled extremity severity score
MH	malignant hyperthermia
mL	milliliter
MOCHA	markers of coagulation hemostatic activation
MODS	multi-organ dysfunction syndrome
MR	mitral regurgitation
MRA	magnetic resonance angiography
MRI	magnetic resonance imaging
MRSA	methicillin-resistant *Staphylococcus aureus*
MS	mitral stenosis
MVT	mesenteric venous thrombosis
NCSE	nonconvulsive status epilepticus
NF-1	neurofibromatosis type 1
NIV	noninvasive ventilation

NMS	neuroleptic malignant syndrome
NNT	number needed to treat
NOMI	nonocclusive mesenteric ischemia
NPO	nothing by mouth
NPPV	noninvasive positive-pressure ventilation
NRB	non-rebreather mask
NS	normal saline
NSTI	necrotizing soft tissue skin infection
OG	osmolal gap
OR	operating room
PA	posteroanterior
PAC	pulmonary artery catheter
$PaCO_2$	partial pressure of carbon dioxide
PAP	proximal airway pressure
PC	pressure control
PCC	prothrombin complex concentrate
PCI	percutaneous coronary intervention
PCP	*Pneumocystis jirovecii* pneumonia
PCWP	pulmonary capillary wedge pressure
PE	pulmonary embolism
PEA	pulseless electrical activity
PEEP	positive end-expiratory pressure
PIP	peak inspiratory pressure
PMH	past medical history
PPI	proton pump inhibitor
PPV	pulse pressure variation
PRBC	packed red blood cells
PS	pressure support
PT	prothrombin time
PTT	partial thromboplastin time
PVC	premature ventricular contraction
RBC	red blood cell
RCA	right coronary artery
ROSC	return of spontaneous circulation
RR	respiratory rate
RRT	renal replacement therapy
RSI	rapid sequence intubation
RTA	renal tubular acidosis
RV	right ventricle
SA	sinoatrial
SAH	subarachnoid hemorrhage
SaO_2	arterial oxygen saturation
SBP	systolic blood pressure
SCD	sickle cell disease

ScvO$_2$	central venous oxygen saturation
SDH	subdural hemorrhage
SGOT	serum glutamic oxalo-acetic transaminase (same as AST)
SIADH	syndrome of inappropriate antidiuretic hormone secretion
SIMV	synchronized intermittent mandatory ventilation
SIRS	severe/systemic inflammatory response syndrome
SLED	sustained low-efficiency dialysis
SMA	superior mesenteric artery
SpO$_2$	pulse oximeter saturation estimate
SPV	systolic pressure variation
ST	sinus tachycardia
STEMI	ST-segment elevation myocardial infarction
SVC	superior vena cava
SvO$_2$	mixed venous oxygen saturation
SVR	systemic vascular resistance
SVT	supraventricular tachycardia
TB	tuberculosis
TBI	traumatic brain injury
TBSA	total body surface area
TCA	tricyclic antidepressant
T_i	inspiratory time
TIPS	transjugular intrahepatic portosystemic shunt
TLS	tumor lysis syndrome
tPA	tissue plasminogen activator
TSCI	traumatic spinal cord injury
TSH	thyroid-stimulating hormone
TTKG	transtubular potassium gradient
TTP/HUS	thrombotic thrombocytopenic purpura/hemolytic uremic syndrome
TXA	tranexamic acid
UA	unstable angina
Uk	urine potassium
UOP	urine output
Uosm	urine osmolality
US	ultrasonography, ultrasound
VAP	ventilator-associated pneumonia
VATS	video assisted thoracic surgery
VBG	venous blood gases
VF	ventricular fibrillation
VHL	von Hippel-Lindau disease
VILI	ventilator-induced lung injury
VL	video laryngoscope/laryngoscopy
VO$_2$	oxygen consumption
VOC	vaso-occlusive crisis

V_t	tidal volume
VT	ventricular tachycardia
VTE	venous thromboembolic events
vWF	von Willebrand factor
WBC	white blood cell

Shock

Kenneth R. L. Bernard

Introduction

- Shock is the pathological state of circulatory collapse resulting in tissue hypoperfusion.
  - At a cellular level there is inadequate delivery of metabolic substrates (i.e., oxygen and glucose) to sustain aerobic metabolism. This leads to anaerobic metabolism and a buildup of lactic acid. As ATP stores are depleted, cell membrane integrity is lost, leading to cellular dysfunction and cell death.
  - At a systemic level, there is activation of compensatory mechanisms to augment cardiac output (CO) and systemic vascular resistance (SVR).
    - Blood flow is preferentially shunted to the brain and heart from splanchnic and renal vascular beds to the detriment of these organ systems.
    - Eventually, compensatory mechanisms are overwhelmed leading to the multiple organ dysfunction syndrome (MODS).
- The circulatory system can be thought of as having three major components: a pump (the heart), fluid (blood), and tubing (blood vessels). The etiologies of shock can be categorized as a malfunction of one or more of these components.
- Conventionally shock is classified as distributive (tubing malfunction), hypovolemic (fluid loss), cardiogenic (pump failure), obstructive (obstruction to the inflow or outflow of the pump), or undifferentiated (Table 1.1).
- A clinician must accurately identify the appropriate category as certain etiologies call for specific interventions (e.g., pericardiocentesis for cardiac tamponade).
- Treatment of shock is dependent on reversing tissue hypoxia by improving oxygen delivery and decreasing oxygen demand, as well as correcting the underlying cause.

Practical Emergency Resuscitation and Critical Care, ed. Kaushal Shah, Jarone Lee, Kamal Medlej, and Scott D. Weingart. Published by Cambridge University Press. © Kaushal Shah, Jarone Lee, Kamal Medlej, and Scott D. Weingart 2013.

Table 1.1. Categories of shock and differential diagnosis

Distributive	Severe inflammatory response syndrome (SIRS) and sepsis, neurogenic, anaphylaxis, adrenal insufficiency/Addisonian crisis, drug or toxin reaction, hepatic failure
Hypovolemic	Hemorrhage (trauma, GI bleed, ruptured AAA), GI losses (diarrhea, vomiting, fistula), insensible losses, third spacing (pancreatitis, burns)
Cardiogenic	Myocardial infarction, myocarditis, arrhythmia, cardiac contusion, valve dysfunction, thyrotoxicosis, end-stage cardiomyopathy
Obstructive	Tension pneumothorax, cardiac tamponade, pulmonary embolism (PE), constrictive pericarditis, aortic coarctation, excessive PEEP or auto-PEEP

- Shock may be difficult to diagnose given subtle presentation in the early stages and rapid decline in late stages, and may encompass more than one category of shock (i.e., septic shock can also result in septic cardiomyopathy, adding a cardiogenic component to the shock state).
- A thorough history and examination along with certain diagnostic modalities can assist with categorizing shock.

Presentation

- A patient in shock presents with a wide variety of signs and symptoms related to both the precipitating event and the resultant cellular dysfunction.
- On presentation to the ED, a patient in shock may be very ill and have difficulty giving a history, which may necessitate obtaining collateral information from emergency medical services personnel, family, or friends.
- In general, a patient will appear toxic, in distress, with pale, clammy skin, with tachypnea, and with tachycardia as a result of the body's stress response to injury.
- Subtle clues from the patient's history including past medical conditions, preceding events, and appearance can help clinicians categorize a patient's shock state (Table 1.2).
- Patients often present in early shock, which will quickly progress from compensated to decompensated, and finally, refractory or irreversible shock.
  - A commonly held misbelief that often leads to delayed treatment and poorer outcomes is that shock necessitates hypotension.
  - Compensated or cryptic shock patients may appear relatively normal and asymptomatic as compensatory mechanisms resulting in tachycardia or vasoconstriction have yet to be overwhelmed.
  - Decompensated shock patients often appear ill, pale, diaphoretic, tachypneic, tachycardic, and with altered mental status.
  - The critical state refractory shock is recognized by manifestations of MODS such as obtundation or coma, refractory hypotension, renal failure, disseminated intravascular coagulation (DIC), and the acute respiratory distress syndrome (ARDS).

Table 1.2. Presentations of shock

Category	History	Past medical history	Appearance
Distributive	Fever, chills, headache, dyspnea, wheezes, stridor, meningismus, malaise, myalgias, cough, dysuria, diarrhea	Immunocompromised, allergies, adrenal insufficiency	Diaphoretic, distressed, flushed, warm skin
Hypovolemic	Poor intake, excessive vomiting or diarrhea, GI bleed or evidence of trauma	Coagulopathy (acquired or inherited), upper or lower GI bleed	Rapid and weak pulses, cool skin, delayed capillary refill, tachypneic, dry mucous membranes, poor skin turgor
Cardiogenic	Syncope, dyspnea, chest pain, palpitations	Coronary artery disease, myocardial infarction, dysrhythmia, congestive heart failure	Tachypneic, jugular venous distension, new murmur, delayed capillary refill, wheezes, rales, cool skin, murmur
Obstructive	Trauma	COPD, connective tissue disorder	*See Cardiogenic, Beck's triad, asymmetric breath sounds, tracheal deviation

Diagnosis and evaluation

- **Vital signs** are nonspecific.
  - Any single vital sign in isolation is not helpful in diagnosing shock or the possible etiology of shock.
  - Shock should be suspected when patients present with a constellation of signs including ill-appearance, tachycardia, tachypnea, hypotension, and oliguria.
  - Tachycardia is seen in the hyperdynamic state of shock. However, bradycardia may also be present in the setting of drug overdose (e.g., beta-blockers, calcium channel blockers, digoxin).
  - Hypotension is usually a late finding in a previously healthy individual, and noninvasive blood pressure monitoring can be inaccurate. Also, normotension in a previously hypertensive patient can be indicative of shock.
- **Signs of shock** are a result of the compensatory mechanisms, organ dysfunction, and the precipitant etiology. They can be helpful in providing clues to the cause of shock.

- Warm extremities can be caused by vasodilation present in distributive shock.
- Cold extremities can be caused by vasoconstriction present in hypovolemic or cardiogenic shock.
- Jugular venous distension in the setting of shock can be caused by cardiogenic or obstructive shock.
- Low jugular venous pressure is indicative of hypovolemic shock.
- Other findings will be present in specific causes of shock:
  - Absent breath sounds in tension pneumothorax
  - Muffled heart sounds in cardiac tamponade
- Signs of organ dysfunction include oliguria/anuria, encephalopathy and hypoxia.
- **Laboratory tests:**
  - A complete blood count will identify leukocytosis or bandemia in the setting of SIRS. It will also identify anemia (Hct <30% or Hgb <10). However, a normal value may be misleading in the acute stage of blood loss.
  - Serum chemistry will assess renal function, hydration status, and detect electrolyte derangements.
  - Cardiac biomarkers will identify myocardial injury.
  - Lactate and base deficits are markers for tissue hypoperfusion.
  - Arterial or venous blood gases will identify oxygenation or ventilation disorders and severe acid–base disturbances.
  - Urine or serum hCG (human chorionic gonadotropin) should be obtained in female patients of child-bearing age to evaluate for potential ruptured ectopic pregnancy as a source of hemorrhage and shock.
- **Electrocardiogram (ECG):**
  - Useful for the early diagnosis of acute coronary syndromes, arrhythmias, or electrolyte disturbances.
- **Imaging:**
  - **Chest radiography** may show edema, effusion, consolidation, pneumothorax, or an enlarged mediastinum and cardiac silhouette.
  - **Pelvic radiography** as a screening tool in blunt trauma may reveal a clinically significant pelvic fracture as a source of hemodynamic instability.
  - **Point-of-care ultrasonography (US)** can be very useful in the management of undifferentiated shock.
    - The Focused Assessment with Sonography in Trauma (FAST) examination can quickly identify free fluid in the abdomen as a potential source of bleeding in a hemodynamically unstable patient.
    - Cardiac views can reveal pericardial effusion and tamponade physiology.
    - Bedside echocardiography can also be used to assess for globally reduced ventricular function, a severely enlarged right ventricle (RV), or preload responsiveness by evaluating the inferior vena cava (IVC).

Table 1.3. Differentiating categories of shock

	CVP	ScvO$_2$	CI	SVR
Distributive	↓	↑ or ↓	↑ or ↓	↓
Hypovolemic	↓	↓	↓	↑
Cardiogenic	↑	↓	↓	↑
Obstructive	↑	↓	↓	↑

- The extended FAST examination with lung views may reveal a pneumothorax or pleural effusion.
  - Additionally, bedside US of the abdomen can identify a ruptured abdominal aortic aneurysm (AAA) as the cause of shock.
- **Conventional echocardiography (transthoracic or transesophageal)** will identify ventricular dysfunction, regional wall motion abnormalities, valvular pathology, aortic pathology, tamponade physiology, or RV strain pattern suggestive of massive pulmonary embolism or other causes of right heart failure.
- **Computed tomography (CT) scanning** may be helpful in identifying the source of shock in specific cases such as pulmonary embolism, aortic dissection, intra-abdominal sepsis, or intra-abdominal hemorrhage.
- **Invasive hemodynamic monitoring** by way of an arterial line, central venous catheter, or pulmonary artery catheter can further differentiate shock categories by determining values such as mean arterial pressure (MAP), central venous pressure (CVP), pulmonary capillary wedge pressure (PCWP), cardiac output (CO), cardiac index (CI), systemic vascular resistance (SVR), and oxygen transport variables. Different categories of shock have different hemodynamic profiles (Table 1.3).
  - **Central venous catheter:** a catheter placed into a central vein, either the internal jugular, subclavian, or femoral vein. It allows one to administer vasoactive medications and obtain the following measurements (a femoral line does not allow for accurate measurements):
    - **CVP** is an indicator of volume status and cardiac pump function. The target range in septic patients is 8–12 mmHg.
    - **Central venous oximetry:** the **ScvO$_2$** value is an indicator of tissue oxygenation and utilization. It is obtained by sampling blood from the superior vena cava (SVC) via a central venous catheter. Low central venous oxygen saturation (<70%) suggests that tissues are extracting more oxygen because of hypoperfusion and hypoxia.
  - **Arterial line:** an invasive catheter placed in the artery (common sites are radial or femoral) that allows for direct measurement of arterial blood pressure. It is more accurate for determining MAP and is helpful in a patient who requires multiple blood draws.
  - **Pulmonary artery catheter (PAC):** an invasive catheter placed in the pulmonary artery that allows a clinician to directly measure PCWP (surrogate

for left atrial pressure) and pulmonary artery pressure to assess pump function. It also allows one to measure other hemodynamic parameters including CO, CI, and SVR. The use of a PAC has not been shown to provide a mortality benefit. This procedure is almost never performed in the emergency department.

Critical management

- **Principles of shock management** include specific therapy for treating the underlying cause, and general therapy to manage the shock syndrome.
  - Specific therapies also referred to as source control include
    - Antibiotics in sepsis
    - Operative repair of traumatic injuries
    - Thrombolysis in massive PE
    - Revascularization in acute coronary syndrome
    - Pericardiocentesis in tamponade
    - Tube thoracostomy in tension pneumothorax
- The general treatment of shock is focused on restoring and maintaining adequate organ perfusion. This is accomplished by increasing oxygen delivery and decreasing oxygen demand.
- **ABCs (airway, breathing, circulation):**
  - As with all critically ill patients, secure the airway early if necessary. If the situation permits, rapid sequence intubation (RSI) is the method of choice.
  - Ensure adequate oxygenation with a goal SaO_2 of >90%.
  - Obtain large-bore intravenous (IV) access to allow infusion of crystalloids or transfusion of blood products. If peripheral IV access fails, consider central venous access if time permits, or emergent intraosseous line placement.
- **Increase oxygen delivery:**
  - **Volume resuscitation:**
    - In some categories of shock, patients have a decreased intravascular volume as a result of blood or fluid loss, or because of vascular dilation or leakage.
    - 20–30 mL/kg bolus of normal saline or lactated Ringer's solution is the preferred initial resuscitation treatment. This bolus may have to be repeated if the patient does not respond adequately.
    - In hemorrhagic shock from trauma, crystalloid administration should be limited and blood products such as packed red blood cells (PRBCs), fresh frozen plasma (FFP), and platelets should be transfused during resuscitation. Excessive crystalloid administration can dilute the important blood constituents that are already depleted and lead to worse outcomes.
  - **Vasopressors (Table 1.4):**
  - Hypotensive patients who do not respond to volume resuscitation may benefit from vasopressor support.

Table 1.4. Vasopressors and inotropes

Agent	Receptors	Mechanism of action	Effective dose
Vasopressors			
Epinephrine	α, β	Vasoconstriction, inotropy, chronotropy	1–10 micrograms/minute
Norepinephrine	$\alpha_1 > \beta_1$	Vasoconstriction, mild inotropy and chronotropy	2–30 micrograms/minute
Phenylephrine	α_1	Vasoconstriction	10–300 micrograms/minute
Vasopressin	V_1	Vasoconstriction	0.01–0.04 U/minute
Dopamine	D, α, β	Inotropy and chronotropy at lower doses, vasoconstriction at high doses	2–20 micrograms/kg/minute
Inotropes			
Dobutamine	$\beta_1 = \beta_2$	Inotropy, chronotropy, vasodilation at high doses	2–20 micrograms/kg per minute
Milrinone	Phosphodiesterase-inhibitor	Inotropy, chronotropy, vasodilation at high doses	0.375–0.75 micrograms/kg per minute

- A MAP of ≥65 mmHg should be targeted to ensure proper perfusion of the vital organs.
- Norepinephrine is the vasopressor of choice in septic shock.
- Epinephrine or vasopressin can be added to norepinephrine in cases of refractory septic shock.
- **Inotropes (Table 1.4):**
  - Patients with low cardiac output secondary to decreased myocardial contractility or cardiogenic shock benefit from inotropic support to improve tissue perfusion.
  - Dobutamine is the preferred agent in decompensated heart failure in patients that are normotensive or mildly hypotensive. It may need to be given in conjunction with vasopressors.
  - Dopamine use is controversial as recent studies have suggested increased mortality in cardiogenic shock due to its arrhythmogenic properties.
- **Blood products:**
  - Hemoglobin is the primary mode of delivering oxygen to tissues and should be transfused in patients with hemorrhagic shock, anemia, or low central venous saturation (<70%).

- In the hemorrhagic shock patient, PRBCs should be transfused based on the patient's clinical status, as hemoglobin and hematocrit levels may not accurately represent blood loss early on.
- In the nonbleeding patient with shock, goal hematocrit levels are controversial but lie somewhere between 21% and 30%.
- **Decrease oxygen demand:**
  - Treat fever with antipyretics to decrease metabolic demand and insensible losses.
  - Initiate mechanical ventilation early to decrease the work of breathing, prevent aspiration, improve oxygenation, and manage acidosis.
- **Assessing resuscitation efforts:**
  - Once appropriate intravenous access, definitive airway, and hemodynamic monitors have been acquired, it is imported to continually assess resuscitation efforts and maintain a goal-oriented approach.
  - Volume resuscitate to achieve a CVP of 8–12 mmHg for optimal preload in nonintubated patients, and 12–15 mmHg in intubated patients. Using CVP as a preload surrogate is controversial as studies have shown that CVP may not be indicative of preload responsiveness. Alternative techniques to CVP monitoring are described in the following chapter.
  - Maintain a MAP >65 mmHg by using vasopressors once the patient is appropriately volume-resuscitated.
  - Keep $ScvO_2$ >70% by administering PRBCs if the patient is anemic, and/or initiating inotropes.
  - Serially assess lactate levels. Clearance of lactate (a decrease of ≥10% of the original value 2–3 hours after initiation of resuscitation) or correction of the base deficit are reliable adjuncts to the measurement of $ScvO_2$.

Special circumstances

- **Pediatric patients:**
  - Recognition of shock is difficult due to variations in age-dependent vital signs, difficulty in assessing mental status, and the nonspecificity of early manifestations of shock such as irritability and poor feeding.
  - Shock should be suspected in children that have signs of poor perfusion such as delayed capillary refill, dry mucous membranes, absent tears, or are ill-appearing.
  - Children have strong compensatory mechanisms and by the time they are hypotensive may already be in an irreversible state of shock.
- **Pregnant patients:**
  - Management is made more difficult due to changes in maternal physiology and due to the considerations for both maternal and fetal well-being.
  - Shock may be caused by pregnancy-specific diagnoses such as peripartum hemorrhage, pulmonary embolism, peripartum cardiomyopathy, or supine hypotensive syndrome.

- Usual monitoring modalities are still employed in addition to cardiotoco-graphic monitoring of the fetus.
- The first resuscitative maneuver, while securing the ABCs, is to have the patient lie in the left lateral decubitus position. This alleviates pressure on the IVC allowing increase venous return to the heart.
- **Geriatric patients:**
  - Elderly patients experience significantly more morbidity and mortality from all causes of shock due to their limited ability to augment cardiac output and maintain vascular tone.
  - Elderly patients often have multiple comorbidities or use multiple medications that distort the diagnosis and management of shock.

REFERENCES

Cheatham ML, Block EFJ, Promes JT, Smith HG, Dent, DL, Mueller DL. Shock: an overview. In: Irwin RS, Rippe JM, eds. *Irwin & Rippe's Intensive Care Medicine.* 5th edn. Philadelphia: Lippincott Williams & Wilkins; 2003.

Gaieski D. Shock in adults: types, presentation, and diagnostic approach. *UpToDate*: Wolters Kluwer Health [updated 2012 December 17]. Available from: www.uptodate.com/contents/shock-in-adults-types-presentation-and-diagnostic-approach (accessed April 30, 2013).

Jones AE, Jeffrey A. Shock. In: Marx JA, Hockberger RS, Walls RM, Adams J, Rosen P, eds. *Rosen's Emergency Medicine: Concepts and Clinical Practice.* 7th edn. Philadelphia, PA: Mosby Elsevier; 2010.

Maier RV. Approach to the patient with shock. In: Longo DL, Fauci AS, Kasper DL, *et al.* eds. *Harrison's Principles of Internal Medicine.* 18th edn. New York: McGraw-Hill; 2012.

Rivers E, Amponsah D. Shock. In: Wolfson AB, Hendey GW, Hendry PL, *et al.*, eds. *Harwood-Nuss' Clinical Practice of Emergency Medicine.* 4th edn. Philadelphia: Lippincott Williams & Wilkins; 2005.

2

Monitoring

Brandy Ferguson

Introduction

Monitoring and understanding of monitoring devices are necessary for proper management of the critically ill patient. The goal of hemodynamic and respiratory monitoring is to ensure and maintain adequate tissue perfusion. This chapter will review the basic methods and principles of monitoring in the emergency setting.

Basic monitoring

Several aspects of a critically ill patient's status can be obtained from the telemetry monitor (Table 2.1).
- Three electrodes (white, black, and red) are used in 3-lead ECG systems, allowing for multiple views of the heart. Lead II is typically displayed on the cardiac monitor. For accurate ECG tracing, the electrodes should be applied in the following manner:
  - The white electrode is placed just below the clavicle on the right shoulder.
  - The black electrode is located on the left clavicle near the shoulder.
  - The red electrode is connected to the left pectoral muscle near the apex of the heart.
- Heart rate is measured as number of beats per minute (bpm). The normal heart rate range is 60–100 bpm.
- Blood pressure is measured as systolic pressure over diastolic pressure.
  - *Systolic pressure* is the peak pressure in the arteries. This occurs when the ventricles contract.

Practical Emergency Resuscitation and Critical Care, ed. Kaushal Shah, Jarone Lee, Kamal Medlej, and Scott D. Weingart. Published by Cambridge University Press. © Kaushal Shah, Jarone Lee, Kamal Medlej, and Scott D. Weingart 2013.

Table 2.1. Basic readings on the telemetry monitor

3-Lead or 5-lead ECG system
Heart rate
Blood pressure
Mean arterial pressure
Respiratory rate
Oxygen saturation
Temperature

- *Diastolic pressure* is the minimum pressure of the arteries. This occurs when the ventricles are filled with blood.
- Noninvasive blood pressure measurements can be obtained via auscultatory or oscillometric measurements.
  - Oscillometric blood pressure is used with telemetry monitoring. Proper cuff size is essential for accurate readings.
- Mean arterial pressure (MAP) is the average arterial pressure during a single cardiac cycle and can be used as indicator of adequate tissue perfusion. MAP = ($\frac{2}{3}$ diastolic pressure) + ($\frac{1}{3}$ systolic pressure).
  - MAP = (cardiac output (CO) × systemic vascular resistance (SVR)) + central venous pressure (CVP).
  - Normal MAP can range between 70 and 110 mmHg.
- Respiratory rate is a measure of the total number of breaths per minute.
- Temperature can be measured via oral, tympanic, axillary, esophageal, or rectal routes. Rectal and esophageal temperatures are more indicative of a patient's core temperature.

Respiratory monitoring

Pulse oximetry

- Pulse oximetry provides continuous measurement of a patient's oxygenation status.
- Measurements are obtained via sensors placed on the patient's fingertip, earlobe, or forehead. These sensors use two light-emitting electrodes.
  - The first emits red light that has a wavelength of 660 nm.
  - The second emits infrared light that has a wavelength of 905, 910, or 940 nm.
  - The difference in absorption of the red light and infrared light determines the oxyhemoglobin to deoxyhemoglobin ratio. This measurement corresponds to the pulse oximeter saturation estimate (SpO_2).
- Pitfalls:
  - Once the arterial oxygen saturation (SaO_2) falls below 70%, the pulse oximetry readings are no longer accurate.

- Pulse oximetry cannot reliably detect hypoxemia in the setting of carbon monoxide poisoning because carboxyhemoglobin has similar light absorption to that of oxyhemoglobin at 660 nm.
- It is also inaccurate in the setting of methemoglobinemia as both red light and infrared light are equally absorbed by methemoglobin. This results in a fixed SpO_2 around 85% regardless of the true SaO_2.
- Oxygenated blood that is redistributed from central to peripheral circulation can cause a delay in saturation readings known as pulse oximetry lag. This lag can be as long as 2–3 minutes in critically ill patients secondary to reduced blood flow.
- A proper waveform must be visualized on the monitor in order to be able to properly determine the SpO_2.
- Hypothermia and peripheral vasoconstriction can lead to inaccurate or unobtainable values.

End-tidal carbon dioxide (EtCO$_2$)

- Capnography measures the partial pressure or concentration of expired carbon dioxide (CO_2), the $EtCO_2$. This concentration is a function of the production of CO_2 at the tissue level and delivery of CO_2 to the lungs by the circulatory system. Therefore, capnography provides important information regarding ventilation, circulation, and metabolism.
- The normal expired CO_2 level is around 5%, which is approximately 40 mmHg.
- There are two different $EtCO_2$ monitoring modalities that are used in the emergency department (ED).
  - Colorimetric capnometry is a filter generally used to confirm endotracheal tube (ET) placement in the trachea.
    - The filter attaches to the ET tube and displays the change in concentration of carbon dioxide by color change.
    - In certain colorimetric capnometers, detection of carbon dioxide is exhibited by filter color change from purple to yellow. This is a semiquantitative mode of monitoring. The color ranges are as follows: purple = $EtCO_2$ <0.5%; tan = $EtCO_2$ 0.5–2%; and yellow = $EtCO_2$ >2%.
    - Pitfalls:
      - The filter can turn yellow when exposed to acidic material such as stomach contents, or medications including lidocaine and epinephrine.
      - In patients in cardiac arrest, color change may not be seen even with tracheal intubation because of the low $EtCO_2$ value resulting from poor or absent blood flow.
  - Quantitative capnography uses infrared technology to provide a continuous numerical value and a continuous waveform display of $EtCO_2$. This measure is plotted graphically on a monitor.
- Some ED applications of quantitative $EtCO_2$ monitoring are listed below.

- Intubation:
  - Quantitative $EtCO_2$ will reliably confirm tracheal placement of endotracheal tube despite low cardiac output states, unlike colorimetric devices.
  - Postintubation continuous capnography can help early identification of airway obstruction or tube dislodgment.
- Procedural sedation:
  - Pulse oximetry provides information about oxygenation, not ventilation. With any amount of supplemental oxygenation, detection of hypoventilation will be significantly delayed. This occurs because patients will start desaturating seconds to minutes after they stop breathing.
  - $EtCO_2$ monitoring provides early detection of airway compromise and can rapidly identify apnea, airway obstruction, bronchospasm, and laryngospasm. Respiratory depression can therefore be identified prior to hypoxia.
- Cardiopulmonary resuscitation (CPR):
  - Monitoring of ventilation:
    - Monitoring of the respiratory rate can be achieved more accurately with an $EtCO_2$ waveform. It is important not to hyperventilate patients during CPR as this leads to worse outcomes.
  - Monitoring of effectiveness of chest compressions:
    - In low flow states, the $EtCO_2$ value is a reflection of the cardiac output to the lungs. The more effective chest compressions are, the higher the $EtCO_2$ value will be.
  - Assessment of return of spontaneous circulation (ROSC):
    - A sudden increase in $EtCO_2$ can represent a return of spontaneous circulation and indicates the need to check for the presence of a pulse.
  - Prognosis:
    - $EtCO_2$ can be used to help determine whether further resuscitation efforts are futile as studies have shown that an $EtCO_2$ <10 mmHg after 20 minutes of CPR is predictive of a failure to resuscitate.
- Monitoring conditions in which arterial $PaCO_2$ levels are critical:
  - Traumatic brain injury or intracerebral hemorrhage with elevated intracranial pressure.
  - Severely acidemic patients prior to intubation.
  - In normal lungs with normal gas exchange, $EtCO_2$ values are usually 3–5 mmHg lower than arterial $PaCO_2$ values. In critically ill patients the values will not correlate. However, if an arterial $PaCO_2$ and $EtCO_2$ values are obtained simultaneously, $EtCO_2$ may be used to trend $PaCO_2$ values.

Noninvasive hemodynamic monitoring

Ultrasonographic assessment of the inferior vena cava (IVC)

Ultrasonography of the IVC can be useful in determining fluid responsiveness. After bringing the IVC into sagittal view, changes in the diameter of the vessel with respiration are recorded. Interpretation of these measurements will depend on whether the patient is mechanically ventilated or breathing spontaneously.

- In a spontaneously breathing patient:
  - Assess the diameter of the IVC and percentage of collapse with inspiratory effort. This provides an estimate of central venous pressure (CVP).
  - An IVC diameter ≤1.7 cm with complete inspiratory collapse demonstrates a low CVP (<5 mmHg).
  - An IVC diameter of >1.7 cm with no inspiratory collapse is indicative of a high CVP (>15 mmHg).
- In a mechanically ventilated patient:
  - Mechanical ventilation causes the diameter of the IVC to increase with inspiration. Therefore the physician should not evaluate for IVC collapse but rather for IVC distension with inspiration.
  - The IVC distensibility index is determined as (Maximum IVC diameter – Minimum IVC diameter)/(Minimum IVC diameter).
  - Values ≥18% are predictive of fluid responsiveness.
- Pitfalls:
  - The IVC may be difficult to visualize in obese patients.
  - Large fluctuations in intrathoracic pressure (i.e., patients in respiratory distress) will cause changes in the IVC diameter that are not a result of the patient's volume status.

Invasive hemodynamic monitoring

This section will highlight invasive monitoring techniques that can be used in the ED setting. Invasive techniques provide data via catheters inserted in central veins or arteries.

Pulmonary artery catheter (PAC)

- The pulmonary artery catheter or Swan–Ganz catheter is a balloon-tipped catheter that is inserted into the internal jugular or subclavian vein. From there it is guided by cardiac blood flow into the right atrium, the right ventricle, and finally into the pulmonary artery.
- It allows to measure a number hemodynamic parameters that are indicators of preload, cardiac output, and oxygen delivery. Central venous pressure (CVP), pulmonary capillary wedge pressure (PCWP), systemic vascular resistance (SVR), cardiac output (CO), cardiac index (CI), and mixed venous O_2 (SvO_2) are some of the commonly used variables that can be obtained from the PAC.
- PAC measures CO via the thermodilution method, which is usually the gold standard for CO measurement in studies.

Table 2.2. Factors that alter the reliability of CVP results

Factors that increase CVP	Factors that decrease CVP
Hypervolemia	Hypovolemia
Pleural effusion	Distributive shock
Tension pneumothorax	
Cardiac tamponade	
Congestive heart failure	
Mechanical ventilation with positive end-expiratory pressure	
Valvular heart disease	

- Preload can be estimated at the level of the right atrium by CVP, or the level of the left atrium by PCWP.
- Global oxygen delivery can be measured by the SvO_2.
- PACs are not typically placed in the ED.
- Pitfall:
  - Studies have not shown a mortality benefit through the use of PACs and their routine placement in critically ill patients has significantly decreased.

Central venous pressure

- CVP is obtained by placing a central venous catheter (CVC) in the internal jugular or subclavian vein. The tip of the CVC should ideally rest at the junction of the superior vena cava (SVC) and the right atrium.
- A normal CVP ranges between 4 and 6 mmHg. A CVP of 8–12 mmHg is targeted in hypotensive septic patients.
- Several factors can affect CVP measurements and these are summarized in Table 2.2.
- Pitfall:
  - A systematic review has demonstrated a poor relationship between CVP and fluid responsiveness. The CVP should be interpreted with caution in critically ill patients that have known heart disease or structural cardiac anomalies.

Pulse and systolic pressure variation

Pulse pressure variation (PPV) and systolic pressure variation (SPV) can be used to determine fluid responsiveness in a mechanically ventilated patient. Both of these methods require an arterial line for continuous measurement of arterial blood pressure.

The pulse pressure and systolic pressure show slight variations with respiration. These are caused by increased blood return to the right heart secondary to the negative intrathoracic pressure generated during inspiration. These variations are exacerbated by hypovolemia and their measurement beyond a certain threshold can be used as an indicator of fluid responsiveness.

- $PPV = (PP_{max} - PP_{min})/[(PP_{max} + PP_{min})/2]$
  - PPV greater than 13% is associated with fluid responsiveness.
- $SPV = SP_{max} - SP_{min}$
  - SPV >10 mmHg is associated with fluid responsiveness.
- Pitfalls:
  - PPV and SPV should be measured in mechanically ventilated patients who are not making an effort to breathe.
  - These patients should also be in sinus rhythm.

REFERENCES

Barbier C, Loubières Y, Schmit C, *et al.* Respiratory changes in inferior vena cava diameter are helpful in predicting fluid responsiveness in ventilated septic patients. *Intensive Care Med.* 2004; **30**: 1740–6.

Bigatello LM, George E. Hemodynamic monitoring. *Minerva Anestesiol.* 2002; **68**: 219–25.

Marik PE, Baram M, Vahid B. Does central venous pressure predict fluid responsiveness? A systematic review of the literature and the tale of seven mares. *Chest.* 2008; **134**: 172–8.

Meyers CM, Weingart SD. Critical care monitoring in the emergency department. *Emerg Med Pract.* 2007; **9(7)**: 1–29.

Nagdev AD, Merchant RC, Tirado-Gonzalez A, *et al.* Emergency Department Bedside Ultrasonographic Measurement of the Caval Index for Noninvasive Determination of Low Central Venous Pressure. *Ann Emerg Med.*; **55**: 290–5.

3

Airway management

N. Seth Trueger

Introduction

- Airway management is one of the core fundamental skills of the emergency medicine or critical care physician.
- Airway management is time-critical and can literally mean the difference between life and death.
- Airway management encompasses the overlapping management of oxygenation, ventilation, and airway protection.

Airway principles (Table 3.1)

- Planning, recognizing failure, and decision-making are top priorities.
- Maintenance of calm permits proper decision-making. Undue haste is detrimental to critical decision-making.
- Specific time-sensitive exceptions include acidosis, impending airway obstruction, and hypoxia.
- Each aspect of airway management is modular. Components can be mixed as needed (e.g., video laryngoscopy with a bougie; awake intubation after preoxygenation with noninvasive ventilation).

Recognizing failure (Figure 3.1)

- When first-line techniques fail to result in intubation, early identification of failure is paramount.

Practical Emergency Resuscitation and Critical Care, ed. Kaushal Shah, Jarone Lee, Kamal Medlej, and Scott D. Weingart. Published by Cambridge University Press. © Kaushal Shah, Jarone Lee, Kamal Medlej, and Scott D. Weingart 2013.

Table 3.1. Principles for safe emergency airway management

Judicious use of rapid sequence intubation (RSI) versus awake technique
Back-up planning
Prioritization of oxygenation
Early recognition of failure
Early use of surgical technique if necessary
Avoidance of ED intubation if necessary

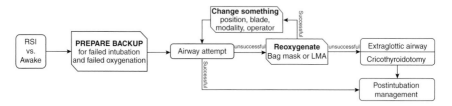

Figure 3.1. (© Reuben Strayer & emupdates.com, used with permission. Adapted from: Reuben Strayer. Emergency Department Intubation Checklist v13. 2012. http://emupdates. com/2012/07/08/emergency-department-intubation-checklist-v13/; accessed July 23, 2012).

- If unsuccessful, laryngoscopy should be abandoned and oxygen restored with mask ventilation.
- Extraglottic airways (EGA) can be placed quickly and may provide better ventilation than bag-mask ventilation.
- If an intubation attempt fails *and* reoxygenation fails, **a cricothyroidotomy must be performed immediately**.
- Failure to recognize a "can't intubate, can't oxygenate" scenario will result in the patient's death.

Decision to intubate (Table 3.2)

- Many factors at play must be balanced, including:
  - Early management of a sick patient
  - Potential danger of paralyzing a patient
  - Limited clinical evaluation of an intubated patient

Noninvasive ventilation

- In patients protecting their airway, noninvasive ventilation (NIV) may be appropriate.
- Many patients will improve dramatically with NIV and avoid intubation.

Table 3.2. Indications for intubation

Indication	Rationale	Comments
Ventilation	The patient is not safely breathing on their own	Circumstances make it difficult to match the patient's inherent drive (e.g., salicylate toxicity)
Oxygenation	Intubation allows high FiO_2 and positive end-expiratory pressure	Noninvasive ventilation may suffice for many patients
Protection	Alterations in mental status may blunt protective airway reflexes, and conditions such as vomiting may result in aspiration	Obstructive processes (e.g., expanding hematoma) may threaten tracheal patency
Expected course	A presently stable patient may be expected to deteriorate	Early intubation is often safer prior to deterioration
Metabolic demand	Decrease work of breathing in critically ill patients (e.g., severe sepsis)	Oxygen consumption from respiration alone can rise from baseline of 5% to 50%

- NIV provides:
  - Up to 100% FiO_2
  - Pressure-support, decreasing the work of breathing
  - PEEP, overcoming shunt physiology (e.g., severe pneumonia, acute pulmonary edema).
- Although alteration in mental status is a traditional relative contraindication to NIV, critically ill emergency department (ED) patients can be closely monitored by experienced airway operators.
- NIV can be used to achieve two simultaneous goals:
  - It can potentially improve the patient sufficiently to obviate the need for intubation.
  - Barring sufficient improvement, NIV will optimize preoxygenation if intubation is necessary.

Oxygenation

- Oxygenation is the primary concern in airway management.
- As hemoglobin and oxygen bind cooperatively, desaturation is slow above SpO_2 90%.
- Below 90%, hemoglobin molecules quickly lose bound oxygen, and critical hypoxia can occur in seconds.
- Due to the technical aspects of pulse oximetry, there is a lag of up to 2 minutes in the measured SpO_2. Therefore, a reading in the 80–90% range may indicate that the actual SpO_2 is much lower.

- Laryngoscopy should be abandoned when SpO_2 reads 90% in order for the patient to be reoxygenated.

Laryngoscopy and intubation

- The following steps are necessary to place an endotracheal tube (or an EGA):
  - Positioning
  - Oxygenation
  - Equipment and discussion of back-up plan
  - Medication administration
  - Laryngoscopy and intubation (or EGA placement)
  - Postintubation management.

Positioning

- Proper positioning is essential for laryngoscopy.
- The same positioning principles will aid in preoxygenation and mask ventilation.
- Proper positioning lifts the anterior pharyngeal structures off the posterior pharynx and optimizes glottis view.
- A combination of head, neck, and body positioning can be used to optimize both of these goals.
  - Jaw thrust: lifting the jaw anteriorly by the angles of the mandible to open the pharynx.
  - Ear-to-sternal-notch: the patient's head should be elevated in order for the external auditory meatus to be at the same level as the manubrium, in a plane parallel to the ceiling (Figure 3.2a).
- Some patients (including: obese, with pleural effusions, at risk for vomiting) may benefit from elevating the head of the bed to 30 degrees while maintaining the same positioning principles (Figure 3.2b).
- Positioning for a video laryngoscope (VL):
  - VL with conventional blades: positioning is unchanged.
  - VL with an angulated blade: completely neutral head and neck position, with the head flat on the bed and the face plane parallel to the ceiling.

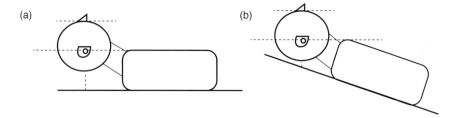

Figure 3.2. Patient positioning.

Preoxygenation

- The goal of preoxygenation is not merely to achieve an SpO_2 of 100%, but also to de-nitrogenate the lungs, completely filling the lungs with oxygen to act as an oxygen reservoir during laryngoscopy.
- Preoxygenate with a non-rebreather mask (NRB) set to 15 liters per minute or higher, for at least 3 minutes.
- If hypoxia persists despite high-flow oxygen, the patient is likely shunting and may require PEEP delivered via NIV.
- Obtunded hypoxic patients, if still ventilating on their own, may be safer to ventilate with NIV under close supervision than with bag-mask ventilation.
- In the apneic patient, bag-mask ventilation (BMV) should be performed.
  - Two-operator technique will provide a better mask seal as one operator can use both hands to secure the mask to the patient's face.
  - Nasal trumpets and oral airways, if tolerated, can be invaluable in maintaining pharyngeal patency.
  - Use slow, smooth, controlled breaths of only half the volume of a standard bag.
  - Patients obtunded due to severe metabolic acidosis will require a much faster respiratory rate, and must be ventilated during the apneic period to avoid cardiac arrest.
  - Most bags accept a PEEP valve if necessary.
  - Ventilators can be attached to masks, allowing for control of tidal volumes, respiratory rate, and PEEP if needed.
- Fully obtunded and apneic patients oxygenate better with the rapid placement of an EGA.

Apneic oxygenation and oxygenation during laryngoscopy

- NRB should be left in place during the apneic period.
- As the oxygen in the lungs is filtered into the body, an O_2-gradient is established allowing passive flow of oxygen from the high-FiO_2 of the NRB to the lungs.
- A nasal cannula set to 15 lpm will similarly provide high-flow oxygen during laryngoscopy.
- If there are insufficient oxygen wall adaptors to provide three sources of oxygen (bag-mask, NRB, and nasal cannula), place a portable oxygen tank under the bed to provide a third source.

Extraglottic airways

- Numerous EGA options exist, primarily laryngeal tubes (mainly used in the prehospital setting) and laryngeal masks.
- EGA are typically used as rescue devices when it is difficult to provide BMV.
- Laryngeal masks do not fully "secure" the airway as vomit may dislodge them.
- Many second-generation laryngeal masks permit intubation through the mask.

Laryngoscopy

- Principles of laryngoscopy are identical for direct and video laryngoscopy, with the exception of different positioning.
- Suction should be available under the patient's right shoulder. Two or more Yankauer suction tips may be necessary if blood, vomit, or copious secretions are expected.
- Various devices exist for video laryngoscopy.
  - Many devices use traditional curved blades and may be used either directly or with the video monitor.
  - Devices with angulated or indirect blades are operated similarly but do not allow for direct visualization.
  - Angulated blades will often insert too far; if the glottis cannot be seen, withdraw slowly.
  - Lifting the handle straight toward the ceiling may also improve the view.
  - Video devices improve views but may be defeated by blood, mucus, or vomit.
  - Tube delivery may be more difficult as the angle of attack to the trachea is steeper.
- Stylets vastly improve tube control and delivery and should be shaped straight to the cuff, then angled to 35 degrees.
- Deliver the tube from the side (3-o'clock): rotation about the long axis will give subtle control in the vertical axis, and the tube will not obscure the glottic view.
- A partial glottic view is sufficient if the tube can be directed above the posterior cartilages (Figure 3.3).
- Tube delivery with angulated VL is often facilitated with malleable stylets shaped similarly to the blade, or with proprietary stylets.

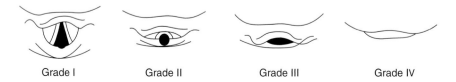

Grade I   Grade II   Grade III   Grade IV

Figure 3.3. View of the vocal cords. Grade I: the entire glottis opening is visualized. Grade II: only the posterior aspect of the glottis opening is visualized. Grade III: only the tip of the epiglottis is visualized. Grade IV: only the soft palate is visualized.

Bimanual laryngoscopy

- Bimanual laryngoscopy includes both external laryngeal manipulation (ELM) and head mobilization.
- ELM is best achieved with the aid of an assistant.
- ELM is not cricoid pressure.

- Cricoid pressure ostensibly occludes the esophagus to avoid passive regurgitation.
- Cricoid pressure is unlikely to work, and may worsen the glottis view.

Bougie

- The bougie is a valuable adjunct, particularly in partial glottis views.
- The bougie is threaded through the glottis and the tube is delivered "over the wire."
- When advanced gently, the bougie will be stopped by a terminal bronchus after 40 cm of insertion if it is properly located in the airway. If in the esophagus, the bougie will advance indefinitely.

Confirmation of placement

- Traditional indicators such as chest rise, auscultation, humidity in the tube, chest radiography, and SpO_2 are helpful but unreliable.
- The preferred method for confirmation of endotracheal intubation is capnography.
- Colorimetric capnography: disposable litmus-paper devices that change color from purple to yellow.
  - Only accurate if color change persists over 6 breaths.
  - Inaccurate if the airway is soiled by vomit.
- Waveform capnography: nearly 100% accurate, end-tidal capnography is near gold-standard.
- Capnography should also be used to confirm ventilation with EGA.

Rapid sequence intubation (RSI)

- RSI is the simultaneous administration of a paralytic and an induction agent.
- The overwhelming majority of ED intubations use RSI.
- Adequate preoxygenation is a prerequisite for safe RSI.
- One goal of RSI is to avoid positive-pressure ventilation during the apneic period to minimize the risk of vomiting by avoiding gastric insufflation.
- RSI has been proven to be safe and effective as paralysis optimizes intubating conditions.

RSI medications (Table 3.3)

- The cornerstone of RSI is the simultaneous use of a potent sedative and fast-acting paralytic.

- Etomidate, propofol, and midazolam may precipitate hypotension. For potential hypotension or hypovolemia, reduce the induction dose by 50% or more.
- Earlier concerns about use of ketamine in elevated intracranial pressure are unfounded.
- Onset of paralysis is 30–45 seconds with either succinylcholine or high dose rocuronium.
- Succinylcholine is widely used but may precipitate hyperkalemia. At-risk populations include:
  - Neuromuscular disorders (acquired and congenital)
  - Sepsis, burns, and crush injuries (generally only vulnerable >3 days after onset)
  - Preexisting hyperkalemia
- While succinylcholine has a shorter duration of action than rocuronium (8–10 minutes vs. 45 minutes), the patient will critically desaturate prior to return of muscle tone if the tube cannot be placed.

Table 3.3. RSI medications

Sedative agents	Dose	Properties
Etomidate	0.3 mg/kg	Linked to adrenal suppression of unclear clinical importance
Ketamine	1.5–2 mg/kg	Releases endogenous catecholamines; avoid in CAD; bronchodilator
Propofol	1.5–2 mg/kg	Antiepileptic; bronchodilator
Midazolam	0.3 mg/kg	Antiepileptic

Paralytic agents	Dose	Properties
Succinylcholine	1.5–2 mg/kg	May precipitate hyperkalemia in vulnerable patients (e.g., neuromuscular disorders)
Rocuronium	1.2 mg/kg	Time of onset and intubating conditions identical to succinylcholine if dosed 1.2 mg/kg

Hemodynamics

- Induction of anesthesia may be detrimental to hemodynamics.
- Sedation blunts the sensation of noxious stimuli, decreasing endogenous catecholamines.
- Intubation and mechanical ventilation results in the shift from physiological negative-pressure ventilation to positive-pressure ventilation, which decreases preload.
- Hemodynamics should be optimized prior to intubation, through fluid resuscitation and/or vasopressors as indicated.

Table 3.4. Technique for increasing levels of risk

Risk scale	Technique	Example
Low risk	RSI	Most patients
Predicted difficult	Awake	Obese patient with short neck
Predicted difficult, potentially unstable	Double setup	Lateral neck trauma
High risk, currently stable	OR	Ludwig's angina, epiglottitis

Assessing airway difficulty (Table 3.4)

- In the potentially difficult airway, awake intubation allows for an increased safety margin.
- Predicting the difficult airway is difficult.
- The gestalt of an experienced physician is likely equal to or superior to specific rules, and is usually informed by similar elements.
- Features that potentially increase intubation difficulty include:
  - Obesity
  - Short neck
  - Decreased neck mobility
  - Small mouth opening
  - Recessed chin
- As most ED intubations utilize RSI, comfort and skill with awake technique may be limited.
- While maintaining the patient's respiratory drive confers a clear level of safety, intubating conditions are not optimized.
- Awake intubation is straightforward, adds only a few minutes of time, and even if unsuccessful, has taken little from the patient.
- A failed awake intubation can easily be converted to an RSI, but a paralyzed patient requires definitive airway control.
- Most patients are safe for RSI.
- Some potentially difficult patients may be safe for paralysis but will benefit from a double setup:
  - Fully prepared for cricothyroidotomy
  - Equipment open at the bedside
  - Cricothyroid membrane marked
  - Neck sterilized
  - While one physician is ready to immediately perform the surgical airway if needed, a separate physician takes a single attempt at RSI
- A double setup will help overcome the cognitive burden of identifying the need for surgical airway if necessary.
- If time allows, some patients may benefit from techniques not possible in the ED and should be considered for definitive control in the operating room (OR).

- Sedative-only intubation, while seemingly attractive, is potentially dangerous.
  - Intubating without paralysis means conditions are not optimized.
  - The dose of sedative necessary for the patient to tolerate laryngoscopy will obliterate respiratory drive, eliminating the benefit of avoiding paralysis.
  - Sedation alone is unlikely to diminish airway reflexes; the risk of vomiting and aspiration caused by laryngoscopy is high.
  - Accordingly, all ED patients undergoing intubation should receive sedation and either paralytics or topicalization.

Alternative airway techniques

Awake intubation

- Awake intubation refers to the use of topical anesthetic instead of paralytic agents to facilitate intubation, while maintaining the patient's respiratory drive and protective airway reflexes.
- "Awake intubation" is a misnomer, as patients require some level of sedation.
- Most sick patients can be intubated awake.
- Awake intubation takes minimal extra time and provides a wide safety margin in the potentially difficult airway.
- Ketamine, ketofol, or dexmedetomidine are optimal agents as they maintain respiratory drive and airway reflexes.
- Video laryngoscopy should be used if available, as the intubating conditions will not be optimized via paralysis.

Delayed sequence intubation (DSI)

- Hypoxic patients may not tolerate preoxygenation due to delirium.
- Under close monitoring, these patients may benefit from delayed sequence intubation; the use of a sedative to allow for proper preoxygenation, followed by paralysis and intubation.
- Sedative dosing should be adjusted to maintain the patient's airway reflexes and respiratory drive.
- Ketamine is the first-line agent for DSI as it will not blunt airway reflexes or respiratory drive.

REFERENCES

Aguilar SA, Davis DP. Latency of pulse oximetry signal with use of digital probes associated with inappropriate extubation during prehospital rapid sequence intubation in head injury patients: case examples. *J Emerg Med.* 2012; **42**: 424–8.

Benumof JL, Dagg R, Benumof R. Critical hemoglobin desaturation will occur before return to an unparalyzed state following 1 mg/kg intravenous succinylcholine. *Anesthesiology.* 1997; **87**: 979–82.

Levitan RM, Everett WW, Ochroch EA. Limitations of difficult airway prediction in patients intubated in the emergency department. *Ann Emerg Med.* 2004; **44**: 307–13.

Weingart SD. Preoxygenation, reoxygenation, and delayed sequence intubation in the emergency department. *J Emerg Med.* 2011; **40**: 661–7.

Weingart SD, Levitan RM. Preoxygenation and prevention of desaturation during emergency airway management. *Ann Emerg Med.* 2012; **59**: 165–75.

4

Mechanical ventilation

Nelson Wong

Introduction

- When a patient in respiratory distress is intubated, the endotracheal (ET) tube by itself does not alleviate or reverse the underlying cause of respiratory distress. Mechanical ventilation, however, can be used to mitigate the effects of the disease process and allow the body time to heal.
- Mechanical ventilation drastically alters normal respiratory physiology. We normally breathe by generating negative pressure in the thoracic cavity, while mechanical ventilation uses positive pressure at the airway opening to create a gradient that drives the flow of gas into the lungs.
- Initiating mechanical ventilation is not without consequence. If done inappropriately, morbidity and mortality can dramatically increase because of the development of certain complications:
  - Ventilator-induced lung injury (VILI):
    - Lung disease does not take place uniformly throughout the lungs.
    - Tidal volumes preferentially inflate healthy lung tissue. Therefore, if the tidal volumes are high, this can cause stress to the alveolar–capillary interface of the normal lungs.
    - Barotrauma occurs as a result of excessive airway pressures and can result in a pneumothorax, a pneumomediastinum, or alveolar rupture.
    - Volutrauma occurs as a result of high tidal volumes.
    - Atelectrauma occurs with the continuous closing and reopening of alveoli.
    - Barotrauma, volutrauma, and atelectrauma can lead to the activation of an inflammatory cascade causing further injury known as biotrauma.

Practical Emergency Resuscitation and Critical Care, ed. Kaushal Shah, Jarone Lee, Kamal Medlej, and Scott D. Weingart. Published by Cambridge University Press. © Kaushal Shah, Jarone Lee, Kamal Medlej, and Scott D. Weingart 2013.

- Ventilator-associated pneumonia (VAP):
  - VAP is defined as a pneumonia that develops within 48 hours of the initiation of mechanical ventilation.
  - The endotracheal tube bypasses many of the body's defenses against pathogens and acts as a direct conduit for bacteria into the lungs.

Definitions

- **Inspiration:** Gas flows into the lungs.
- **Expiration:** Ventilator flow is stopped and the exhalation circuit is opened to allow gas to escape from the lungs.
- **Triggering:** Initiation of breath.
  - Can be machine initiated after a set amount of time has elapsed since the last breath.
  - Can be patient initiated in response to a reduction of airway pressure below a preset threshold, or in response to the detection of inspiratory flow.
- **Limit:** A parameter that is used to control inspiration. Ventilation can be either volume or pressure limited.
- **Cycling:** Switching from inspiration to expiration.
  - Can occur because a certain amount of time has passed, a preset volume has been delivered, or a preset decrease in flow rate has occurred.
- **Minute ventilation (V_E)** = Tidal volume (V_t) × Respiratory rate (RR).

Common ventilator settings

- **Fraction of inspired oxygen (FiO_2):** The percentage of oxygen being delivered to the patient. It ranges between 21% and 100%.
- **Positive end-expiratory pressure (PEEP):** Positive airway pressure applied by the ventilator at the end of expiration. PEEP prevents alveolar collapse at the end of expiration and "recruits" alveoli to participate in respiration, thereby improving gas exchange.
- **Respiratory rate (RR):** Number of breaths delivered per minute.
- **Tidal volume (V_t):** Volume in mL delivered in a single breath.
- **Inspiratory flow rate (IFR):** The rate of air entry in L/minute during inspiration.
- **Inspiratory pressure**: Set pressure used to inflate the lungs during inspiration.
- **Inspiratory time (T_i):** The time over which the V_t is delivered.
- **I:E ratio:** The ratio of inspiratory time to expiratory time. A normal I:E ratio is 1:2 to 1:3. Increasing the I:E ratio can improve oxygenation by increasing the mean airway pressure. A longer inspiration will result in a longer period of high pressure, thus increasing the mean airway pressure over the entire respiratory cycle.

Table 4.1. Ventilator modes

Mode	Trigger	Breaths	Limit	Cycle	Variables set
CMV	Ventilator (time)	Mandatory	Volume	Ventilator (volume)	V_t, RR, IFR, FiO$_2$, PEEP
AC	Ventilator (time) and/or patient (flow or pressure)	Mandatory or assisted	Volume	Ventilator (volume)	V_t, RR, IFR, FiO$_2$, PEEP
SIMV	Ventilator (time) and/or patient (flow or pressure)	Mandatory or assisted; breaths above set RR are spontaneous and unassisted (unless PS used)	Volume, pressure	Ventilator (volume), breaths above set RR are patient cycled (flow)	V_t, RR, IFR, FiO$_2$, PEEP PS (can be used for breaths above set RR)
PC	Ventilator (time) and/or patient (flow or pressure)	Mandatory or assisted	Pressure	Ventilator (time)	Inspiratory pressure, RR, T_i, FiO$_2$, PEEP
PS	Patient (flow or pressure)	Assisted by pressure support	Pressure	Patient (flow)	PS, PEEP

Modes of ventilation (Table 4.1)

- **Controlled mandatory ventilation (CMV)**: The ventilator controls all aspects of ventilation. A set RR and V_t are delivered by the ventilator. This mode is usually a volume-controlled mode but can also be a pressure-controlled mode. The patient has no ability to initiate breaths, breathe over the set RR, or influence the characteristics of the breath. This mode is mostly used in heavily sedated and paralyzed patients in the operating room.
- **Assist volume control**: Commonly referred to just as Assist Control (**AC**). This is a volume-cycled mode of ventilation that delivers the same V_t during every breath. Breaths can be triggered by the patient or the machine. There is a set RR and V_t but the patient can breathe over the set RR. If the patient does not initiate a breath after a set time, the ventilator will initiate the breath. All patient-triggered breaths are assisted by the ventilator to produce the set V_t. This is a commonly used mode for patients in respiratory distress and has become the mode of choice in the ED.
- **Synchronized intermittent mandatory ventilation (SIMV)**: SIMV represents a combination of breathing types. It is a mix of ventilator triggered and controlled

breaths and the patient's spontaneously triggered and controlled breaths. If the patient is breathing below the set RR, then the breaths are machine assisted. If the patient is breathing above the set RR, then the patient's breaths are spontaneous and unassisted. Unlike AC there is no guarantee of a set V_t for every breath because the V_t for the unassisted breaths depends on the patient's respiratory effort and lung mechanics.

- **Pressure control (PC)**: PC is an assist control mode of ventilation in which the desired inspiratory pressure is set. This mode is similar to assist volume control but instead of a set V_t being delivered a set pressure is delivered. Breaths can be triggered by the machine or the patient. In this mode the RR and T_i are set which will determine the I:E ratio. Each breath is assisted by the machine and the set pressure is delivered. An advantage of this mode is the pressure limit can be set to limit barotrauma and this may improve patient ventilator synchrony. A disadvantage of this mode is that V_t will vary with each breath based on the patient's thoracic compliance, airway resistance, and patient effort. Therefore, a set minute ventilation will not be guaranteed.
- **Pressure support (PS)**: This mode of ventilation provides partial support. The patient is spontaneously breathing and the ventilator will augment each breath with a set inspiratory pressure. The patient sets his or her own respiratory rate and V_t. This mode necessitates an intact ventilatory drive and is commonly used as a weaning modality.

Strategies of ventilation

Outlined below are two ventilation strategies that can be used in critically ill patients in the emergency department. Both of these strategies utilize the assist control (AC) volume cycled mode of ventilation.

Lung protective strategy (Figure 4.1)

- This strategy is designed for patients with acute lung injury (ALI) or acute respiratory distress syndrome (ARDS), or who are at risk for lung injury. The majority of patients fit into this category.
- It is believed that all intubated and mechanically ventilated patients are at risk for ALI. This strategy should therefore be employed on most critically ill patients that are on a ventilator.
- This ventilation strategy is derived from the ARDSNet study and has been shown to decrease mortality in patients with ALI/ARDS.
- It prevents VILI by avoiding over-distension of the alveoli and preventing atelectrauma.
- *ARDSNet Protocol*:
  - Use "low" physiological tidal volumes (4–8 mL/kg of ideal body weight).

- Maintain a plateau pressure (P_{plat}) <30 cm H_2O.
- Oxygenation is maintained with protocol driven PEEP and FiO_2 values.

LUNG PROTECTIVE STRATEGY
- Calculate the predicted body weight (PBW).
  - Males = 50 + 2.3 [height (inches) – 60] or Females = 45.5 + 2.3 [height (inches) – 60].
- Select Assist Control Mode.
- Set initial Vt to 8 mL/kg PBW.
  - Reduce Vt by 1 mL/kg at intervals ≤2 hours until Vt = 6 mL/kg PBW.
- Set initial respiratory at 18 and adjust to target pH >7.30 (not >35 bpm).
- Adjust Vt and RR to achieve pH and plateau pressure goals.
- Set inspiratory flow rate above patient demand (usually 60–80 L/min).
- **PLATEAU PRESSURE GOAL: ≤30 cm H_2O.**
  - Check P_{plat} (0.5 – 1 second inspiratory pause), SpO_2, total RR, Vt, and pH (if available) at least every 4 hours and after each change in PEEP and Vt.
  - If P_{plat} >30 cm H_2O: decrease Vt by 1 mL/kg steps (minimum = 4 mL/kg).
  - If P_{plat} <25 cm H_2O and Vt <6mL/kg, increase Vt by 1 mL/kg until P_{plat} >25 cm H_2O or Vt = 6 mL/kg.
  - If P_{plat} <30 cm H_2O and breath stacking or dys-synchrony occurs: may increase Vt in 1 mL/kg increments (maximum = 8mL/kg) if P_{plat} remains <30 cm H_2O.
- **OXYGENATION GOAL: PaO_2 55–80 mmHg or SpO_2 88–95%.**
  - Use incremental FiO_2/PEEP combinations such as shown below to achieve goal.

FiO_2	0.3	0.4	0.4	0.5	0.5	0.6	0.7	0.7	0.7	0.8	0.9	0.9	0.9	1.0	1.0	1.0
PEEP	5	5	8	8	10	10	10	12	14	14	14	16	18	20	22	24

Figure 4.1. Ventilator settings for lung protective strategy. (Courtesy of Scott D. Weingart, MD.)

Obstructive strategy (Figure 4.2)

- This strategy is designed for patients with obstructive lung disease (i.e., asthma or COPD) whose airways are constricted and therefore require a longer time to fully exhale.
- They also require respiratory support for fatigued respiratory muscles during inspiration.
- The basis of this strategy is to decrease the RR and adjust the IFR to achieve a prolonged I:E ratio (1:4 to 1:5). This will allow the patient sufficient time to fully exhale and avoid auto-PEEP or breath stacking.
- Breath stacking is the phenomenon of delivering another breath before the lungs have completely exhaled. This results in an increased intrathoracic pressure and can cause a pneumothorax or hemodynamic instability secondary to a decrease in venous return.
- Decreasing the respiratory rate results in retention of CO_2 which in turn leads to a respiratory acidosis. This is referred to as permissive hypercapnia and is tolerated to a certain extent ($PaCO_2$ <85 mmHg and pH >7.20).

OBSTRUCTIVE STRATEGY
- Select Assist Control Mode.
- Set initial TV to 8 mL/kg PBW.
- Set initial rate to 10 and adjust to achieve I:E ratio of 1:5.
- Set inspiratory flow rate to 80 L/min.
- Set PEEP to 0.
- Titrate FiO_2 to maintain SpO_2 >88–90%.
- **PLATEAU PRESSURE GOAL: ≤30 cmH$_2$O**
- **CHECK EXPIRATORY FLOW CURVE:**
  - Make sure the expiratory flow reaches zero before the next breath is initiated.

Figure 4.2. Ventilator settings for obstructive strategy. (Courtesy of Scott D. Weingart, MD.)

Basic lung mechanics

There are two basic pressures that should be monitored in mechanically ventilated patients:
- Peak inspiratory pressure is automatically measured by the ventilator. It is a function of the resistance in the airways and the compliance of the lung and chest wall.
  - Can be elevated in conditions that increase airway resistance, like asthma, COPD, small ET tubes, and ET tube obstruction.
- Plateau pressure (P_{plat}) is measured after instituting a 0.5–1 second end-inspiratory pause. Since there is no airflow present at this time, the resistive component of the pressure is eliminated. P_{plat} is a reflection of the compliance of the lung and chest wall.
  - It is the more important pressure to monitor for risk of VILI because it is the pressure that is transmitted to the alveoli.
- PIP and P_{plat} can help identify the cause of distress in a mechanically ventilated patient.
  - If PIP is high and P_{plat} is normal, airway resistance is likely high.
  - If PIP is high and P_{plat} is high, lung compliance is likely low.
  - If PIP is low and P_{plat} is low, suspect an air leak or tube dislodgment.

Sudden deterioration

- Use the mnemonic **DOPES** on patients that are deteriorating while on the ventilator:
  - **D**islodgment of tubes:
    - Check the ET tube position by direct visualization or by connecting it to quantitative $EtCO_2$ capnography and looking for a loss of waveform.
  - **O**bstruction:
    - Usually from kinking of the ET tube or from a mucous plug.
    - Confirm with fiberoptic bronchoscopy if available.

- Insert a suction catheter through the ET tube to remove the plug.
- In some cases, the tube will have to be replaced.
- **P**neumothorax:
  - Place a chest tube on the affected side.
  - If the patient is hypotensive and the side of the pneumothorax is not clear, bilateral chest tubes should be placed.
- **E**quipment failure:
  - Disconnect the patient from the ventilator and ventilate with a bag valve apparatus until another ventilator is available.
- **S**tacking of breaths:
  - Remove the patient from the ventilator and allow for a full expiration.
  - Gentle pressure can be applied to the chest to accelerate the exhalation process.

REFERENCES

Acute Respiratory Distress Syndrome Network. Ventilation with lower tidal volumes as compared with traditional tidal volumes for acute lung injury and the acute respiratory distress syndrome. *N Engl J Med.* 2000; **342**: 1301–8.

Marino PL. Modes of assisted ventilation. *The ICU Book.* 3rd edn. Philadelphia: Lippincott Williams & Wilkins; 2006.

Pertucci N, Iacovelli W. Lung protective ventilation strategy for the acute respiratory distress syndrome. *Cochrane Database Syst Rev.* 2007; (3): CD003844.

Weingart, S. Dominating the vent: part I. *EMCrit Blog* 2010 [updated May 24, 2010; cited August 1, 2012]. Available from: http://emcrit.org/lectures/vent-part-1/ (accessed April 30, 2013).

Wilson J, Ablordeppey E. Mechanical ventilation. In: Swaminathan A, ed. *Critical Care Handbook.* Irvin, TX: Emergency Medicine Residents Association; 2012.

5

The boarding ICU patient in the emergency department

Robert L. Sherwin and Bram Dolcourt

Introduction

- Over 2 million patients are admitted to intensive care units (ICUs) from emergency departments (EDs) each year in the United States.
- The common definition of an "ICU boarder" is a patient who remains in the ED after the decision to admit due to the lack of an available ICU bed.
- ED boarding of ICU patients is widely reported and ED lengths of stay (LOS) often range from 4–6 hours to 24 hours or more in extreme circumstances.
- Literature illustrates that ICU patients boarded in the ED have worse outcomes. There is no data to explain exactly why patients with longer ED stays die more frequently, but patient crowding, suboptimal nurse-to-patient ratios, and lack of appropriate resources are often cited as speculative causes.

Fundamentals of shock resuscitation and oxygen delivery

- Shock is best defined as an imbalance between oxygen delivery (DO_2) and oxygen consumption (VO_2).
- Shock occurs when a patient's condition causes a fall in DO_2 (i.e., myocardial infarction) or a marked increase in VO_2 (i.e., septic shock).
- As DO_2 falls below a critical threshold ($DO_2 < VO_2$), cellular respiration halts and pyruvate is shunted to lactate to maintain ATP production.
- All resuscitation principles primarily focus on augmentation of DO_2 (Figure 5.1).
- Little can be done to mitigate VO_2 abnormalities with the exception of antipyretics (to control fever), and intubation (to eliminate the work of breathing).

Practical Emergency Resuscitation and Critical Care, ed. Kaushal Shah, Jarone Lee, Kamal Medlej, and Scott D. Weingart. Published by Cambridge University Press. © Kaushal Shah, Jarone Lee, Kamal Medlej, and Scott D. Weingart 2013.

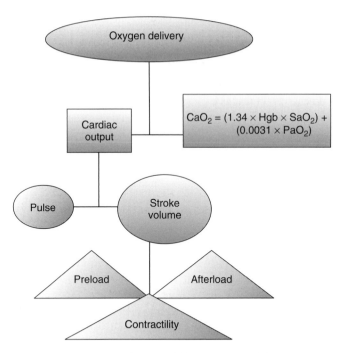

Figure 5.1. Components of oxygen delivery. CaO$_2$, arterial oxygen content; PaO$_2$, partial pressure of oxygen; SaO$_2$, oxygen saturation; Hgb, hemoglobin.

Endpoints of resuscitation

- Endpoints of resuscitation (EOR) are vital to avoid under or over-resuscitation.
  - Identify your endpoints early and assess them often.
  - It is best to target multiple endpoints as no single endpoint is superior to the others.
  - Pulse and blood pressure (BP) are inaccurate predictors of outcome or fluid responsiveness.
    - BP is a product of cardiac output (CO) and systemic vascular resistance (SVR). Patients free of cardiopulmonary disease can compensate for impaired CO and display normal vital signs.
- Lactate is a good indicator of hypoperfusion (<2.0 mmol/dL = normal; 2.0–3.9 = mild elevation; >4.0 = severe elevation).
  - Lactate elevation may be due to a number of factors including hypoperfusion (i.e., shock), cellular metabolic dysfunction (i.e., toxins affecting either the tricarboxylic acid cycle or the electron transport chain), increased production (i.e., seizures), or decreased clearance (i.e., liver dysfunction).
  - Even patients with mild lactate elevation have poorer outcomes.

- Rule of 2s: after 2 hours or 2 L of intravenous fluids (IVF), get a second lactate.
  - The half-life of lactate is 15 minutes so it should be checked often.
  - Any decrease >10% is good, but normalization is best.
- Estimates of preload:
  - A perfect predictor of volume responsiveness does not exist.
  - Central venous pressure (CVP) is the most widely available endpoint and is most accurate in patients without cardiopulmonary disease.
    - A low CVP in a patient with shock is a good indicator of fluid responsiveness.
    - When the initial CVP is elevated, however, it does not mean that the patient is adequately fluid resuscitated. It may be that the patient has cardiopulmonary disease and a baseline elevated CVP. Therefore, an alternative EOR should be selected.
    - When a patient is intubated, the target CVP is 12–15 mmHg due to increased intrathoracic pressures related to mechanical ventilation.
- Additional measures can be obtained from noninvasive monitoring devices such as pulse pressure variation (PPV), stroke volume variation (SVV), or thoracic fluid content (TFC).
  - These also provide imperfect measures, with reported sensitivities of 80–90%.
- Estimates of afterload:
  - In patients presenting with shock, noninvasive blood pressure monitoring can underestimate a patient's central pressure. An intra-arterial catheter should be placed to minimize the amount of vasopressors administered.

Ongoing assessment of the ICU boarder

- Frequent reassessment of ICU boarders is essential. Since mortality starts to increase at about 6 hours, it is reasonable to completely reassess an ICU boarder every 2–4 hours.
- Assessments should focus on fundamentals of care and disease-specific goals.
- Use the mnemonic: Have **MAD LoVE** for your ICU boarders.
  - **M**edications often need to be re-dosed during extended ED stays or titrated down (i.e., vasoactive medications).
  - **A**ncillary rounds: round with the nurse(s) and keep them updated on the plan of care.
  - **D**iagnostic reevaluation can prevent misdiagnosis. The "picture" is often clearer once all the data has been obtained and can be assessed in its entirety.
  - **L**aboratory evaluation: oversights in addressing laboratory deficiencies or rechecking abnormalities are extremely common.
  - **V**olume status is a critical component of resuscitation and management. Accurate "Ins and Outs" are frequently poorly recorded in ICU boarders. This can be remedied by asking the nurses to never take down an empty IV bag, and to number each IV bag with a permanent marker prior to administration.
  - **E**OR review: review and/or repeat your EOR to optimize care.

Septic patients

- Many hospitals have a multidisciplinary sepsis team including an ED champion.
  - Sepsis order sets help streamline care.
  - Completion of the *Surviving Sepsis Resuscitation Bundle* improves outcomes and reduces resource utilization.
- The EORs of early goal-directed therapy (indicated for septic patients with a systolic BP <90 mmHg despite 30 mL/kg of IVF, or a lactate >4.0 mmol/dL) are
  - CVP goal of 8–12 mmHg (spontaneously breathing patients) ← *Preload*
  - MAP goal of ≥65 mmHg
    - Can add norepinephrine as first-line pressor ← *Afterload*
- $ScvO_2$ goal of >70%
  - If not, transfuse to achieve a Hct ≥30% ← *Arterial O_2 content*
- If CVP, MAP and Hct are at goal and $ScvO_2$ is still <70%, dobutamine is recommended to augment contractility (the only component of DO_2 *not* optimized) (Figure 5.1). ← *Contractility*
- Aim to complete the above EOR within 6 hours from patient presentation.

Intubated patients

Mechanically ventilated patients in the ED are vulnerable to suboptimal care.
- Auto-PEEP caused by breath stacking and hyperinflation is dangerous (Auto-PEEP = intrinsic PEEP = dynamic hyperinflation).
  - It is usually due to bronchospasm resulting in retained air. This in turn causes an increase in intrathoracic pressure leading to decreased CO.
  - It also diminishes the efficiency of respiratory muscles, increases the work of breathing, and causes barotrauma and hypotension.
  - The goal is to allow for full expiration and to minimize its occurrence.
    - Reduce the respiratory rate to 10–12 breaths per minute.
    - Set the tidal volume at 6 mL/kg.
    - Increase the flow rate.
    - Add extrinsic PEEP (50–80% of measured intrinsic PEEP).
- Patients often require deep sedation and paralysis to tolerate these settings.
- These measures may result in retained CO_2 (i.e., permissive hypercapnia; keep $PaCO_2$ <85 mmHg and pH >7.20).
- Proximal airway pressures (PAP) should be regarded as a vital sign in intubated patients and monitored regularly (normal <30 cmH_2O).
  - Troubleshooting an intubated patient in distress requires an assessment of PAP (Figure 5.2).
  - The peak inspiratory pressure (PIP) represents resistance to flow inside the airways. If elevated (with a normal plateau pressure), it suggests bronchospasm or secretions resulting in airway plugging, and should be managed with suction and bronchodilators.

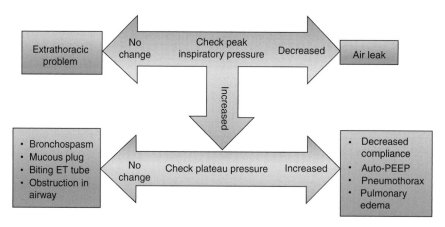

Figure 5.2. Suggested algorithm to assess PAP in troubleshooting a deteriorating intubated patient.

- Plateau airway pressure (Pplat) represents the compliance of the system. If elevated, the underlying cause should be identified and treated.
- Compliance with analgesia and sedation recommendations for intubated patients is generally poor in the ED. There is little data to support any single strategy.
  - Analgesia: fentanyl or morphine.
  - Sedation: propofol, lorazepam, or midazolam.
  - Intermittent boluses or continuous infusions can be used.
  - ED nurses should be trained to assess pain and sedation in mechanically ventilated patients.
- Ventilator associated pneumonia (VAP) increases hospital LOS, mortality, and hospitalization cost. Certain interventions have been shown to help decrease the incidence of VAP:
  - Elevate the head of bed to 30–40 degrees.
  - Perform daily oral care with chlorhexidine mouthwash.
  - Maintain the endotracheal tube cuff pressure between 25 and 30 cmH_2O.
  - Perform daily sedation holidays.
- Deep vein thrombosis (DVT) prophylaxis by subcutaneous injection of unfractionated or low molecular weight heparin should be initiated as these patients are at increased risk of developing DVT.
- These patients are also at increased risk of gastrointestinal stress ulcers and an H_2-blocker or a proton pump inhibitor should be administered as well.
- Most intubated patients do not need 100% FiO_2 and it should be weaned appropriately to maintain an oxygen saturation ≥93%. Prolonged exposure to 100% O_2 potentiates reperfusion injuries (i.e., patients post–cardiac arrest) and lowers the seizure threshold.

Specific strategies to manage ICU boarders in the ED

- **Management models:** It is helpful to define the model most applicable to your hospital to clearly define responsibilities and guide plans of action.
  - *ED-centric model:* The ED is completely responsible for patient care with minimal input from the ICU team. The ICU team takes over care when a bed is available in the ICU.
  - *ICU-centric model:* The ICU is completely responsible for patient care, orders, and management. The emergency physician is still available for emergent interventions and acute deterioration while the patient is located in the ED.
  - *Mixed-model:* Shared responsibility of care is often dictated by a consensus interdepartmental policy. This may include agreements to send available ICU nurses or staff to help with ICU boarders.
- **ED-based Critical Care Rotations:** Several emergency medicine residency programs have ED-based critical care rotations during which the resident's shift duties focus solely on the care of critically ill patients including ICU boarders.
- **MAD LoVE** checklist to improve the care of ICU boarders.
  - Pronovost *et al.* reported that a checklist intervention helped decrease the rate of iatrogenic infections due to central venous line insertion to near zero. Checklists are used in various forms to augment care.

REFERENCES

Bonomo JB, Butler AS, Lindsell CJ, *et al.* Inadequate provision of postintubation anxiolysis and analgesia in the ED. *Am J Emerg Med.* 2008; **26**: 469–72.

Chalfin DB, Trzeciak S, Likourezos A, *et al.* Impact of delayed transfer of critically ill patients from the emergency department to the intensive care unit. *Crit Care Med.* 2007; **35**: 1477–83.

Dellinger RP, Levy MM, Carlet JM, *et al.* Surviving Sepsis Campaign: international guidelines for management of severe sepsis and septic shock: 2008. *Crit Care Med.* 2008; **36**: 296–327.

Nguyen HB, Rivers EP, Knoblich BP, *et al.* Early lactate clearance is associated with improved outcome in severe sepsis and septic shock. *Crit Care Med.* 2004; **32**: 1637–42.

Pronovost P, Needham D, Berenholtz S, *et al.* An intervention to decrease catheter-related bloodstream infections in the ICU. *N Engl J Med.* 2006; **355**: 2725–32.

Resar R, Griffin FA, Haraden C, Nolan TW. Using care bundles to improve health care quality. IHI Innovation Series white paper. Cambridge, Massachusetts: Institute for Healthcare Improvement; 2012 [updated May 23, 2012; cited July 11, 2012]. Available from: www.ihi.org/knowledge/Pages/IHIWhitePapers/UsingCareBundles.aspx (accessed April 30, 2013).

Shapiro NI, Howell MD, Talmor D, *et al.* Serum lactate as a predictor of mortality in emergency department patients with infection. *Ann Emerg Med.* 2005; **45**: 524–8.

General trauma principles

Benjamin Schnapp

On arrival

- The emergency medical services (EMS) can provide invaluable information on a trauma patient if you take the time to obtain it.
- Gather a brief history from EMS ("the bullet") initially. Important aspects of the scene history include mechanism of injury, vital signs, mental status, IV access, or any changes or interventions en route.
- Attempt to obtain more details (e.g., amount of damage to the vehicle, size of knife, etc.) once the patient is stabilized. If necessary, appoint one of your team members to gather the prehospital history.

Primary survey

The primary survey aims to identify life-threatening and reversible causes of life-threatening injury. The primary survey should be completed in a consistent and thorough manner for every trauma patient.

Airway

- A talking patient is usually a good indication of airway patency, but be mindful of voice changes or other abnormal sounds, which can indicate upper airway obstruction.
- Reasons to consider early intubation in a trauma patient include

Practical Emergency Resuscitation and Critical Care, ed. Kaushal Shah, Jarone Lee, Kamal Medlej, and Scott D. Weingart. Published by Cambridge University Press. © Kaushal Shah, Jarone Lee, Kamal Medlej, and Scott D. Weingart 2013.

- Head injury with GCS ≤8
- Penetrating neck trauma
- Significant burns
- Need for transport to higher level of care
- Significant chest trauma
- Agitation/uncooperativeness.

- If the patient needs to be intubated immediately, try to obtain a brief neurological examination before the patient is sedated and paralyzed.
- Rapid sequence intubation is the preferred method of securing the airway.
- Trauma patients are different from medical patients. Trauma patients are using their sympathetic response to maintain their blood pressure, and may drop their blood pressure quickly with induction agents. Consider dose reduction of non–hemodynamically stable induction agents.
- Distribution of drugs may take longer in cases of poor perfusion. Therefore you may need a larger than usual dose of paralytic.
- Several airway adjuncts are available to assist in endotracheal intubation, including the gum elastic bougie, supraglottic airway devices, videolaryngoscopy, or fiberoptic scopes.
- A cricothyrotomy kit should be readily available for instances when endotracheal intubation fails.

Breathing

- The breathing evaluation includes visualization of chest rise, auscultation of breath sounds, palpation of the chest wall feeling for crepitus or flail segments, and assuring that the trachea is midline.
- If there is concern about tension pneumothorax (severe shortness of breath, unilateral decreased breath sounds, jugular venous distension [JVD], hypotension), a chest tube should be placed immediately on the affected side. If there is any delay in tube thoracostomy, decompress the lung with a needle thoracostomy in the second intercostal space, midclavicular line.
- For patients who have signs or symptoms of a pneumothorax or hemothorax but are hemodynamically stable with no signs of tension, confirmation may be obtained with either chest radiography or ultrasound before placing a chest tube.
- Ultrasound of the lungs as part of the extended FAST (eFAST) examination is quickly becoming commonplace for early detection of a pneumothorax, even in patients with low suspicion and should be considered.

Circulation

- Examine the patient for signs of hemorrhage, including all compartments that can hold life-threatening amounts of blood loss.

Sources of hypotension in trauma

Bleeding	Nonbleeding
Chest	Tension pneumothorax
Abdomen	Pericardial tamponade
Pelvis (retroperitoneal)	Spinal cord injury (neurogenic shock)
Long bones (femur fracture)	Cardiac dysfunction (infarction, arrhythmia)
Street (external)	Toxic ingestion

- Look for other signs of poor perfusion, such as cool extremities, duskiness, pulseless extremity, and slow capillary refill.
- Place two large-bore (18-gauge or larger) peripheral IVs to facilitate the administration of fluids and medications; if access proves to be difficult, consider placement of an intraosseous line or central access.
- Obtain a complete set of vital signs.
- Assess pelvis stability by squeezing in firmly from the sides of the pelvis with both hands. If there is movement, maintain inward pressure and notify the team that the pelvis is unstable; there should be no more examinations of the unstable pelvis, and a pelvic binder or bedsheet should be immediately placed around the greater trochanters to prevent the possibility of worsened pelvic bleeding.
- Many patients with circulation problems may initially show no evidence of blood loss (class I shock) or little evidence of blood loss, such as isolated tachycardia (class II shock). Only when the patient has lost 1.5–2 L of blood do they begin to manifest the classic signs of shock, such as low blood pressure (class III shock), and altered mental status (class IV shock). Maintain a high index of suspicion if the mechanism of injury is suggestive of blood loss or vital signs are trending in the wrong direction.

Classes of shock

	Class I	Class II	Class III	Class IV
Blood loss	<750 mL	750–1500 mL	1500–2000 mL	>2000 mL
Pulse	–	↑	↑	↑↑
Blood pressure	–	–	↓	↓↓
Respirations	–	↑	↑↑	↑↑
Mental status	Normal/mild anxiety	Anxious	Anxious/mild confusion	Lethargic/significant confusion
Capillary refill	–	↓	↓	↓

- If the patient does not appear to be perfusing well, or demonstrates evidence of shock, consider the need for rapid volume replacement with blood and consider activating your massive transfusion protocol. Most importantly, you need to identify the source of bleeding as soon as possible. Uncrossmatched type O+ should be used for men and uncrossmatched type O- should be used for women because of the risk of Rh sensitization.
- Obtain a baseline set of laboratory tests, including lactate, complete blood count, coagulation studies, basic metabolic panel, and most importantly, a type and cross. The initial hematocrit is of little value when assessing whether your patient has lost a large volume of blood. The result may be falsely reassuring since the body has not had time to equilibrate to its losses.
- Elevated lactate levels indicate inadequate tissue oxygenation (production of lactate through anaerobic metabolism) and suggest the need for further resuscitation. Levels above 2 mmol/L are correlated with longer ICU and hospital stays. Serial lactate levels demonstrating lactate clearance are helpful in guiding resuscitation.
- Be sure to send a type and screen for possible later matched transfusions and a coagulation panel, especially for patients who are suspected to be coagulopathic (warfarin use, liver disease, etc.). Other baseline labs should be drawn but are generally not helpful in the immediate management of a trauma patient and empiric treatment should not be withheld pending lab results.
- If you suspect large volume blood loss, initiate your massive transfusion protocol. Normal saline should be considered only a *brief* stopgap in trauma resuscitations until blood is available. Massive transfusion protocol should bring a mix of products, including packed red blood cells (PRBC), fresh frozen plasma (FFP), and platelets that need to be replaced in the bleeding trauma patient as well.
- If FFP is not available, or will be delayed, prothrombin complex concentrate (PCC) should be considered because it can be given rapidly without the need to thaw. If the patient is on warfarin, PCC may be superior to FFP because it can provide maximally effective reversal.
- Your goal in trauma resuscitation should be to prevent the **"trauma triad of death"** – hypothermia, acidosis, and coagulopathy. This can be accomplished by resuscitating the patient with blood products to a normal vascular tone (they should not be relying on their sympathetic drive to maintain blood pressure).
- Aim your resuscitation for a goal mean arterial pressure (MAP) of 65 mmHg, or if the patient has a head injury, a MAP of 80 mmHg. Patients sustaining *penetrating trauma* should be resuscitated only to these bare minimum normal blood pressures (also referred to as "permissive hypotension"). Organ perfusion is adequate at these pressures and aiming for higher pressures appears to increase the possibility of dislodging a clot that may be controlling bleeding without conferring any advantages. In general, judicious use of crystalloid is indicated because crystalloids have drawbacks – e.g., dilution of coagulation factors – increasing hypothermia if fluids are not warmed and they can cause increase in hydrostatic pressure that may dislodge a clot.

- There is no indication for pressor agents in the acutely bleeding patient. They have been shown to increase hemorrhage and do not appear to increase perfusion to the end organs. If the patient's blood pressure is low, they likely need additional blood products until source control is obtained.
- In patients receiving large volume resuscitation, ionized Ca^{2+} is likely to be low due to dilution and chelation effects by preservatives in transfused blood. $CaCl_2$ 1–2 g can be given for repletion, and may have positive effects on ionotropy and the clotting cascade with little risk to the patient.
- Tranexamic acid (TXA) is a newer agent in the United States (used extensively in Europe) that has shown promise in preventing excessive blood loss in trauma based on the CRASH-2 Trial. The dose is 1 g (and can be repeated once), administered within 3 hours of the onset of bleeding. There are few apparent complications.

Disability

- Evaluation for disability in the primary survey should include GCS, neurological examination to rule out neurological deficit, and pupil examination for signs of intracranial injury.
- All patients should be assumed to have cervical spine injury until demonstrated otherwise. c-Spine immobilization should be maintained until clinical or radiographic clearance is obtained. Remember that penetrating trauma to the neck with no clear signs of neurological injury does not require c-spine immobilization. If a c-collar was placed by EMS in a penetrating trauma, and there are no signs of neurological deficit, it should be removed for better access to the area.
- Examine the patient for obvious signs of injury, such as grossly deformed limbs that may need prompt reduction for neurovascular compromise.
- For patients being emergently intubated, be sure to obtain a baseline neurological examination so the patient's mental status can be followed over time.

Expose

- Remove all clothing from the patient to look for any injuries that may be easily missed.

Secondary survey

- Examine the patient in detail, beginning at the head and proceeding towards the feet.
- Do not forget easily missed areas such as the axilla, back of the patient, the ears, and the nose. These can hide significant injuries.

Imaging

- Obtain portable films of the chest and pelvis to assess for occult but potentially important injuries that may need to be addressed urgently.
- Perform an eFAST examination to assess for free fluid in the abdomen, thorax and in the pericardium as well as for pneumothorax. If the patient is unstable with a positive abdominal FAST, then the patient should be brought immediately to the operating room (OR). If the patient is hemodynamically stable with a positive FAST, further imaging with CT scan may be obtained.

Disposition

- Ultimately, a bleeding trauma patient needs their source of bleeding controlled. This often occurs in the OR, but may also occur in the interventional radiology suite.
- With increasing noninvasive management of trauma (e.g., low-grade spleen/liver lacerations), patients are often stabilized in the surgical ICU and operations are avoided successfully.
- Emergency department thoracotomy (EDT) is a resuscitative procedure that has a low survival rate and should be performed in unique circumstances. The highest survival is in patients with stab wounds to the chest. The current recommendations for patients to undergo EDT, assuming a trauma surgeon is available within 45 minutes, are
  - Penetrating trauma to the chest with CPR <15 minutes
  - Blunt trauma with CPR <10 minutes.

7

Severe traumatic brain injury

Jacob D. Isserman

Introduction

- Severe traumatic brain injury (TBI) should be considered in the unconscious patient (GCS ≤8) following head trauma with either
  - Significant mechanism of injury (fall from height, high speed MVC), or
  - Significant physical examination findings (depressed skull fracture, facial trauma, scalp lacerations).
- Severe TBI patients have a very high mortality rate. In the United States, there are 52 000 deaths each year from head trauma. Unlike other conditions, severe TBI often affects the young and able-bodied. Worldwide, it is the leading cause of mortality and disability in children and young adults.
- Always consider reversible causes of altered mental status in the trauma patient: toxicological, infectious, pulmonary, cardiac, hypoglycemia.
- The goals of early resuscitation should focus on identifying and treating the initial injuries and limiting the negative cascade of secondary injuries such as hypotension and hypoxia.
- All patients with suspected severe TBI need an emergent computed tomography (CT) scan of the brain to identify hemorrhage immediately following initial stabilization.
- 10% of severe TBI patients have concomitant c-spine injury.
- See Table 7.1 for common patterns of TBI.

Management

Glasgow Coma Scale

- Calculate concurrently with other resuscitation efforts.

Practical Emergency Resuscitation and Critical Care, ed. Kaushal Shah, Jarone Lee, Kamal Medlej, and Scott D. Weingart. Published by Cambridge University Press. © Kaushal Shah, Jarone Lee, Kamal Medlej, and Scott D. Weingart 2013.

- Preferably before administration of any sedative or paralytic medications.
- Also perform pupillary reflex examination.

Score	Eyes	Verbal response	Motor response
1	Closed	None	No response to painful stimuli
2	Open to pain	Incomprehensible sounds	Decerebrate (extension) to painful stimuli
3	Open to voice	Inappropriate words	Decorticate (flexion) to painful stimuli
4	Open spontaneously	Disoriented, confused speech	Withdraws to painful stimuli
5		Oriented, normal speech	Localizes painful stimuli
6			Follows commands

Add the total of each column.

Airway

- Early intubation is indicated in all severe TBI patients.
- Maintain c-spine precautions until clearance is possible (i.e., rigid cervical collar, logroll the patient, do not allow them to flex or extend the neck).

Rapid sequence intubation (RSI)

- The cerebral perfusion of severe TBI patients is tenuous, and first pass intubation is critical.
- The RSI medications should include a sedative and a paralytic agent with these objectives:
  - Maintenance of hemodynamic stability and CNS perfusion
  - Maintenance of adequate oxygenation
  - Prevention of increases in intracranial hypertension
  - Prevention of vomiting and aspiration.
- Pretreatment may help minimize increase in intracranial pressure (ICP) during intubation (no strong evidence to support its use and not universally used):
  - Lidocaine (1.5 mg/kg) intravenous push 3 minutes prior to induction
  - Fentanyl (3 micrograms/kg) slow intravenous push 3 minutes prior to induction, after lidocaine.

Table 7.1. Common traumatic brain injury patterns

Diagnosis	Findings	Management	Images
Traumatic SAH	Clinical: spectrum of mental status from asymptomatic to coma, with or without neurologic deficits CT imaging: localized bleeding in superficial sulci, adjacent skull fracture, and cerebral contusion as well as external evidence of traumatic injury	Neurosurgical evacuation recommended if: (1) Volume >30mL (2) GCS <8 with pupil abnormalities Medical: (1) CTA brain to check for aneurysmal bleed (2) BP goal, 160 systolic if obtunded, 140 (or patient's baseline if normal MS). Agents: nicardipine or labetalol (3) Aminocaproic acid 4 g ×1	
Epidural	Clinical: spectrum of AMS. Classically transient LOC, then lucid interval, followed by deterioration CT imaging: bright, lens-shaped collection because spread is contained by dural attachments at the cranial sutures	Neurosurgical evacuation recommended if: (1) Volume >30 mL (2) GCS <8 with pupil abnormalities	

Table 7.1. (cont.)

Diagnosis	Findings	Management	Images
Subdural hematoma	Clinical: spectrum of mental status for asymptomatic to coma, with or without neurologic deficits CT imaging: bright, crescent shaped collection along the hemispheric convexity, collection crosses suture lines	Neurosurgical evacuation recommended if: (1) Hematoma >1 cm thickness (2) Midline shift >5 mm (3) GCS <8 or decreases by 2 from presentation (4) ICP >20	
Intraparenchymal hemorrhage	CT imaging: hyperdense areas, surrounded by hypodense rings of edema	Neurosurgical intervention recommended if: (1) Volume >50 mL (2) GCS <8 and midline shift >5 mm (3) Posterior fossa location with mass effect or hydrocephalus	

DAI (diffuse axonal injury)	CT imaging: acutely may be normal, later edema, atrophy, loss of grey-white differentiation	Medical: (1) ICP precautions and monitoring (2) Avoid causes of secondary brain injury: hypotension, hypoxia, fever, hyperglycemia, and seizures
Basilar skull fx	Clinical: (1) Battle sign (2) Raccoon eyes (3) Hemotympanum (4) CNS otorrhea/rhinorrhea	Medical: (1) Steroids for delayed cranial nerve palsies (2) Admission for observation (3) Antibiotics for immunocompromised
Depressed skull fx	Clinical: palpable deformity on exam, either with or without overlying laceration	Neurosurgical debridement recommended if: (1) Dural penetration (2) Significant intracranial hematoma (3) Frontal sinus involvement (4) Cosmetic deformity (5) Wound infection or contamination (6) Pneumocephalus

Induction agents

- Etomidate (0.3 mg/kg) has been demonstrated to be hemodynamically stable and not increase ICP.
- Ketamine (1.5 mg/kg) should be considered if hypotensive or normotensive (avoid if the patient is already hypertensive).

Paralytic agents

- Rocuronium (RSI dose 1.2 mg/kg), onset of action 45–60 seconds.
- Succinylcholine (1.5 mg/kg IV), onset of action 45–60 seconds (avoid in patients with crush injuries).
- Vecuronium (0.1–0.2 mg/kg), onset of action 60–90 seconds.

Breathing

- Avoid hypoxemia and hyperoxemia (goal pulse oximeter of 95%).
- Monitor with quantitative end-tidal $PaCO_2$.
- Maintain $PaCO_2$ levels of 35–38 mmHg.

Circulation

- The goal is to maintain blood flow to the brain. The important measure is cerebral perfusion pressure (CPP), as opposed to systolic blood pressure (SBP). CPP = MAP – ICP. Systemic hypotension causes a decrease in CPP and must be avoided. If someone has increased ICP they need a higher blood pressure to maintain cerebral perfusion.
- 500 mL to 1 L boluses of isotonic crystalloid should be given to maintain SBP >90.

Intracranial pressure

- Intracranial pressure is normally ≤15 mmHg. ·
- Traumatic causes of increased ICP:
  - Intracranial mass lesions (hematomas)
  - Cerebral edema (acute hypoxic ischemic encephalopathy, large cerebral infarction, severe traumatic brain injury)
  - Obstructive hydrocephalus.
- See the table below for clinical signs of increased ICP and impending herniation.

Clinical signs of increased ICP and impending herniation
Unilateral or bilateral fixed and dilated pupil(s)
Decorticate or decerebrate posturing
Cushing reflex: bradycardia, hypertension, and/or respiratory depression
Decrease in GCS >2

Ocular ultrasound
- Can assist in detection of ICP by measuring the optic nerve sheath diameter.
- Measure transverse length approximately 3 mm posterior to globe.
- The average of two measurements >5 mm is suspicious for increased ICP.

Management of increased ICP
- The goal is to maintain cerebral perfusion pressure of at least 60 mmHg (CPP = MAP − ICP).
- Treatment is aimed at decreasing ICP first, then increasing MAP.

Decrease ICP
- Mechanical:
  - Elevate head of bed to 30 degrees.
  - Optimize venous drainage by keeping the neck in neutral position and loosening neck braces if too tight.
- Osmotic therapy:
  - Mannitol 20% (1 g/kg) over 5 minutes, works in the short term as a temporizing measure to obtain CT imaging or definitive surgical management. Causes hypotension, so avoid in patients with SBP <90.
  - Hypertonic saline (3%) 150–250 mL through a peripheral line. This is preferable if the patient is hypotensive.
- Hyperventilation:
  - In a patient with clinical signs of herniation, MILD hyperventilation may be beneficial.
    - Goal $PaCO_2$ of 28–35 mmHg.
- If an external ventricular drain (EVD) is in place, CSF can be removed at 1–2 mL/minute (pause drainage every 2–3 minutes). Continue until ICP is <20 or fluid is not easily withdrawn.

Increase mean arterial pressure (if MAP <80)
- Isotonic crystalloid boluses.
- Vasopressors to maintain CPP >60 (consider phenylephrine or norepinephrine).
- Packed red blood cells if active hemorrhage or hemoglobin <7 g.

Anticoagulation reversal

- Warfarin:
  - Reverse if INR >1.5 (goal is INR ≤1.4).
  - Vitamin K 10 mg IV over 10 minutes.
  - Prothrombin complex concentrate (PCC) 50 U/kg over 20 minutes or FFP 15 mL/kg.
  - Recheck INR 10 minutes after infusion.

- Antiplatelet agents (ASA or clopidogrel):
  - Desmopressin (DDAVP) 0.3 microgram/kg (~20 micrograms in 50 mL NS) over 15–30 minutes.
  - Platelet transfusion.
- Dabigatran (Pradaxa):
  - Management is controversial with no single reversal agent available.
  - If PTT is in normal range, it is unlikely that a significant drug effect is present.
  - Activated charcoal will adsorb this drug if the patient took it within 2 hours.
  - Can potentially be dialyzed and ~60% will be removed within 2–3 hours.
- Liver failure with known coagulopathy or elevated PT or INR >1.5:
  - Vitamin K 10 mg IV over 10 minutes (monitor for hypotension/anaphylaxis).
  - FFP 15 mL/kg IV or PCC 50 U/kg IV.

Neurosurgical issues

- All severe TBI patients should have a neurosurgical evaluation early in their ED course.
- If the patient has a seizure, treatment and loading with 1 g of phenytoin or fosphenytoin is indicated.
- The decision to place invasive ICP monitoring should generally be made in conjunction with neurosurgery.
- Indications for invasive ICP monitoring (external ventricular drain or intraparenchymal monitor):
  - Severe TBI and a CT showing hematomas, contusions, swelling, herniation, or compressed basal cisterns.
  - Severe TBI and a normal CT scan *if* two or more of the following apply: age >40 years, posturing (unilateral or bilateral), or SBP <90 mmHg.
- Sedation:
  - Propofol or pentobarbital coma may be induced for severe, but nonsurgical TBI.
  - The goal is to reduce cerebral activity and oxygen demand.
  - These agents cause hypotension and decreased CPP and should only be initiated with neurosurgical input.

Pitfalls to avoid in severe TBI

Hypoxemia/hyperoxemia (goal O_2 95%)
Hyperventilation (goal $PaCO_2$ 35–38 mmHg)
Hypotension (goal SBP >90 mmHg)
Coagulopathy (goal INR >1.4 or platelets <75 000/microliter)
Anemia (Hgb <8)
Hypo/hyperthermia (goal 36–38°C)
Hypo/hyperglycemia (goal 80–180 mg/dL; 4.44–9.99 mmol/L)

REFERENCES

Al-Rawi PG, Tseng MY, Richards HK, *et al.* Hypertonic saline in patients with poor-grade subarachnoid hemorrhage improves cerebral blood flow, brain tissue oxygen, and pH. *Stroke.* 2010; **41**: 122–8.

Blaivas M, Theodoro D, Sierzenski PR. Elevated intracranial pressure detected by bedside emergency ultrasonography of the optic nerve sheath. *Acad Emerg Med.* 2003; **10**: 376–81.

Bourgoin A, Albanèse J, Léone M, *et al.* Effects of sufentanil or ketamine administered in target-controlled infusion on the cerebral hemodynamics of severely brain-injured patients. *Crit Care Med.* 2005; **33**: 1109–13.

Brain Trauma Foundation; American Association of Neurological Surgeons; Congress of Neurological Surgeons; Joint Section on Neurotrauma and Critical Care, AANS/CNS, Bratton SL, Chestnut RM, Ghajar J, *et al.* Guidelines for the management of severe traumatic brain injury. *J Neurotrauma.* 2007; **24** Suppl 1: S1–106.

Bullock M, Chesnut R, Ghajar J, *et al.* Guidelines for the surgical management of traumatic brain injury. *Neurosurgery.* 2006; **58**(3) Supplement: S2-47–S2-55.

Crashingpatient.com [homepage on the Internet]. New York, NY: Scott Weingart; ©2006–2012 [updated 2012; cited August 1, 2012]. Available from: www.crashingpatient.com/ (accessed April 30, 2010).

Eisenberg HM, Frankowski RF, Contant CF, Marshall LF, Walker MD. High-dose barbiturate control of elevated intracranial pressure in patients with severe head injury. *J Neurosurg.* 1988; **69**: 15–23.

Emcrit.org [homepage on the Internet]. New York, NY: Scott Weingart; c2008–2012 [updated 2012; cited 2012 Aug 1]. Available from: www.emcrit.org/ (accessed April 30, 2010).

Fredriksson K, Norrving B, Strömblad LG. Emergency reversal of anticoagulation after intracerebral hemorrhage. *Stroke.* 1992; **23**: 972–7.

Kelly DF, Goodale DB, Williams J, *et al.* Propofol in the treatment of moderate and severe head injury: a randomized, prospective double-blinded pilot trial. *J Neurosurg.* 1999; **90**: 1042–52.

Kerr ME, Sereika SM, Orndoff P, *et al.* Effect of neuromuscular blockers and opiates on the cerebrovascular response to endotracheal suctioning in adults with severe head injuries. *Am J Crit Care.* 1998; **7**: 205–17.

Samama CM. Prothrombin complex concentrates: a brief review. *Eur J Anaesthesiol.* 2008; **25**: 784–9.

Swadron SP, Leroux P, Smith WS, Weingart SD. Emergency neurological life support: traumatic brain injury. *Neurocrit Care.* 2012; **17** Suppl 1: 112–21.

Vigué B. Bench-to-bedside review: Optimising emergency reversal of vitamin K antagonists in severe haemorrhage – from theory to practice. *Crit Care.* 2009; **13**: 209.

8

Spinal cord trauma

Ani Aydin

Introduction

- Traumatic spinal cord injury (TSCI) refers to the disruption of the neural structures that result in temporary or permanent loss of motor and/or sensory function.
- Spinal cord trauma can be a devastating event, with associated severe morbidity and mortality.
- Due to its flexibility, the cervical spine is the most commonly injured region of the spinal column. C2 is the most commonly injured vertebra, followed by the C5–C7 region.
- This section describes the most common and significant injuries to the cervical, thoracic, and lumbar spinal columns and the spinal cord.
- The most common causes of death in TSCI patients, following the initial injury, include sepsis and pneumonia.

Pathophysiology of traumatic spinal cord injuries

Mechanisms of injury

Most spinal cord injuries are associated with one of the following types of injuries to the spinal column:
- Bony injury – fracture of bones (see Table 8.1 for common vertebral fractures) and dislocation of joints
- Ligamentous injury via subluxation
- Intervertebral disk herniation
- Vascular injury (resulting in spinal cord ischemia)

Practical Emergency Resuscitation and Critical Care, ed. Kaushal Shah, Jarone Lee, Kamal Medlej, and Scott D. Weingart. Published by Cambridge University Press. © Kaushal Shah, Jarone Lee, Kamal Medlej, and Scott D. Weingart 2013.

Table 8.1. Some of the most common unstable vertebral fractures

Mechanism	Injury
Flexion	Teardrop fracture
	Atlanto-occipital dislocation (AOD)
	Odontoid fracture, Type III
	Chance fracture
Extension	Hangman's fracture (C2)
Vertical compression, axial load	Jefferson fracture (C1)
	Burst fracture

- Direct spinal cord trauma
  - Contusion
  - Compression (transient versus permanent)
  - Distraction – forcible stretching of the spinal cord
  - Transection or laceration.

Primary spinal cord injury

- The immediate trauma that results in the contusion, compression, low blood flow state, distraction, transection, or laceration of the spinal cord.
- Penetrating injuries can result in a complete or partial spinal cord transection.
  - Gunshot wounds may injure the spinal cord via the transferred kinetic energy, in addition to the direct missile injury.
  - Knife wounds usually create a more defined trajectory of injury.
- Blunt injuries, such as motor vehicle collisions, can result in more variable levels and severities of injury.

Secondary spinal cord injury

- Following the immediate trauma, secondary injury can occur to the spinal cord within minutes to hours.
- Mechanisms of secondary injury to the spinal cord include
  - Hypoxia
  - Ischemia
  - Inflammation
  - Edema
  - Necrosis
  - Electrolyte and ion disturbances
  - Excitotoxicity and apoptosis.
- Following a spinal cord injury, all efforts should be made to minimize any secondary injury to the spinal cord, which can result in progression of neurological deterioration.

Clinical presentations and grading systems

- Universal spinal immobilization after significant trauma continues to be an important practice. All patients are assumed to have TSCI until safely demonstrated otherwise.
- Physicians should have a high level of suspicion of TSCI in patients who present with multiple injuries, patients with head injuries, and those who are unconscious.
- Patients with spinal vertebrae fractures may complain of pain at the site of injury. However, head or associated injuries may limit a patient's ability to reliably identify TSCIs.
- **American Spinal Injury Association (ASIA) Scale**
  - *Complete spinal cord injury*
    - A complete spinal cord injury patient is given an ASIA Scale A.
    - Patients with a complete spinal cord injury will present with:
      - Sensation spared above the level of injury
      - Reduced muscle strength and tone below the level of injury; flaccid muscle tone more caudally
      - Reduced or absent reflexes
      - Priapism
      - Absent bulbocavernous reflex
      - Urinary retention, bladder distension.
  - *Incomplete spinal cord injury*
    - Incomplete spinal cord injuries are given ASIA Scale scores of B through E, depending on the severity of the injury and the extent of neurological dysfunction.
    - These patients would present with varying degrees of motor function.
    - Sensation is often spared more than motor function.
    - The bulbocavernous reflex and anal sensation are present.
      - The importance of the rectal examination in a trauma patient is to characterize the severity of TSCI and the patient's prognosis of neurological recovery.
- **Incomplete traumatic spinal cord injury syndromes**
  - These patients present with incomplete spinal cord injuries, and would be classified as ASIA Scale B through E.
  - *Central cord syndrome*
    - Motor function deficits are greater in the upper extremities, as opposed to the lower extremities.
    - There is a variable loss of sensation below the level of injury
    - There may be associated bladder dysfunction
    - Most common in elderly patients with underlying cervical canal narrowing after hyperextension injury.
  - *Anterior cord syndrome*
    - Occurs after injury to the anterior two-thirds of the spinal cord.
    - May occur after direct trauma to the anterior spinal artery.
    - More commonly is due to bony fragments or intervertebral disk impingement on the spinal artery.

- Spares the dorsal column; intact light touch and proprioception.
- *Brown–Séquard syndrome*
  - Often secondary to a spinal cord transection.
  - Loss of motor function ipsilateral to the side of the injury.
  - Loss of pain, temperature, and sensation contralateral to the injured side.
- *Cauda equina syndrome*
  - Decreased anal tone causing fecal incontinence
  - Saddle anesthesia
  - Lower extremity pain or weakness
  - Decreased or absent ankle reflexes
  - Sphincter weakness resulting in urinary retention and postvoid residual incontinence.
- **Clinical examination findings**
  - *Neurogenic shock*
    - Life threatening; true shock state.
    - Inadequate perfusion resulting from spinal cord injury.
    - Decreased vascular resistance due to interrupted autonomic pathways.
    - Presents with:
      - Hypotension
      - Bradycardia
      - Decreased cardiac output
      - Warm, dry extremities
      - Peripheral vasodilation
      - Temperature dysregulation.
  - *Spinal shock*
    - *Not* a true shock state.
    - A transient phenomenon lasting minutes to hours.
    - Temporary loss of sensation, motor paralysis, and diminished reflexes.
    - Often results from complete transection.
    - There is no cardiovascular compromise.
  - *Autonomic dysreflexia*
    - Due to a significant sympathetic discharge from afferent stimuli below the level of injury.
    - Presents with:
      - Hypertension
      - Bradycardia
      - Sweating, flushing.

Initial evaluation

- Follow the Trauma Assessment Algorithm, as outlined in the Advanced Trauma Life Support (ATLS) course, and discussed in other sections of this manual.

- Always remember to protect the cervical spine (c-spine) in all trauma patients with a rigid collar, especially those with head injuries, multiple injuries, neurological deficits, or in those who are unconscious.
- Immobilize the spine during transportation with a rigid long board. During the hospital assessment, remove the long board by log-rolling the patient until spinal injuries have been excluded.
- Consider and evaluate for any life-threatening injuries associated with the trauma.
  - The evaluation and treatment of life-threatening injuries, such as significant hemorrhage, pneumothorax, or airway compromise, take precedence over spinal cord injuries. Such injuries can lead to secondary spinal cord trauma, and therefore should be treated quickly to minimize further neurological deterioration.
- **Airway and breathing**
  - One-third of all patients with cervical spine injuries will require intubation within the first 24 hours.
  - Hypoxia can lead to secondary spinal cord injury, and should be quickly corrected.
  - Monitor the patient with pulse oximetry and use supplemental oxygen as needed.
- **Circulation**
  - Hypotension in a trauma patient should be assumed to be due to hemorrhagic shock until proven otherwise.
  - Hypotension can also be due to neurogenic shock.
  - Spinal shock does not result in hypotension.
- **Neurological examination**
  - A complete examination should be conducted to determine the level and severity of injury.
  - A mental status examination should be conducted, including an initial Glasgow Coma Scale (GCS), as explained in other sections of this manual.
  - Cranial nerve examination should be conducted, if possible, as many TSCI patients also sustain significant head trauma.
- **Imaging of spinal cord injuries**
  - *National Emergency X-Radiography Utilization Study (NEXUS)*
    - Allows the clinical clearance of c-spine injuries (no radiography).
    - NEXUS criteria for clinical c-spine clearance:
      - Alert, with no confusion
      - No distracting injuries
      - Not intoxicated
      - No neurological deficits
      - No midline c-spine pain or tenderness.
    - These five criteria for clinical clearance had a 99.8% negative predictive value, with a sensitivity of 99% and specificity of 12.9%.
  - *Plain radiographs*

- A complete set of images of the cervical spine includes the following:
  - The anteroposterior (AP) view, lateral view, and open-mouth odontoid view.
  - To be able to evaluate all possible injuries, images should include C1 through T1.
  - In patients whose body habitus obstructs the view of the lower cervical vertebrae, a swimmer's view can be obtained to better evaluate this region.
  - Based on the most recent Eastern Association for the Surgery of Trauma (EAST) guidelines in 2009, CT scanning has replaced radiography as the primary screening tool for cervical spine injury in the trauma patient.
  - Thoracic and lumbar images can be obtained in patients with pain, tenderness to palpation, or neurological deficits.
- *Computed tomography (CT)*
  - With coronal and sagittal reconstructions, the CT is better at identifying bone fractures in the spinal column with a sensitivity of almost 100%.
  - Patients with persistent pain despite normal radiographs should be considered for CT imaging.
  - CT remains the diagnostic method of choice in most trauma centers for diagnosis of c-spine injury after major trauma. For patients with mild to moderate mechanism of injury, there are no clear recommendations and practitioners must weigh the risks and benefits of plain radiographs versus CT scan.
- *Magnetic resonance imaging (MRI)*
  - MRI is able to identify injuries to the spinal cord, in addition to ligamentous, intervertebral disk, and soft tissue injuries.
  - There are several contraindications to emergent MRIs:
    - Patients who are transported for MRI must be clinically stable, as these images take longer to acquire, and the machines are often located farther away from the treatment area.
    - Pacemakers, cochlear implants, metallic implants or foreign bodies (such as bullets), and certain stents also pose contraindications to MRI scanning.

Critical management

- **Airway and breathing**
  - Consider early intubation for all patients with cervical spinal cord injuries who demonstrate any signs of inadequate ventilation or oxygenation in order to minimize secondary spinal cord injuries.
  - High cervical spine injuries may result in chest wall weakness, and inability to take deep breaths. Some patients may display paradoxical breathing, with the chest going inward and the abdomen distending during inspiration.

Such patients should be intubated early to minimize the work of breathing and fatigue that can result.

- Care should be taken during the intubation of patients with cervical spine injuries to minimize any movement of the neck that may cause worsening of the injury. The use of airway adjuncts, such as video laryngoscopy or fiber-optic techniques, may be preferable to direct laryngoscopy.

- **Cardiovascular**
  - *Hemorrhagic shock*
    - Hypotensive, hemodynamically unstable trauma patients should be presumed to have a hemorrhagic shock until proven otherwise.
    - These patients should be treated quickly with intravenous fluids, followed by blood products and source control, to minimize further neurological deterioration due to secondary spinal cord injury.
  - *Neurogenic shock*
    - Neurogenic shock can result in hypotension and bradycardia.
    - Treatment includes intravenous fluid, followed by vasopressors as needed to ensure perfusion of the spinal cord.
  - *Autonomic dysreflexia*
    - Patients with spinal cord injuries above the level of the sympathetic outflow (T5–T6) may suffer from autonomic dysreflexia, with episodic bouts of significant hypertension, diaphoresis, flushing of the skin, and bradycardia.
    - Care of these episodes is supportive, including treatment of reversible causes, such as bladder distension, fecal impaction, or any irritating stimulus below the level of the injury.

- **Glucocorticoids**
  - This topic is controversial; however, multitrauma patients with spinal injuries should not receive high-dose steroids.
  - While some animal studies found that steroids can decrease spinal cord edema and improve neurological function, such experiments have not been replicated in humans.
  - The National Acute Spinal Cord Injury Study (NASCIS) II study found no significant difference in neurological function between traumatic spinal cord injured patients treated with methylprednisolone, naloxone, or placebo. However, there were modest improvements in those treated within 8 hours.
  - The NASCIS III study found that patients treated between 3 and 8 hours after their injury had modest motor, but no significant functional recovery. Those with longer infusion of steroids had a higher rate of sepsis and pneumonia.
  - While steroids remain a treatment option, this decision should be made in conjunction with the trauma and neurosurgical services that will provide continued care for the patient.

- **Surgical options**
  - *Closed reduction*
    - Considered in patients with cervical spine injuries with subluxation and neurological deficits.

- Not used in thoracic or lumbar injuries.
- *Surgical indications*
  - Spinal cord compression with neurological deficits
  - Unstable vertebral fracture or dislocation
  - Penetrating injuries with imbedded foreign bodies in tissues, to prevent wound infection
- **Experimental treatments**
  - Spinal cord cooling
  - Electrical stimulation
  - Neural stem cells

REFERENCES

Braken MB, Sheppard MJ, Collins WF, *et al.* Methylprednisolone or naloxone treatment after acute spinal cord injury: 1-year follow-up data. Results of the second National Acute Spinal Cord Injury Study. *J Neurosurg.* 1992; **76**: 23–31.

Braken MB, Sheppard MJ, Holford TR, *et al.* Administration of methylprednisolone for 24 or 48 hours or tirilazad mesylate for 48 hours in the treatment of acute spinal cord injury. Results of the Third National Acute Spinal Cord Injury Randomized Controlled Trial. National Acute Spinal Cord Injury Study. *JAMA.* 1997; **277**: 1597–604.

Como JJ, Diaz JJ, Dunham CM, *et al.* Practice management guidelines for identification of cervical spine injuries following trauma: update from the Eastern Association for the Surgery of Trauma Practice Management Guidelines Committee. *J Trauma.* 2009; **67**: 651–9.

Dumont RJ, Okonkwo DO, Verma S, *et al.* Acute spinal cord injury, Part I: Pathophysiologic mechanisms. *Clin Neuropharmacol.* 2001; **24**: 254–64.

Hoffman JR, Mower WR, Woldson AB, *et al.* Validity of a set of clinical criteria to rule out injury to the cervical spine in patients with blunt trauma. National Emergency X-Radiography Utilization Study Group. *N Engl J Med.* 2000; **343**: 94–9.

NSCISC. Spinal Cord Injury Facts and Figures at a Glance. Birmingham, AL: National SCI Statistical Center; February 2012. Available at: www.nscisc.uab.edu/PublicDocuments/fact_figures_docs/Facts%202012%20Feb%20Final.pdf (accessed April 30, 2013).

9

Neck trauma

Vishal Demla

Introduction

- Most penetrating neck trauma is due to stab, slash, or gunshot wounds.
- Most blunt trauma is due to motor vehicle collisions.
- The incidence of penetrating neck trauma is reported to be approximately 1–5% of all traumatic injuries; blunt injuries are less common, approximately 5% of all neck traumas; they are also easily completely overlooked.
- Clinicians need to be particularly concerned about injuries to the larynx and trachea, lungs, vascular structures, nervous system, and esophagus.
- Innocuous-appearing neck injuries have the potential to cause either immediate or delayed life-threatening injuries and complications.
- The zones of the neck (see Table 9.1) are important because they help define the potentially injured structures and they allow for a common nomenclature. With the development and high utilization of multidetector CT scanners, the zones are less important for management decisions; virtually all neck trauma patients with suspicion of injury receive CT imaging as the first-line diagnostic modality.

Presentation

- In **penetrating injuries**, it is important to look for hard and soft signs of injury (see Table 9.2).
- Any hard or soft signs are concerning for significant neck trauma.
- Screening guidelines exist to determine the presence of blunt cerebrovascular injury (see Table 9.3).

Practical Emergency Resuscitation and Critical Care, ed. Kaushal Shah, Jarone Lee, Kamal Medlej, and Scott D. Weingart. Published by Cambridge University Press. © Kaushal Shah, Jarone Lee, Kamal Medlej, and Scott D. Weingart 2013.

Table 9.1. Zones of the neck

Zones	Landmarks	Structures/considerations
I	Defined inferiorly by clavicles and superiorly by the cricoid cartilage	In addition to neck structures (e.g., trachea, esophagus, neck vessels), consider injuries to thoracic structures, i.e., lung, subclavian vessels, common carotid artery, thoracic duct
II	Extends from the cricoid cartilage inferiorly to the angle of the mandible superiorly	Easily accessible surgically with ability to obtain proximal and distal control of bleeding. Includes carotid vessels, internal jugular veins, pharynx, esophagus
III	Includes the area superior to the angle of the mandible to the base of the skull	In addition to neurovascular injury (e.g., distal carotid, vertebral artery, cranial nerves), consider as a head injury

Table 9.2. Hard and soft signs of injury

Hard signs	Soft signs
Expanding hematoma	Hemoptysis/hematemesis
Severe active bleeding	Oropharyngeal blood
Shock not responding to fluids	Dyspnea
Decreased/absent radial pulse	Dysphonia/dysphagia
Vascular bruit/thrill	Subcutaneous/mediastinal air
Cerebral ischemia	Chest tube leak
Airway obstruction, stridor	Nonexpanding hematoma
Air bubbling through wound	Focal neurological deficit (contralateral side)
	Carotid: sensory or motor deficits, ipsilateral Horner syndrome
	Vertebral: ataxia, vertigo, emesis, or visual field deficit
	Carotid–cavernous sinus fistula: orbital pain, decreased vision, diplopia, proptosis, seizures, epistaxis
	Cervicothoracic seat belt sign

Diagnosis and evaluation

- High-resolution CT-angiography (CTA) is the initial diagnostic study of choice in the stable patient with penetrating neck trauma or blunt neck trauma when blunt cerebrovascular injury is suspected.
  - CTA can be the initial diagnostic study of choice regardless of zone of injury.
  - CTA is particularly useful for zone I and III penetrating injuries, which are more difficult to evaluate by physical examination.

Table 9.3. 2011 Denver Health Medical Center Blunt Cerebrovascular Injury Screening Guidelines

Signs/symptoms
- Arterial hemorrhage from neck/nose/mouth
- Cervical bruit in patient <50 years old
- Expanding cervical hematoma
- Focal neurological defect (including TIA)
- Neurological deficit inconsistent with head CT
- Stroke on CT/MRI

Risk factors
- LeFort II or III mid-face fracture
- Mandible fracture
- Complex skull fracture, basilar skull fracture/occipital condyle fracture
- Diffuse axonal injury and GCS <6
- Cervical subluxation or ligamentous injury/transverse foramen fracture/fracture C1–C3/any body fracture
- Near hanging with anoxic brain injury
- Clothesline injury or seat belt abrasion with altered mental status/significant swelling/pain
- Traumatic brain injury with thoracic injuries
- Scalp degloving
- Thoracic vascular injuries
- Blunt cardiac rupture

- Historically, stable, symptomatic patients with zone II penetrating injury required mandatory exploration but with the capabilities of CTA, there has been a paradigm shift and selective exploration is recommended.
- Injuries can be categorized into laryngotracheal (airway), pharyngoesophageal (digestive tract), and vascular.
  1. Laryngotracheal:
     - Symptoms include hoarseness, dyspnea, stridor, subcutaneous air, hemoptysis, and tenderness of the laryngeal area.
     - Plain radiographs are recommended as an initial screening tool but if clinical suspicion is high, plain films are not definitive to rule out injuries.
       - May show extraluminal air, edema, or fracture of laryngeal structures.
     - Direct laryngoscopy or flexible nasopharyngoscopy should be performed to rule out laryngeal injury if CTA is positive or inconclusive.
       - Indicated in stable patients with penetrating injuries to zone I and blunt neck trauma with symptoms.
  2. Pharyngoesophageal:
     - Symptoms include dysphagia, odynophagia, hematemesis, and blood in nasogastric tube or orogastric tube. However, even patients with significant injuries may present with no clinical signs.

- Esophageal injuries are the leading cause of delayed mortality, especially if there is a delay in diagnosis >24 hours.
- Broad-spectrum antibiotics are recommended for esophageal injuries.
- Similar to laryngotracheal injuries, plain radiographs are recommended as an initial screening tool. May show subcutaneous emphysema, retropharyngeal air, or pneumomediastinum if a perforation is present.
- Esophagoscopy or esophagraphy is the gold standard for diagnosing esophageal injury and should be used when there is high suspicion of injury and negative CT. Indicated in stable but symptomatic patients with penetrating zone I injury and blunt neck injury.

3. Vascular:
- Symptoms include shock, evidence of cerebral stroke, vascular bruit, upper extremity ischemia, expanding hematoma, pulsatile hematoma, or large hemothorax.
- Angiography/four-vessel cerebrovascular angiography (FVCA), still considered the gold standard for any vascular injury, should be considered when CTA is positive, inconclusive, or more information is needed (e.g., occasionally requested by surgeons for preoperative planning).
- CTA must be eight-slice or greater to rule out blunt cerebrovascular injury, and has similar sensitivity to FVCA. Four-slice CTA is neither sensitive nor specific enough to assess for blunt cerebrovascular injury.
- Duplex ultrasonography is not adequate for screening for blunt cerebrovascular injury and is particularly limited for nonocclusive injury.
- Magnetic resonance angiography (MRA) has not been shown to be superior to CTA.

Critical management

- Unstable patients with penetrating injuries require immediate surgical consultation and exploration in the OR. Unstable patients include those patients with hard signs: clear airway injury (air bubbling through wound), hemodynamic instability despite resuscitation, uncontrolled bleeding (including expanding hematoma), or evolving neurological deficit. See suggested clinical management pathways (Figure 9.1).

Airway

- Indications for immediate airway management in the context of neck trauma include stridor, respiratory distress, shock, and rapidly expanding hematoma.
- Indications for urgent or prophylactic airway management include: progressive neck symptoms (especially swelling), need to transfer a symptomatic patient, voice changes, extensive subcutaneous emphysema, edema or tracheal shift, alteration in mental status, and an anticipated prolonged period away from the ED.

Clinical pathway for management of penetrating neck trauma, zones I, II, or III

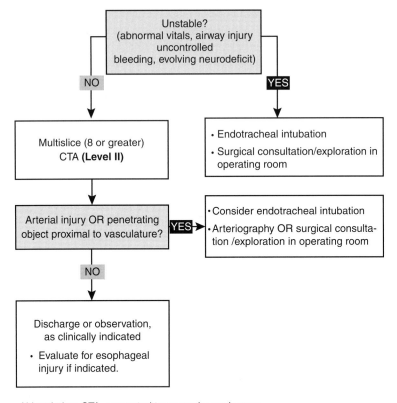

Abbreviation: CTA, computed tomography angiogram

Figure 9.1. Clinical pathway for management of penetrating neck trauma.

- Rapid sequence intubation (RSI) has a very high success rate and should be initiated early in the appropriate circumstances.
- The presence of neck trauma, by itself, is not a contraindication to RSI.
- Consider RSI if patient is not difficult to bag and there is no anatomical disruption.
- If oral rapid sequence intubation is planned it should be under a double setup with preparations and personnel in place to perform immediate surgical cricothyrotomy if oral intubation is not possible.
- Consider an awake intubation if difficulty is anticipated in bagging or suspected tracheal disruption. Awake intubation is preferably done with a fiberoptic scope, if available, which would allow better visualization if anatomy is distorted.
- Consider needle cricothyrotomy if a child is <10 years of age.

- Tracheostomy should be considered if the patient cannot receive/has failed RSI and contraindications to cricothyrotomy exist.
- Consider direct tracheal intubation for open trachea but be wary of potentially completely transecting the trachea.

Breathing

- Patients with zone I injury are especially prone to pneumothoraces and hemothoraces.
- Tension pneumothorax should be considered in a patient with hypotension, respiratory distress and decreased breath sounds.
- Prompt needle decompression or open thoracostomy should be performed.

Circulation

- Bleeding should be managed by direct compression.
- If central venous access is necessary, place a large-bore single lumen catheter through the subclavian (on opposite side of injury) or femoral vein.
- If the patient is unstable or hard/soft signs are present, the patient needs emergent surgical consultation and should proceed to the OR regardless of zone of injury.

Special considerations

- Immobilization is not necessary in penetrating neck trauma unless there is an overt neurological deficit or an adequate physical examination cannot be performed.
- Cervical spine injuries are extremely rare in penetrating neck trauma. There is an abundance of literature (but no randomized trials) corroborating the safety of removing the cervical collar for penetrating neck trauma. Removal of the collar facilitates the physical examination and is highly recommended to rule out penetrating injuries to the posterior neck.

REFERENCES

Bromberg WJ, Collier B, Diebel L, *et al.* Blunt cerebrovascular injury practice management guidelines: East Practice Management Guidelines Committee. *J Trauma.* 2010; **68**; 471–7.

Demla V, Shah K. Neck trauma: current guidelines for emergency physicians. *Emerg Med Pract Guidelines Update.* 2012;**4**(3):1–9.

Newton K. Neck. In: Marx JA, Hockberger RS, Walls RM, Adams J, Rosen P, eds. *Rosen's Emergency Medicine: Concepts and Clinical Practice.* 7th edn. Philadelphia, PA: Mosby Elsevier; 2010.

Schaider J, Bailitz J. Neck trauma: don't put your neck on the line. *Emerg Med Pract.* 2003; **5**(7): 1–28.

Sutijono D. Blunt neck trauma. In: Shah K, ed. *Essential Emergency Trauma*. Philadelphia, PA: Lippincott Williams & Wilkins; 2011.

Tisherman AT, Bokhari F, Collier B, *et al.* Clinical practice guidelines: penetrating neck trauma. *J Trauma.* 2008; **64**: 1392–1405.

Walls RM, Vissers RJ. The traumatized airway. In: Hagberg CA., ed. *Benumof's Airway Management*. Philadelphia, PA: Mosby Elsevier, 2007.

10

Thoracic trauma

Samantha Wood

Introduction

- As with any trauma patient, the evaluation of the patient with suspected thoracic trauma begins with an organized, stepwise evaluation and stabilization of the ABCDEs.
- Initial evaluation of possible thoracic trauma includes obtaining a brief but accurate history to understand the mechanism of injury and to elicit the patient's symptoms.
- A careful physical examination must be conducted including inspection (with careful attention to visualization of the axillae and back, where injuries may be missed), palpation for deformity and crepitus, and auscultation for breath sounds and heart murmur.
- Bedside ultrasound is useful in the initial assessment of the patient with chest trauma to rapidly evaluate for pneumothorax and pericardial effusion.
- Initial imaging of the patient with thoracic trauma typically includes portable chest radiography, followed by case-specific imaging.
- Trauma to the thorax may be categorized as penetrating (i.e., gunshot wound, stab wound) or blunt (i.e., motor vehicle collision, fall).
- Penetrating injuries to "the box" (the area defined by the clavicles superiorly, nipple lines laterally, and costal margins inferiorly) are of particular concern because of the high likelihood of injury to the heart and mediastinal structures.
- The diaphragm may elevate as high as the fourth intercostal space on exhalation, so concurrent abdominal injury must be considered when penetrating trauma is located at or below the fourth intercostal space.
- Patients with thoracic trauma may be stable on initial presentation and may lack obvious signs and symptoms of thoracic trauma. A high level of suspicion and thorough workup is required to evaluate for life-threatening injuries.

Practical Emergency Resuscitation and Critical Care, ed. Kaushal Shah, Jarone Lee, Kamal Medlej, and Scott D. Weingart. Published by Cambridge University Press. © Kaushal Shah, Jarone Lee, Kamal Medlej, and Scott D. Weingart 2013.

Pneumothorax

- Pneumothorax is the most common thoracic injury associated with penetrating trauma.
- It occurs when air enters the pleural space, causing the lung to collapse.
- Tension pneumothorax results from increasing air collection in the pleural space, causing high intrathoracic pressures and impeding venous return to the heart, which results in hypotension and hemodynamic collapse. A pneumothorax also can compromise respiration as the lungs are compressed.

Presentation

Classic presentation
- Patient with traumatic pneumothorax may present with complaints of pleuritic chest pain and/or dyspnea.
- Physical examination findings in pneumothorax include decreased or absent breath sounds, hyperresonance to percussion, and crepitus on the side of the injury.

Critical presentation
- Tension pneumothorax presents with hypotension, tachypnea, tachycardia, distended neck veins, diminished or absent breath sounds on the affected side, and tracheal deviation away from the side of injury.

Diagnosis and evaluation

- Tension pneumothorax is a clinical diagnosis; obtaining a chest radiograph will only delay treatment of this critical condition.
- All patients at risk for any thoracic trauma should receive a chest radiograph as an initial screening tool.
- However, chest radiography is insensitive for pneumothorax and may miss up to half of pneumothoraces in trauma patients. Detection of pneumothorax by supine chest radiography is particularly insensitive as air in the pleural space tends to accumulate anteriorly in patients in this position. If a patient is able to sit upright, an upright PA film is preferred.
- Because of the poor sensitivity of chest radiography for pneumothorax, there should be a low threshold to pursue further imaging with CT scan.
- Ultrasound performed by a trained provider looking for lung sliding and comet tails has superior sensitivity and specificity to supine chest radiography and similar sensitivity to chest CT in detecting pneumothorax.
- In patients with apparently minor penetrating chest trauma who are asymptomatic and have an initial chest radiograph negative for pneumothorax, 12% will develop a delayed pneumothorax requiring intervention. These patients should be monitored and undergo repeat chest radiography at 3–6 hours.

Critical management

- Suspected tension pneumothorax must be treated immediately.
- Traditional teaching is that tension pneumothorax should be treated by performing immediate needle decompression using a 14-gauge angiocatheter inserted at the second intercostal space at the midclavicular line, followed immediately by tube thoracostomy. However, needle decompression has a significant rate of failure as a standard catheter is often too short to reach the parietal pleura. If tube thoracostomy can be performed immediately, this may be preferable.
- Tube thoracostomy is also indicated for any patient with pneumothorax who has dyspnea, hypoxia, or chest pain or when the pneumothorax is >15% of the chest cavity. Classic teaching recommends that a large chest tube (36 French or greater) should be used in traumatic pneumothorax because many patients will have concurrent hemothorax; however, more recent data suggests that smaller tubes may be equally effective.
- Administration of prophylactic antibiotics after tube thoracostomy is controversial. A recent meta-analysis supports the use of prophylactic antibiotics to decrease infectious complications, with this effect most pronounced in penetrating trauma. However, recent guidelines acknowledge that there is insufficient evidence to support recommendations for or against this practice.
- Asymptomatic patients with an occult or small pneumothorax may be observed; tube thoracostomy should be performed if the patient becomes symptomatic or the pneumothorax enlarges.

Sudden deterioration

- Sudden deterioration in a patient with known or suspected pneumothorax must raise concern for the development of tension physiology.
- Positive-pressure ventilation can convert a simple pneumothorax to a tension pneumothorax. The trauma patient who decompensates shortly after intubation must be evaluated for pneumothorax. Hypovolemia, medications, and incorrect endotracheal tube placement can also cause the recently intubated patient to decompensate.

Hemothorax

- Hemothorax results when injury to thoracic, mediastinal, chest wall, or abdominal structures cause blood to collect in the pleural cavity.

Presentation

Classic presentation

- Physical examination findings include decreased breath sounds and chest movement on the side of the hemothorax, dullness to percussion on the affected side, evidence of rib fractures, and findings of concurrent pneumothorax.

Critical presentation
- Massive hemothorax is defined as hemothorax of >1500 mL is defined as massive hemothorax and may cause hypoxia secondary to lung collapse, as well as hypotension secondary to hypovolemia and impedance of venous return (tension hemothorax).

Diagnosis and evaluation

- A hemothorax must be 400–500 mL in volume to be visible on an upright chest radiograph.
- Hemothorax will appear on a supine chest radiograph as opacification of the affected hemithorax (not as a fluid level); for this reason even a substantial hemothorax can be missed on a supine radiograph.
- Bedside ultrasonography can reveal fluid in the pleural space suggesting hemothorax and is comparable to portable radiography in making the diagnosis.
- CT scan has the highest sensitivity and specificity for detection of hemothorax.

Critical management

- Hemothorax should be drained with a large (36 French or greater) chest tube; retained hemothorax can consolidate and result in infection and fibrosis.
- Initial drainage of >1500 mL or continued drainage of >200 mL/hour should prompt consideration of surgical thoracotomy.
- Retained hemothorax following tube thoracostomy is a risk factor for infection, and should generally prompt early video assisted thoracic surgery (VATS); however, recent data indicates that small retained hemothoraces <300 mL may be considered for observation.

Sudden deterioration

- The development of massive hemothorax can cause sudden hemodynamic instability. If this is suspected, immediate tube thoracostomy must be performed to drain the hemothorax. Hemorrhagic shock should be treated with resuscitation using crystalloids and blood products. Surgical intervention is recommended for the indications described above and should be considered in any patient who shows signs of continuous bleeding or persistent instability.

Cardiac tamponade

- Cardiac tamponade is the accumulation of fluid in the pericardial space under pressure, causing pressure on the heart chambers and decreased cardiac output.

Presentation

Classic presentation
- Beck's triad (hypotension, distant heart sounds, jugular venous distension) describes the classic presentation of cardiac tamponade.
- Pulsus paradoxus (inspiratory systolic fall in blood pressure of 10 mmHg or more) may be present.

Critical presentation
- Tamponade can impede cardiac output to the point of cardiac arrest.

Diagnosis and evaluation

- Pericardial effusion may be diagnosed on FAST examination with the finding of fluid surrounding the heart.
- Chest radiography may show an enlarged cardiac silhouette.
- Cardiac tamponade is identified on ultrasound by collapse of the right atrium and/or ventricle; even if these findings are not observed, the presence of a pericardial effusion in a hemodynamically unstable patient with a thoracic injury and no alternative explanation strongly suggests tamponade physiology.

Critical management

- Traumatic pericardial tamponade must be treated with immediate surgical thoracotomy to address the cause of the bleeding into the pericardium.
- Emergency department thoracotomy is indicated in the patient with traumatic arrest due to penetrating chest trauma who had recent signs of life (such as pupillary response, spontaneous ventilation, palpable pulse, measurable blood pressure, or cardiac electrical activity). This procedure allows the physician to perform pericardotomy to release tamponade, repair cardiac lacerations, cross-clamp the aorta to prevent exsanguination from abdominal injuries, and perform internal cardiac massage and defibrillation.
- Patients with blunt chest trauma who have undergone >10 minutes of prehospital CPR without response, penetrating chest trauma with >15 minutes of prehospital CPR without response, or presenting rhythm of asystole without pericardial tamponade are unlikely to have meaningful survival with ED thoracotomy. There should be consideration of withholding the procedure in these settings.
- Factors that predict survival after ED thoracotomy include penetrating injury (8.8% survival), especially stab wounds (16.8% survival), and signs of life on arrival at the hospital (11.5% survival). Survival is extremely low in patients with blunt trauma, multiple injuries, and those who had no signs of life in the field (1–2%).

Sudden deterioration

- In-hospital cardiac arrest due to pericardial tamponade is an indication for ED thoracotomy.
- Pericardiocentesis or pericardial window in traumatic pericardial tamponade may briefly stabilize the patient if surgical management is not immediately possible; however, it will not fix the underlying cause of the tamponade and surgical thoracotomy must follow.

Aortic injury

- Blunt aortic injury carries a very high mortality and 75–90% of patients with this condition die immediately at the scene of the accident.
- Patients with blunt aortic injury who survive transport to the emergency department will often be hemodynamically stable initially, so the clinician must be alert to the possibility of this critical injury in the stable patient with a concerning mechanism.

Presentation

Classic presentation
- The classic mechanism for blunt aortic injury is sudden deceleration (such as a fall from >3 m or high-speed head-on motor vehicle collision). Front seat occupants, unbelted drivers or passengers, and people over 60 years old are at particularly high risk.
- However, lower-speed collisions may account for many cases of traumatic aortic rupture, especially in patients over 60 years old and in cases of lateral impact.
- Patients may complain of chest pain, back pain, and dyspnea and will frequently have multiple associated injuries.
- Steering wheel or seat belt contusion on the chest, flail chest, unequal extremity pulses, hoarseness, and paraplegia raise concern for aortic injury; however, physical examination is not sensitive in the evaluation of aortic injury and the physician must have a low threshold to pursue diagnostic imaging.

Critical presentation
- The critical patient with aortic injury who survives transport to the emergency department has a high probability of aortic rupture resulting in complete hemodynamic collapse and death if not immediately diagnosed and treated.

Diagnosis and evaluation

- See Figure 10.1 for an example of blunt aortic injury on plain film and CT.

(a)

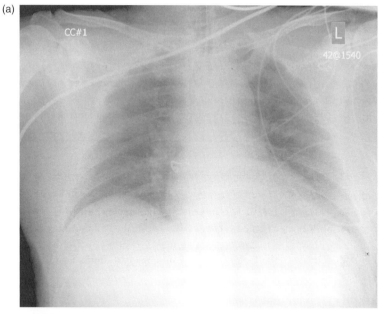

(b)

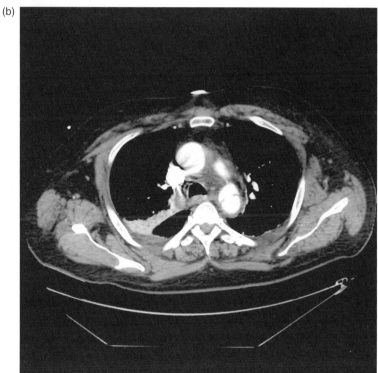

Figure 10.1. (a) demonstrates a wide mediastinum suspicious for blunt aortic injury on portable chest radiograph. The diagnosis is confirmed on CT (b). (Image courtesy of Michael A. Gibbs, MD.)

Chest radiography findings concerning for blunt aortic injury

---

Widened mediastinum (>8 cm on supine or >6 cm on upright film)
Obscured aortic knob
Left apical cap (blood above apex of lung)
Large left hemothorax
Rightward deviation of nasogastric tube
Rightward deviation of trachea or downward deviation of right mainstem bronchus
Wide left paravertebral stripe

- CT scan of the chest should be performed if any of these findings are present on chest radiography.
- A negative chest radiograph is not sufficient to exclude aortic injury, and CT scan should be performed if there is any clinical suspicion for this injury.
- Transesophageal echocardiogram by a skilled operator can accurately identify aortic injury and may be performed if a patient is unable to undergo CT scan.

Critical management

- Immediate surgical repair is necessary in patients who are unstable due to traumatic aortic injury.
- Medical management of the stable traumatic aortic injury patient or those in whom surgical repair must be delayed centers on the reduction of wall tension and shearing forces. Use a short-acting beta-blocker, such as esmolol, to reduce heart rate to a goal of 60 bpm, followed by an arterial vasodilator such as nicardipine or sodium nitroprusside to reduce blood pressure to 100–120 mmHg. These measures minimize risk of rupture prior to repair and can allow delay of repair while other more critical injuries are treated. Patients with significant traumatic head injury are an exception to this recommendation.

Sudden deterioration

- The patient with traumatic aortic injury is at extremely high risk for deterioration.
- Rapid surgical consultation at the first suspicion of traumatic aortic injury must be obtained to expedite repair.

Tracheobronchial injury

- Injury to the tracheobronchial tree is relatively uncommon.

Presentation

Classic presentation
- May present with dyspnea, subcutaneous emphysema, sternal tenderness, and Hamman's sign (a "crunching" sound heard on auscultation of the precordium due to mediastinal emphysema).
- Tracheobronchial injury should be suspected in the presence of a large air leak from a chest tube, or a rapidly reaccumulating pneumothorax or pneumomediastinum.
- Diagnosis of tracheobronchial injury is frequently delayed and may present as retained lung secretions, poor lung expansion, persistent air leak or recurrent pneumothorax, or bronchial obstruction in the days to weeks following the injury.

Critical presentation
- Tracheal transection is usually associated with multiple other severe injuries and is generally fatal.
- Missed tracheobronchial injury can result in mediastinitis, bronchial stenosis, and recurrent pulmonary infections.

Diagnosis and evaluation

- Definitive diagnosis may be established by bronchoscopy or operative evaluation.
- High-quality CT scan may also diagnose tracheobronchial injury.

Critical management

- Most tracheobronchial injuries should be surgically repaired; however, observation may be considered in hemodynamically stable patients in whom ventilation is not difficult, there is no accumulating subcutaneous or mediastinal emphysema, and there is no involvement of the esophagus.

Flail chest

- Flail chest occurs when three or more ribs are each fractured in two or more places resulting in a "floating" segment of the rib cage. The floating segment paradoxically moves inward with inhalation and outward with exhalation and can greatly increase work of breathing.

Presentation

Classic presentation
- The patient with flail chest may present with pain, dyspnea, tachypnea, chest wall tenderness and crepitus, and visible flail segment on observation of breathing.

Critical presentation
- Patients with a significant flail chest, especially older patients or those with underlying lung disease or multiple other injuries, may present with respiratory distress or arrest.

Diagnosis and evaluation

- Chest radiograph shows multiple rib fractures.
- Patients who present with flail chest should receive CT of the chest to evaluate for other injuries including blunt aortic injuries, pulmonary contusions and pneumothorax.

Critical management

- External stabilization of the flail segment restricts chest expansion and is not recommended.
- Positive-pressure ventilation, either invasive or noninvasive, may be used in patients with hypoxia, hypercapnea, or respiratory distress. However, obligatory mechanical ventilation in flail chest should be avoided as it may increase complications and many patients will do well with pain control and pulmonary toilet alone.
- As with all chest wall injuries, pain management is critical to prevent splinting and the development of atelectasis or pneumonia. An epidural catheter is preferred for pain control in severe chest injury.
- Elderly trauma patients who sustain blunt chest trauma with rib fractures have twice the mortality and morbidity of younger patients with similar injuries. For each additional rib fracture in the elderly, mortality increases by 19% and the risk of pneumonia by 27%. Aggressive pain control with epidural catheter placement is recommended in these patients.
- Surgical fixation of rib or sternal fractures is controversial but may be considered.

Sudden deterioration

- Patients with flail chest can deteriorate rapidly to the point of respiratory arrest due to increased work of breathing combined with hypoxia caused by underlying lung contusion.
- Endotracheal intubation and mechanical ventilation is indicated for the decompensating patient with flail chest.

REFERENCES

Ball CG, Kirkpatrick AW, Laupland KB, *et al.* Factors related to the failure of radiographic recognition of occult posttraumatic pneumothoraces. *Am J Surg.* 2005; **189**: 541–6; discussion 546.

Bosman A, de Jong MB, Debeij J, van den Broek PJ, Schipper IB. Systematic review and meta-analysis of antibiotic prophylaxis to prevent infections from chest drains in blunt and penetrating thoracic injuries. *Br J Surg*. 2012; **99**: 506–13.

DuBose J, Inaba K, Demetriades D, *et al*. Management of post-traumatic retained hemothorax: a prospective, observational, multicenter AAST study. *J Trauma Acute Care Surg*. 2012; **72**: 11–22; discussion 22–4; quiz 316.

Fabian TC, Richardson JD, Croce MA, *et al*. Prospective study of blunt aortic injury: Multicenter Trial of the American Association for the Surgery of Trauma. *J Trauma*. 1997; **42**: 374–80; discussion 380–3.

Fabian TC, Davis KA, Gavant ML, *et al*. Prospective study of blunt aortic injury: helical CT is diagnostic and antihypertensive therapy reduces rupture. *Ann Surg*. 1998; **227**: 666–76; discussion 676–7.

Leigh-Smith S, Harris T. Tension pneumothorax – time for a re-think? *Emerg Med J*. 2005; **22**: 8–16.

Moore EE, Knudson MM, Burlew CC, *et al*. Defining the limits of resuscitative emergency department thoracotomy: a contemporary Western Trauma Association perspective. *J Trauma*. 2011; **70**: 334–9.

Moore F, Duane TM, Hu CK *et al*. Presumptive antibiotic use in tube thoracostomy for traumatic hemopneumothorax: An Eastern Association for the Surgery of Trauma practice management guideline. *J Trauma Acute Care Surg*. 2012; **73**: S341–4.

Mowery NT, Gunter OL, Collier BR, *et al*. Practice management guidelines for management of hemothorax and occult pneumothorax. *J Trauma*. 2011; **70**: 510–18.

Neff MA, Monk JS, Jr., Peters K, Nikhilesh A. Detection of occult pneumothoraces on abdominal computed tomographic scans in trauma patients. *J Trauma*. 2000; **49**: 281–5.

Ordog GJ, Wasserberger J, Balasubramanium S, Shoemaker W. Asymptomatic stab wounds of the chest. *J Trauma*. 1994; **36**: 680–4.

Rhee PM, Acosta J, Bridgeman A, *et al*. Survival after emergency department thoracotomy: review of published data from the past 25 years. *J Am Coll Surg*. 2000; **190**: 288–98.

Rowan KR, Kirkpatrick AW, Liu D, *et al*. Traumatic pneumothorax detection with thoracic US: correlation with chest radiography and CT – initial experience. *Radiology*. 2002; **225**: 210–14.

Sastry P, Field M, Cuerden R, Richens D. Low-impact scenarios may account for two-thirds of blunt traumatic aortic rupture. *Emerg Med J*. 2010; **27**: 341–4.

Simon B, Ebert J, Bokhari F *et al*. Management of pulmonary contusion and flail chest : an Eastern Association for the Surgery of Trauma practice management guideline. *J Trauma Acute Care Surg*. 2012; **73**: S351–61.

Spodick DH. Acute cardiac tamponade. *N Engl J Med*. 2003; **349**: 684–90.

11

Solid organ abdominal trauma

Jayaram Chelluri

Introduction

- The solid organs of the abdomen include the liver, pancreas, kidneys, and spleen. They are most often affected during injury to the abdomen, back, and flank.
- When injured, these organs have a tendency to bleed given their abundant vascular supply.
- Injuries are generally classified based on mechanism into either blunt or penetrating due to differing means of evaluation and treatment for each.
- *Penetrating injuries*
  - Stab wounds:
    - Stabbings are less likely to penetrate the peritoneum or cause intra-abdominal injury requiring surgical treatment than are projectile wounds.
    - The liver is the most commonly injured solid organ given its surface area in the abdominal cavity.
  - Projectile wounds or gunshot wounds (GSW):
    - Degree of injury is highly related to velocity of projectile
      - Medium- and high-velocity projectiles create explosive type injuries and create a secondary zone of injury through tissue.
      - High-velocity projectiles have a tendency to fragment internally, which may cause closure along the tract of injury, leading to difficulty assessing tissue damage. Also, they are complicated by contaminants in the wound.
  - GSW are associated with greater mortality.
  - Shotgun wounds receive special consideration given the nature of the projectile.

Practical Emergency Resuscitation and Critical Care, ed. Kaushal Shah, Jarone Lee, Kamal Medlej, and Scott D. Weingart. Published by Cambridge University Press. © Kaushal Shah, Jarone Lee, Kamal Medlej, and Scott D. Weingart 2013.

- *Blunt injuries*
  - Solid organs are commonly injured with acceleration/deceleration injuries (i.e., motor vehicle collisions [MVC]) and crush injuries.
  - Blunt injuries are associated with greater mortality than penetrating ones because of difficulties in diagnosis leading to potential delays.
  - They are often associated with severe mechanisms.
  - The spleen is the most commonly injured solid organ followed by the liver.

Presentation

- There is a range of presentations from stable with seemingly insignificant injuries to severe hemorrhagic shock.
- History may be difficult to obtain or deferred based on the clinical condition of the patient.
- The ability to adequately identify injuries on physical examination may be compromised by concomitant injuries (i.e., head trauma) or confounding factors (i.e., intoxication).
- Emergency responders or other observers may provide crucial information.
- Common symptoms are abdominal, back or flank pain, nausea, vomiting, confusion, or dizziness.
- Common signs are tenderness to palpation and ecchymosis (e.g., seat-belt sign) but they are not universally present.

Diagnosis and evaluation

- The primary survey should be aimed at determining which patients need immediate laparotomy versus those that are stable for further diagnostic workup.
- Vital signs provide a key to hemodynamic stability. Unstable patients with blunt or penetrating trauma to the abdomen require immediate laparotomy.
- **Physical examination**
  - May be the only clues to injuries if history is unobtainable.
  - Look for abdominal tenderness and skin lesions (i.e., bruising patterns, entry/exit wounds).
  - Pain is often focal in solid organ injury but can be referred (i.e., hemoperitoneum).
  - Serial abdominal examinations in awake and alert patients can provide valuable information since the patients can be initially asymptomatic with symptoms developing over time. However, distracting injuries, particularly in blunt trauma, may obfuscate the examination.
  - Ecchymosis of flank and umbilicus (Gray Turner's sign or Cullen's sign, respectively) may represent retroperitoneal or intraperitoneal hemorrhage.

- **Laboratory tests**
  - Hematological laboratory tests should not be used solely for diagnosis and are only adjuncts to clinical picture. Complete blood count may not reflect blood loss initially.
  - Lactate level is nonspecific but has been demonstrated to be a useful marker of severity of illness illustrating deficits in organ perfusion. Lactate clearance is also a useful marker of resuscitation.
  - Pancreatic enzymes, liver function tests and chemistry are unreliable in the setting of trauma.
  - Urinalysis may be useful to evaluate for the presence of hematuria indicating possible renal injury.
  - Sending a blood type and crossmatch is essential in the setting of significant trauma.
- **Radiology**
  - Resuscitation efforts should take precedence over imaging studies. Hemodynamic stabilization is the priority.
  - All patients after significant trauma, both blunt and penetrating, should receive screening AP chest radiography.
  - Abdominal radiographs are of limited value in solid organ blunt trauma.
  - *Focused Assessment with Sonography for Trauma* (FAST) – helps to determine whether there is free fluid in the abdomen.
    - Blood on ultrasound will be visualized as anechoic areas, best viewed when contrasted against the solid organ. Like abdominal examinations, the diagnostic sensitivity of the FAST examination improves when done serially, particularly in blunt abdominal trauma.
    - Positive FAST examination in a hemodynamically stable patient will still need abdominal CT imaging to identify the location and severity of hemorrhage; nonoperative management may still be an option.
    - Pros:
      - Can be done rapidly at the bedside. Ideal for unstable patients because you do not have to leave the trauma bay.
      - No radiation exposure.
      - Sensitive for detecting typically 500 mL of fluid. Sensitivity can be improved by placing the patient in Trendelenburg position.
      - Noninvasive.
    - Cons:
      - Quality of examination is dependent on examiner experience.
      - Does not evaluate solid parenchymal damage (i.e., splenic capsular injury) or retroperitoneum (e.g., pancreatic injuries).
      - May not be accurate in obese or uncooperative patients. Images can be obscured by bowel gas or subcutaneous air.
  - *Computed tomography* (CT) has virtually replaced diagnostic peritoneal lavage. Generally done with IV contrast only; little information is added with oral contrast.

- Pros:
  - CT is very accurate for identification of solid visceral organ injuries.
  - Active bleeding from the liver/spleen can be visualized by extravasation of IV contrast (often called a "blush").
  - The retroperitoneum can be visualized.
  - CT can guide nonoperative management by aiding in grading of lacerations and contusions.
  - Noninvasive.
- Cons:
  - It requires leaving the trauma resuscitation area, so the patient should be stabilized before transport to the radiology department.
  - It is not sensitive for pancreatic injuries.
  - The quantity of blood or presence of isolated free fluid on CT cannot guide surgical management.
  - Radiation exposure (8–15 millisieverts depending on the scanner and protocol). For reference, a portable chest radiograph delivers ~0.02 millisieverts.
- *Diagnostic peritoneal lavage* (DPL) is useful for determination of intra-abdominal bleeding when the patient is unstable and unable to obtain CT, FAST is negative or inconclusive, and source of hemorrhage is unclear.
  - DPL is particularly useful for penetrating trauma in equivocal cases and to assess for diaphragmatic injury. It can be limited in assessing damage to the liver, spleen, and bowel and can reduce the number of unnecessary laparotomies.
  - Relative contraindications
    - Prior abdominal surgery or infections
    - Coagulopathy
    - Obesity
    - Second/third trimester pregnancy.
  - Absolute contraindications
    - Indications are present to go directly to laparotomy.
- **Other diagnostic modalities**
  - Angiography is rarely used in diagnostic evaluation but may be a useful therapy in management of bleeding, particularly in splenic and liver lesions.
    - Indications
      - Higher grades of injury
      - Active extravasation of contrast
      - Presence of pseudoaneurysm and increased amount of hemoperitoneum.
  - Magnetic resonance imaging (MRI) is generally not helpful in solid organ abdominal trauma.
  - Local wound exploration in the abdominal region is useful in determining the depth of a wound and to determine whether the wound has penetrated the peritoneum.

The following tables demonstrate grading systems for blunt injuries to various solid abdominal organs (adapted from the American Association of Surgery for Trauma).

Spleen injury grading scale

Grade	Hematoma	Laceration
I	Subcapsular, <10% surface area	Capsular tear, <1 cm parenchymal depth
II	Subcapsular, 10–50% surface area; intraparenchymal <5 cm in diameter	Capsular tear, 1–3 cm parenchymal depth that does not involve a trabecular vessel
III	Subcapsular, >50% surface area or expanding; ruptured subcapsular or parenchymal hematoma; intraparenchymal hematoma 5 cm or expanding	>3 cm parenchymal depth or involving trabecular vessels
IV	Involves the hilum	Involves segmental or hilar vessels leading to devascularization >25% of spleen
V	Shattered spleen	Hilar vascular injury devascularizing spleen

Liver injury grading scale

Grade	Hematoma	Laceration
I	Subcapsular <10% surface area	Capsular tear, <1 cm parenchymal depth
II	Subcapsular 10–50% surface area; intraparenchymal <10 cm in diameter	Capsular tear, 1–3 cm parenchymal depth, <10 cm in length
III	Subcapsular, >50% surface area of ruptured subcapsular or parenchymal hematoma; intraparenchymal hematoma >10 cm or expanding	>3 cm parenchymal depth
IV	Involves segmental or hilar vessels leading to devascularization >25% of spleen	Parenchymal disruption involving 25–75% hepatic lobe or 1–3 Couinaud's segments
V	Hilar vascular injury devascularizing spleen	Parenchymal disruption involving >75% of hepatic lobe or >3 Couinaud's segments within a single lobe; vascular injury – juxtaheptatic venous injuries
VI		Vascular injury – hepatic avulsion

Renal injury grading scale

Grade	Characteristics
I	Contusion: microscopic or gross hematuria, urological studies normal
	Subcapsular hematoma: nonexpanding without parenchymal lacerations
II	Nonexpanding perirenal hematoma confined to renal retroperitoneum
	Laceration <1 cm parenchymal depth of renal cortex without urinary extravasation
III	>1 cm parenchymal depth of renal cortex without collecting system rupture or urinary extravasation
IV	Parenchymal laceration extending through renal cortex, medulla, collecting system; vascular – main renal artery or vein injury with contained hemorrhage
V	Completely shattered kidney

Pancreas injury grading scale

Grade	Characteristics
I	Minor contusion without duct injury or superficial laceration without duct injury
II	Major contusion without duct injury or tissue loss, or major laceration without duct injury or tissue loss
III	Distal transection or parenchymal/duct injury
IV	Proximal transection or parenchymal injury involving ampulla
V	Massive disruption of the pancreatic head

Critical management

- Evaluation and resuscitation should be done simultaneously.
- Assess hemodynamic stability and signs of shock:
  - Altered mental status
  - Dizziness
  - Cool, clammy skin
  - Worsening urine output
  - Hypotension
  - Tachycardia.
- ABCDEs
  - Place the patient on cardiac monitoring and pulse oximetry.
  - Airway
    - Be cognizant of indications for intubation including changes in mental status from shock or airway compromise from other injuries.
  - Breathing

- Based on mechanism, thoracic injuries may be involved. For example, penetrating trauma may violate the diaphragm depending on trajectory of implement.
- Circulation
  - Place two large-bore IVs.
  - Goal mean arterial pressure >65 mmHg.
  - An initial fluid bolus of 1–2 L of crystalloid. Be judicious because aggressive use of crystalloid solution will worsen the lethal triad: hypothermia, acidosis, and coagulopathy (by diluting the clotting factors).
  - Patients who remain hemodynamically unstable after initial crystalloid infusion should receive uncrossmatched blood. Consider activating massive transfusion protocol, as necessary. These protocols generally entail infusion of red blood cells, platelets and fresh frozen plasma. Remember to administer calcium to counteract the citrate effect in the packed RBCs.
  - Consider administering tranexamic acid (antifibrinolytic) for significant hemorrhage requiring massive transfusion if the patient arrives within 3 hours of trauma.
- Disability
  - Establish GCS and monitor for changes to assess neurological status.
- Exposure
  - Examine the patient completely without clothing to find subtle signs of injury (e.g., penetrating wound in axilla).
- Imaging studies
  - FAST or e-FAST examination should be performed initially especially if patient is unstable.
  - CT abdomen/pelvis if patient is stable.
- Consider antibiotics in penetrating trauma.
  - Should be aimed at covering anaerobic and aerobic organisms (i.e., piperacillin-tazobactam)
- Laparotomy
  - The decision will ultimately involve discussion with general or trauma surgery based on grade and type of injury, as well as hemodynamic status.
  - Indications for laparotomy in solid organ trauma:
    - Hemodynamic instability or shock
    - Evidence of continued bleeding
    - Free fluid as indicated on initial FAST/e-FAST examination.

Special circumstances

- Pediatrics
  - Blunt trauma is the most common mechanism of solid organ injury.
  - Given small anteroposterior diameter and developing abdominal musculature children are more vulnerable to blunt forces.

- History and physical may be complicated by age, fear, and difficulty in following instructions.

Sudden deterioration

- Reassess vital signs and look for signs of hypovolemia, poor organ perfusion, and shock.
- Repeat abdominal examination to assess for change.
- Repeat an e-FAST examination to determine other occult sources of hypotension.
- The most likely reason for sudden deterioration in a trauma patient with solid organ injury is hemorrhagic shock; therefore consider more aggressive resuscitation and facilitate the process to get patient to the OR for laparotomy.

REFERENCES

American Association for the Surgery of Trauma. *Trauma Source:* Injury scoring scale. Chicago, IL: American Association for the Surgery of Trauma; 2013. Available from www.aast.org/Library/TraumaTools/InjuryScoringScales.aspx (accessed April 30, 2013).

American College of Radiology. Expert panel on Urologic Imaging. ACR Appropriateness Criteria® renal trauma. Reston, VA: American College of Radiology; Last review date 2012. Available from www.guideline.gov/content.aspx?id=15770&search=abdominal+trauma (accessed April 30, 2013).

Jansen, J, Yule, S, Loudon, M. Investigation of blunt abdominal trauma. *BMJ.* 2008; **336**, 938–42.

Spinella P, Holcomb J. Resuscitation and transfusion principles for traumatic hemorrhagic shock. *Blood Rev.* 2009; **23**, 231–40.

12

Severe pelvic trauma

Jeffrey Pepin

Introduction

- Severe pelvic fractures are a major cause of morbidity and mortality in trauma patients.
- The most common mechanisms that lead to major pelvic fractures are motor vehicle and motorcycle collisions, falls from height, and pedestrians being struck by motor vehicles.
- As hemorrhage is the main cause of mortality in pelvic trauma, it is critical to assess hemodynamic stability and identify ongoing bleeding in the chest, abdomen, and long bones. If no clear source of hemorrhage is identified and patient remains unstable, suspicion for primary pelvic hemorrhage should be high.
- Suspect pelvic fracture in all cases of serious or multi-trauma patients.
- In pelvic trauma, there is a high incidence of associated injuries that may cause long-term complications; therefore, special attention should be paid to the rectal and urogenital examinations.
- *Classification:* The most commonly used classification system for pelvic fractures is the Young–Burgess system (Table 12.1; Figure 12.1). This system categorizes injuries on the basis of mechanism of injury and can be used to predict the risk of blood loss.

Practical Emergency Resuscitation and Critical Care, ed. Kaushal Shah, Jarone Lee, Kamal Medlej, and Scott D. Weingart. Published by Cambridge University Press. © Kaushal Shah, Jarone Lee, Kamal Medlej, and Scott D. Weingart 2013.

Table 12.1. Young–Burgess classification system for pelvic fractures

Mechanism and type	Characteristics	Hemi-pelvis displacement	Stability
APC-I	Pubic diastasis <2.5 cm	External rotation	Stable
APC-II	Pubic diastasis >2.5 cm, anterior sacroiliac joint disruption	External rotation	Rotationally unstable, vertically stable
APC-III	Type II plus posterior sacroiliac joint disruption	External rotation	Rotationally unstable, vertically unstable
LC-I	Ipsilateral sacral buckle fractures, ipsilateral horizontal pubic rami fractures (or disruption of symphysis with overlapping pubic bones)	Internal rotation	Stable
LC-II	Type I plus ipsilateral iliac wing fracture or posterior sacroiliac joint disruption	Internal rotation	Rotationally unstable, vertically stable
Vertical shear	Vertical pubic rami fractures, sacroiliac joint disruption ± adjacent fractures	Vertical (cranial)	Rotationally unstable, vertically unstable

Presentation

Classic presentation
- Patients (who can verbalize) with severe pelvic trauma may complain of pain at the fracture site, low back, abdominal, or hip pain, though they may be altered or have other distracting injuries.
- They are frequently hypotensive and require rapid fluid resuscitation.
- It is important to keep pelvic fractures high in the differential diagnosis when evaluating any patient with multiple injuries.

Critical presentation
- Severely injured patients are often hypotensive and require early intubation and fluid resuscitation.

Diagnosis and evaluation

- **Vital signs** are often an early indicator of severity of hypovolemic shock.

(a)

(b)

(c)

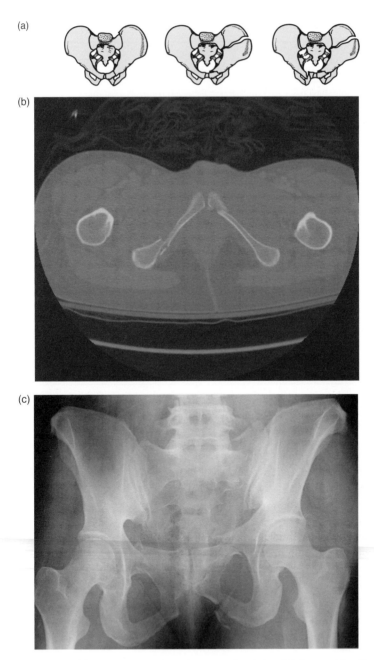

Figure 12.1. (a) Young–Burgess lateral compression (LC) pelvic fracture classifications; (b) computed tomography (CT) of LCI fracture pattern; (c) radiograph of LCI fracture pattern. (Reprinted with permission from Hammel J. Pelvic fracture. In: Legone, E, Shockley, L, Traum, W. *A Comprehensive Emergency Medicine Approach*. Cambridge University Press. 2011.)

- Tachycardia is usually the first abnormal vital sign that may lead to the diagnosis of acute blood loss.
- Hypotension is a late finding and a sign of significant hemorrhage.
- **Signs of pelvic trauma**
  - Ecchymosis, abrasions, or hematomas
  - Pelvic and leg deformity or asymmetry
  - Bony tenderness to palpation
  - Instability with gentle lateral pressure on the iliac wings
  - Peripheral neurovascular deficit
  - Difficulty with active and passive range of motion of the hip
  - Blood at urethral meatus
  - Rectal bleeding and poor sphincter tone
  - "High-riding prostate" is a theoretical finding for possible urethral injury.
- **Diagnostic tests**
  - *Laboratory tests:*
    - Type and cross
    - Serum electrolytes
    - CBC
    - Lactic acid
    - Coagulation panel
    - Urinalysis
    - Beta human chorionic gonadotropin for women of childbearing age.
  - *eFAST examination*
    - All trauma patients should have an extended focused assessment with sonography for trauma to investigate for internal bleeding and pneumothorax.
    - eFAST examinations are not sensitive or specific for retroperitoneal injuries but they are highly sensitive in detecting clinically significant hemoperitoneum.
  - *Chest radiography*
    - Portable chest radiography is complementary to the e-FAST to determine the extent of other chest injuries.
  - *Pelvic radiography*
    - Anteroposterior (AP) pelvic radiography is the initial imaging modality of choice; it identifies up to 90% of fractures.
    - Posterior sacroiliac ligament disruption may be difficult to diagnose.
    - In the past, inlet and outlet pelvic views (taken with beam 45 degrees caudally or cephalad, respectively) were used to demonstrate posterior dislocation of pelvic ring and opening of pubic symphysis; these views are now replaced by CT imaging.
  - *Abdominal/pelvic CT*
    - Provides optimal imaging for evaluation of bony pelvic anatomy, while also providing information on pelvic, retroperitoneal, and intra-abdominal bleeding.

- In patients with a significant mechanism of injury, CT of the abdomen/pelvis is often performed.
- Intravenous contrast is necessary to highlight active hemorrhage.
- CT scan can also confirm hip dislocation associated with an acetabular fracture.

Critical management

ABCs
Correct hemodynamic instability
FAST examination and pelvic radiograph
Pelvic binding, if indicated
Pain control
Avoid hypothermia
Invasive/operative management

- **Manage ABCs**
  - In acute trauma, attention to airway, breathing, and circulation/hemorrhage is the primary focus.
- **Correct hemodynamic instability**
  - Intravenous access should be above the diaphragm.
  - In hypotensive patients IV crystalloids should be initiated at a high rate but quickly replaced with blood products as soon as they are available.
  - Consider initiation of massive transfusion protocols as hemodynamically unstable patients may require high volumes of blood products.
- **eFAST examination and pelvic radiograph**
  - Evidence of intra-abdominal free fluid is an indication for emergent laparotomy prior to pelvic repair.
  - Always obtain an AP radiograph of the pelvis when history/mechanism suggests pelvic injury or in an unconscious trauma patient.
  - Pelvic radiographs should not delay pelvic binding.
- **Pelvic binding**
  - The primary goal is early reduction of pelvic volume, which decreases venous hemorrhage through tamponade and clot formation, thereby improving mortality.
  - Noninvasive methods are preferred initially.
  - Circumferential wrapping of the pelvis with a sheet is an easy and inexpensive option. Commercially available pelvic binders are also an excellent option.
  - Other methods of stabilization, more complicated and less commonly used, include military anti-shock trousers (MAST), spica casting, applications of a posterior C-clamp, or external fixation.

- **Pain control** is important in painful traumatic resuscitations and will help in patient cooperation.
- **Avoid hypothermia**
  - Use warm fluids and keep warm sheets/blankets on the patient
- **Invasive/operative management. There are three accepted strategies for controlling pelvic bleeding:**
  - Angiography with selective arterial embolization
  - Mechanical stabilization via external fixation
  - Surgical preperitoneal packing.

Sudden deterioration

- **Hypotension**
  - If pelvic binding and resuscitative efforts seem to be failing, the pelvic bleeding is likely ongoing.
  - Suspicion for arterial bleeding should prompt activation of the interventional radiology suite to initiate arterial embolization via angiography.
  - Suspicion should be higher for venous bleeding and should initiate operative management for tamponade of venous bleeding that cannot be addressed via angiography. In many cases, patients need both modalities.

13

Compartment syndrome

Katrina L. Harper and Kaushal Shah

Introduction

- Compartment syndrome is a rare but serious complication of trauma, surgery, or repetitive muscle use that leads to muscle swelling and results in increased pressure within a fascial compartment.
- As compartment pressure increases, circulation is compromised leading to tissue hypoxia and loss of viability of nerve and muscle tissue.
- The increased pressure can occur from three basic scenarios: increase in content of the compartment, decrease in the volume of the compartment, or external pressure on the compartment.
- Normal compartment pressure <10 mmHg.

Presentation

Classic
- The hallmark presentation is pain that is out of proportion to injury or findings.
- Patients will describe the pain as "deep", "burning," and "unrelenting" with difficulty in localization.
- Pain with passive stretching of the muscle groups or tightness of the compartment is also common.
- Compartment syndrome can occur when the compartment is seemingly open, such as open fractures and stab wounds.

Practical Emergency Resuscitation and Critical Care, ed. Kaushal Shah, Jarone Lee, Kamal Medlej, and Scott D. Weingart. Published by Cambridge University Press. © Kaushal Shah, Jarone Lee, Kamal Medlej, and Scott D. Weingart 2013.

- In trauma, the anterior compartment of the leg is the most common location of compartment syndrome; however, it is possible for it to occur in any extremity compartment.
- Symptoms commonly arise within 2 hours of injury but can also present up to 6 days later.

Presentation

Critical presentation

- The additional findings of paresthesias, anesthesia, paralysis, poikilothermia, and pulselessness are very late findings and should not be relied upon in the initial evaluation.
- It is estimated that muscles and nerves can tolerate ischemia for 4–6 hours without significant sequelae. After this there is risk of permanent nerve damage, myonecrosis and muscle contractures.
- After 8 hours, necrosis of tissue is certain and a nonfunctional limb is likely.
- Rarely, rhabdomyolysis, renal failure, and disseminated intravascular coagulation (DIC) can result from tissue necrosis secondary to the failure to relieve compartmental pressure.
- Delay in diagnosis correlates directly with worse outcomes.

Diagnosis and evaluation

- **Physical examination** is paramount as the physician must rely on clinical judgment for diagnosis. See the table below for lower leg compartment syndrome findings.

Lower leg compartment syndrome findings

General findings
- Pain out of proportion to injury
- Analgesia use out of proportion to injury

Anterior compartment
- Weakness of toe extension
- Pain on passive toe flexion
- Diminished sensation in the first web space

Deep posterior compartment
- Weakness of ankle inversion and toe flexion
- Pain on passive toe extension referred to the posterior leg
- Diminished sensation over medial sole of foot

- **Measurement of compartmental pressures**
  - Commercially available devices exist (e.g., Stryker) that easily and accurately measure pressures.
  - Compartmental pressures >25 mmHg are diagnostic.
- **Doppler ultrasound**
  - Not indicated because arterial blood flow can appear normal in cases of clear compartment syndrome.
- **Laboratory findings**
  - There is no blood test to diagnose compartment syndrome.
  - Necrotic muscle tissue will produce lactic acid and creatine phosphokinase but these are not specific and they are late findings.

Critical management

- The treatment of compartment syndrome is **immediate relief of the pressure**.
- This starts with removing any constricting devices, bandages or casts.
- **Surgical intervention** is the definitive treatment in which complete **fasciotomy** is performed in the operating room (OR) by trauma, vascular, or orthopedic surgeons.
- **Neutral elevation** is the preferred position. Raising the limb above the heart decreases perfusion without decreasing compartment pressures.
- In addition to a rapid diagnosis and facilitating OR fasciotomy **within 6 hours ideally**, the emergency physician should administer timely prophylactic **antibiotics and analgesia**.

ED interventions in compartment syndrome

Rapid diagnosis of compartment syndrome
Remove casts and occlusive dressings
Place extremity in neutral position
Prophylactic antibiotics
Analgesia
Emergent fasciotomy or facilitating OR fasciotomy

Sudden deterioration

Patients can progress to **DIC**, which can lead to acute worsening of their clinical status.

REFERENCES

Frykberg ER, Schinco MA. Peripheral vascular injury. In: Feliciano DV, Mattox KL, Moore EE, eds. *Trauma*, 6th edn. New York: McGraw-Hill; 2008.

Gillooly J, Hacker A, Patel V. Compartment syndrome as a complication of a stab wound to the thigh: a case report and review of the literature. *Emerg Med J*. 2007; **24**:780–1.

Matsen FA, 3rd, Wyss CR, Krugmire RB, Jr., Simmons CW, King RV. The effects of limb elevation and dependency on local arteriovenous gradients in normal human limbs with particular reference to limbs with increased tissue pressure. *Clin Orthop Relat Res*. 1980; **150**: 187–95.

Newton EJ, Love J. Acute complications of extremity trauma. *Emerg Med Clin North Am*. 2007; **25**: 751–61.

Siefert JA. Acute compartment syndrome. In: Wolfson AB, ed. *Clinical Practice of Emergency Medicine*. Philadelphia: Lippincott Williams & Wilkins. 2005.

14

Soft tissue injury: crush injury, arterial injury, and open fractures

Katrina L. Harper and Kaushal Shah

Introduction

- A **crush injury** occurs when a limb is compressed, resulting in direct tissue injury and disruption of vascular supply that may lead to tissue necrosis, muscle swelling, and neurological disturbances. The severity of injury is directly related to the force applied to an extremity and to the degree and duration of the compression.
- Approximately 85% of **arterial injuries** are caused by penetrating trauma, which tends to be more discrete or focal. The most common vessels involved are the popliteal and femoral arteries in the lower extremity and the brachial and axillary arteries in the upper extremity.
- **Open fractures** are complex injuries of not only bone but the surrounding neurovascular structures. The communication with the outside world results in contamination and the gross deformity may result in compromised vascular supply. This combination places the wound at very high risk of infection and wound healing complications.
- Table 14.1 gives a classification of fractures with soft tissue injuries.

Presentation

Classic presentation

- While motor vehicle collisions, pedestrians being struck by motor vehicles, and industrial accidents are the most common causes of a **crush injury**, a large number of life-threatening crush injuries occur as a result of natural disasters. Injury is often clear from chief complaint and mechanism.

Practical Emergency Resuscitation and Critical Care, ed. Kaushal Shah, Jarone Lee, Kamal Medlej, and Scott D. Weingart. Published by Cambridge University Press. © Kaushal Shah, Jarone Lee, Kamal Medlej, and Scott D. Weingart 2013.

Table 14.1. Tscherne classification of fractures with soft tissue injuries

Fracture type	Description
0	Minimal soft tissue damage; indirect violence; simple fracture patterns (e.g., torsion fracture of the tibia in skiers)
I	Superficial abrasion or contusion caused by pressure from within; mild to moderately severe fracture configuration (e.g., pronation fracture-dislocation of the ankle joint with a soft tissue lesion over the medial malleolus)
II	Deep contaminated abrasion associated with localized skin or muscle contusion; impending compartment syndrome; severe fracture configuration (e.g., segmental bumper fracture of the tibia)
III	Extensive skin contusion or crushing injury; underlying muscle damage may be severe; subcutaneous avulsion; decompensated compartment syndrome; associated major vascular injury; severe or comminuted fracture configuration

- **Arterial injuries** can present broadly, from a simple hematoma to profound hemorrhagic shock. The clinical presence of **"the 5 Ps"** (pain, pallor, pulselessness, paresthesias, and paralysis) should be attributed to arterial injury.
- **Open fractures** are typically obvious with significant disruption of the original anatomy and visible bony structures. The main concerns are arterial injury compromising the viability of the extremity and deep tissue and joint space contamination that can lead to long-term complications, such as osteomyelitis.

Critical presentation

- The **"crush syndrome"** comprises the systemic manifestations that arise as a result of a crush injury once the external force is removed. The patient can develop hypovolemia, shock, compartment syndrome, lactic acidosis, or renal failure from traumatic rhabdomyolysis. Rhabdomyolysis can cause acute renal failure in up to 40% of patients with crush injuries.
- **Arterial injury** can lead to hypotension if the hemorrhage is not addressed aggressively with source control and resuscitation with fluids.
- The mangled extremity severity score (MESS) is the most widely validated classification system of the lower extremity when evaluating the severity of **open fractures**. Limb viability is related to vascular status, patient age, duration of ischemia, and absorbed energy. A score of 6 or less predicts limb viability while a score of 7 or higher predicts the need for amputation. MESS has high specificity but low sensitivity. As yet, there is no scoring system that reliably predicts the need for amputation.

Mangled extremity severity score (MESS)	
Points	Component
Skeletal and soft tissue injury	
1	Low energy (stab, simple fracture, civilian gunshot wound)
2	Medium energy (open or multiplex fractures, dislocation)
3	High energy (close-range shotgun/military gunshot wound; crush injury)
4	Very high energy (same as above plus gross contamination, soft tissue avulsion)
Limb ischemia (doubled if >6 hours)	
1	Pulse reduced or absent but perfusion normal
2	Pulseless, paresthesias, diminished capillary refill
3	Cool, paralyzed, insensate, numb
Shock	
0	Systolic blood pressure always >90 mmHg
1	Hypotensive transiently
2	Persistent hypotension
Age (years)	
0	<30
1	30–50
2	>50

Diagnosis and evaluation

- **Crush injury**
  - *Electrolyte abnormalities* such as low calcium and elevated serum potassium, phosphate, and uric acid that results from massive cellular damage.
  - *Venous (or arterial) blood* gas will reveal metabolic lactic acidosis.
  - *Creatine phosphokinase (CPK),* as the surrogate marker to assess the extent of muscle damage.
  - *Urine studies* will determine the presence of myoglobin indirectly. Myoglobin in the urine will be detected as "blood" on the urine dipstick but there will be no red blood cells noted on the urine analysis.
  - Evaluate for manifestations of hyperkalemia by obtaining an *ECG*. The increase in serum potassium is most severe in the first 12–36 hours after muscle injury. Initially, there may be peaked T waves and prolonged PR interval. At levels between 7–8 mEq/L, the ECG may reveal a widened QRS and flattened P waves. For potassium levels >8 mEq/L, the ECG may degenerate into a sine wave pattern (see Figure 14.1), then ventricular fibrillation, followed by cardiac arrest.

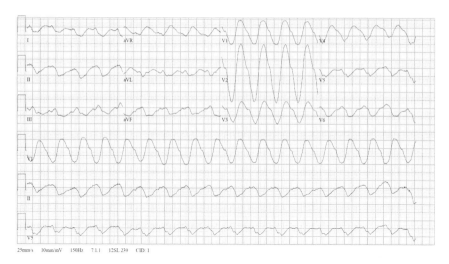

Figure 14.1. Severe hyperkalemia on ECG.

Severe hyperkalemia on ECG (Figure 14.1)

- **Arterial injury**
  - If an arterial injury is suspected, the initial goals of the emergency physician are to diagnose the injury by considering the "hard" and "soft" signs as outlined in the table below.
  - There should be a low threshold for angiography to rule out arterial injury in shotgun wounds.
  - There is up to a 30% incidence of injury to the popliteal artery in patients with traumatic knee dislocation. These patients should undergo serial vascular examinations, ABI, followed by angiography in patients with abnormal findings.
  - Supracondylar humerus fractures can be associated with brachial artery injury.
  - **Imaging** studies should be considered for evaluation of limbs with soft findings.
    - *Ankle-brachial index (ABI)* is determined by checking the pulse pressure of the injured lower extremity with that of the upper extremity. An ABI of <0.9 is considered abnormal.
    - *Duplex ultrasound* detects both venous and arterial blood flow and can be performed at the bedside.
    - *Computed tomography angiography (CTA)* has 100% sensitivity and specificity for detection of clinically relevant vascular injury.
    - *Arteriography* is the gold standard in the diagnosis of vascular injury; however, CTA has proved to be an acceptable alternative.

Hard findings of arterial injury
Pulsatile or rapidly expanding hematoma
Obvious pulsatile arterial bleeding
Bruit or thrill with arterial palpation
"The 5 Ps" of arterial insufficiency: pulseless, pallor, pain, paresthesia, paralysis

Soft findings of arterial injury
Diminished pulse compared to opposite limb
Delayed capillary refill
Isolated peripheral nerve injury
Nonpulsatile, stable hematoma

- **Open fractures**
  - Obtain radiographs to better understand the internal disruption and identify fractures which may not be obvious on physical examination.
  - Wounds in the vicinity of a fracture should be considered an "open fracture" until proven otherwise. Wound cultures prior to debridement are not necessary.
  - A thorough sensory and motor examination is necessary to identify a peripheral nerve injury. Evaluate capillary refill time, temperature and color of skin, and presence or absence of distal pulses.

Gustilo open fracture classification system

Grade	Injury	Risk of infection
I	Puncture wound <1 cm with minimal contamination or crushing	0–2%
II	Laceration >1 cm with moderate soft tissue injury	2–10%
IIIA	Extensive soft tissue damage, severe crush component, massive contamination. Bone coverage adequate	10–50%
IIIB	Extensive soft tissue damage with periosteal stripping and exposure. Severe contamination and bone comminution. Flap coverage required	10–50%
IIIC	Arterial injury requiring repair	10–50%

Critical management

- **Crush injury**
  - **Intravenous (IV) fluids resuscitation** should be the first priority. The majority of the metabolic derangements can be addressed with intravenous fluid hydration as this will reduce the lactic acidosis and flush out the myoglobin and CPK. If rhabdomyolysis develops, early hydration is the key to prevent or lessen the severity of acute renal failure.
  - Consider **placement of a Foley catheter** to monitor urine output carefully. Low urine output suggests ongoing hypovolemia or acute renal failure.
  - **Alkalinization of urine** with sodium bicarbonate is controversial. Some argue alkaline urine with a pH of 7.0 or higher helps to prevent renal failure and reduces the crystallization of uric acid, decreasing damage to renal tubules. However, a recent meta-analysis demonstrated no added benefit for bicarbonate infusion versus normal saline.
- **Arterial Injury**
  - Apply **direct pressure** for hemorrhage control. If a bleeding vessel can be identified, it should be isolated and a non-crushing **vascular clamp** should be utilized to control the bleeding. Blind clamping of bleeding vessels should never be attempted.
  - **Reduce and splint** angulated/dislocated fractures as soon as possible to decrease hemorrhage and correct pulse deficits.
  - **Emergent surgery** by trauma or vascular surgeon is necessary if "hard signs" of arterial injury are present.

Arterial injury algorithm (Figure 14.2)

- **Open fracture**
  - Dislocations with concern of arterial injury should be reduced emergently.
  - The simplest method to reduce hemorrhage from a long bone deformity is to apply traction and splint the extremity.
  - Intravenous analgesia with narcotics is often necessary.
  - Early irrigation should be performed to minimize bacteria count.
  - Tetanus toxoid is the standard treatment for patients who have completed the primary tetanus immunization series. Those who have not received the series or particularly tetanus-prone wounds should receive the tetanus immune globulin in addition to the toxoid.
  - Prophylactic intravenous antibiotics should be started in the emergency department within 3 hours. The risk of infection is stratified by the severity of injury.
    - Cephalosporins have been demonstrated to reduce the infection rate significantly.

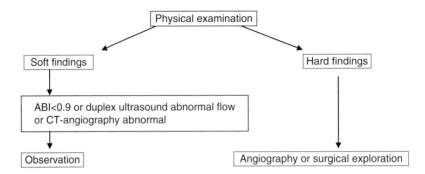

Figure 14.2. Arterial injury algorithm.

- The addition of an aminoglycoside for grades II and III fractures is recommended for adequate Gram-negative coverage.
- Many authors recommend high-dose penicillin to cover *Clostridium* for any fracture with suspected soil contamination.

ED open fracture treatment
Analgesia
Reduction of the fracture/dislocation
Antibiotics intravenously
Tetanus prophylaxis
Orthopedic consultation for possible surgical debridement
Surgical open fracture treatment
Irrigation and debridement
Wound closure
Soft tissue reconstruction
Fracture stabilization
Secondary procedures: bone grafting to stimulate healing

Sudden deterioration

- **Hypovolemic shock** is the leading cause of death after soft tissue injury. Placement of two large-bore IVs and aggressive fluid resuscitation is necessary in the hypotensive individual. Consider early administration of uncrossmatched blood and instituting massive transfusion protocol.
- **Cardiac arrhythmias and cardiac arrest** contributes to a large percentage of early deaths in crush injury patients, occurring due to life-threatening hyperkalemia. It should be addressed quickly and effectively.

- Calcium administration to stabilize the cardiac membranes is first-line treatment for severe hyperkalemia defined either with ECG changes or serum potassium >7 mEq/L.
- Temporary reduction in the potassium can be achieved with intravenous insulin with glucose, intravenous sodium bicarbonate, and inhaled beta-2 agonists; all of which act to drive extracellular potassium into the intracellular compartment.

REFERENCES

Gonzalez D. Crush syndrome. *Crit Care Med.* 2005; **33**: S34–41.

Gustilo RB, Anderson JT. Prevention of infection in the treatment of one thousand and twenty-five open fractures of long bones: retrospective and prospective analyses. *J Bone Joint Surg Am.* 1976; **58**: 453–8.

Malinoski DJ, Slater MS, Mullins RJ. Crush injury and rhabdomyolysis. *Crit Care Clin.* 2004; **20**: 171–92.

Pons PT. Peripheral vascular injuries. In: Wolfson AB, ed. *Clinical Practice of Emergency Medicine.* 4th edn. Philadelphia: Lippincott Williams & Wilkins; 2005: 1018.

Seamon MJ, Smoger D, Torres DM, *et al.* A prospective validation of a current practice: The detection of extremity vascular injury with CT angiography. *J Trauma.* 2009; **67**: 238–43.

White PW, Gillespie DL, Feurstein I, *et al.* Sixty-four slice multidetector computed tomographic angiography in the evaluation of vascular trauma. *J Trauma* 2010; **68**: 96–102.

Zalavras CG, Marcus RE, Levin LS, *et al.* Management of open fractures and subsequent complications. *J Bone Joint Surg Am.* 2007; **89**: 884–95.

15

Burns

Jonathan Friedstat, Jeremy Goverman, and Shawn Fagan

Introduction

- Approximately 450 000 patients are evaluated annually for the treatment of thermal injury and approximately 70 000 will require hospitalization.
- The majority of patients hospitalized with thermal injuries have burns affecting less than 10% of total body surface area (TBSA) and require a relatively short hospital stay. Even among the subset of patients who suffer a major thermal injury and manifest significant physiological derangements, the majority of such patients survive, including those with greater than 90% TBSA involvement.
- Improvement in mortality rates is directly related to advances in resuscitation, control of infection, modulation of the hypermetabolic response to traumatic injury, and early excision and grafting.
- Burn resuscitation is a continuous process that should be goal directed to achieve optimal outcomes.

Initial assessment

- **Safety:** All individuals attending to the care of a thermally injured patient should wear proper protective equipment. The protective equipment serves not only to protect the caregiver from contamination (body fluids, chemicals exposure from chemical burns) but also to prevent early nosocomial infections.
- **Airway:** The thermally injured patient may be at risk for early airway compromise secondary to a progressive edematous state.

Practical Emergency Resuscitation and Critical Care, ed. Kaushal Shah, Jarone Lee, Kamal Medlej, and Scott D. Weingart. Published by Cambridge University Press. © Kaushal Shah, Jarone Lee, Kamal Medlej, and Scott D. Weingart 2013.

- Clinical symptoms (stridor, hoarseness) or signs (carbonaceous sputum, singed facial hair) of upper airway injury warrant close observation and/or evaluation.
  - Endoscopic visualization of the posterior oral pharynx should be performed for all patients at risk to determine the need for early intubation.
  - Maximum edema secondary to thermal injuries occurs at 24 hours; obvious clinical signs of deterioration should be managed with early controlled intubation.
  - Emergent intubations should be avoided due to the association with early pneumonias.
- **Breathing:** Respiratory insufficiency or failure may result from mechanical or physiological mechanisms following a thermal injury.
  - *Mechanical failure:* A subset of thermally injured patients present with circumferential thermal injuries to the torso affecting the ability of the chest cavity to expand properly with inspiration. The clinical situation results in an ineffective minute ventilation secondary to limitations in tidal volume.
    - Treatment begins with early recognition of the pathophysiological process.
    - If not already performed, the airway should be controlled with endotracheal intubation.
    - Inability to provide effective tidal volume with mechanical ventilation (increasing peak airway pressures, hypercarbia) should be treated with bilateral mid-axillary line escharotomies.
    - Occasionally, a secondary escharotomy needs to be performed along the subcostal margin to completely decompress the chest cavity and allow for proper chest wall expansion with inspiration.
  - *Physiological failure:* Rarely a result of direct thermal injury to the lung, physiological failure is most commonly associated with the inhalation of toxic substances resulting in a "chemical pneumonitis" or inhalation injury. The incidence of inhalation injury increases with the size of thermal injury. The treatment is early recognition and support.
    - All patients at risk for inhalation injury should have a bronchoscopy performed and documented in order to grade, and identify, the extent of burn.
    - All patients should be supported early with lung-protective ventilation. Low tidal volume, low pressure, and prevention of atelectasis should be instituted in the Emergency Center to prevent additional ventilator-associated injury.
- **Circulation:** Thermal injuries can result in a significant impact to the cardiovascular system. The cardiovascular insufficiency observed following thermal injury may result from direct cardiac suppression via inflammatory mediators, alterations in preload, cardiac contractility, or peripheral vascular tone. Cardiovascular insufficiency should be evaluated and treated in a goal-directed manner.

Initial management

- **Vital signs:** A complete set of vital signs including height and weight should be obtained on all thermally injured patients. Large thermal injuries (TBSA >10%) require continuous vital sign monitoring.
- **IV access:** Early intravenous access should be established to begin the resuscitative process. Delayed resuscitation increases mortality.
  - Access can be obtained through thermally injured areas that have been properly prepped with an aseptic technique. Early thermal injuries are not infected or colonized with bacteria.
  - Failure to obtain peripheral access requires central venous or intraosseous access. Intraosseous access is effective for administration of fluids and medications but limited by a maximum infusion rate. Large thermal injuries may require several points of intraosseous access.
- **Estimation of burn size:** A gross determination of total body surface area affected by the partial and full thickness (second and third degree) thermal injury should be established to assist in guiding the initial resuscitation. Do not include superficial (first degree) injury in fluid calculations.
  - TBSA <20%: initiate maintenance fluids.
  - TBSA >20%: initiate Parkland formula.
- **Parkland formula:** The Parkland formula provides an estimate of the fluid requirements during the initial 24 hours following thermal injuries as 2–4 mL × TBSA (%) × Ideal Body Weight (kg).
  - The first half is administered over the first 8 hours *after injury* (time is based on time from injury, not time from arrival at the emergency room); the second half is administered over the second 16 hours.
  - Preferred fluid: Ringer lactate.
  - Special consideration: A source of glucose should be considered in patients less than 2 years old to prevent hypoglycemia due to a lack of glycogen stores.

Example: Parkland Formula Calculation

Patient: Age 50 years; weight 75 kg
10% TBSA superficial (first degree)
50% TBSA partial and full thickness (2nd/3rd degree)
4 mL × 50% TBSA × 75 kg = 15 liters
Half is administered over the first 8 hours:
Total volume: 15 L/2 = 7.5 L
Hourly rate: 7.5 L/8 hours = 940 mL/hour
Half is administered over the remaining 16 hours:
Total volume: 7.5 L/16 hours
Hourly rate: 469 mL/hour

- Adjustments to initial volume resuscitation should be based on the patient's physiological response. Fluid adjustments should be made cautiously with the goal of gentle normalization of global perfusion and resuscitation parameters.

- Over-resuscitation should be avoided as it has been shown to increase morbidity and mortality. Patients are at risk for compartment syndromes and over resuscitation even with close and appropriate following of the Parkland formula.
  - Normalization of lactate levels, base deficit, pH.
  - Urine output (0.5 mL/kg/hour).
- **Failure of initial resuscitation:** Evaluate the patient for proper preload (intravascular volume).
  - Consider central venous access or advanced hemodynamic monitoring.
  - Evaluate the patient for proper myocardial contractility/cardiac output:
    - Cardiac insufficiency has been observed following major thermal injuries and may persist for several months.
    - Cardiac insufficiency should be addressed with the appropriate inotrope to support the abnormal physiological condition.
  - Evaluate the patient for proper peripheral vascular tone. Thermal injuries are associated with a significant systemic inflammatory response, which may result in decreased peripheral vascular tone. After ensuring appropriate intravascular volume (preload), peripheral vascular tone should be supported with an appropriate vasopressor (e.g., levophed). Decreased peripheral vascular tone should not be treated with volume since this may lead to over-resuscitation and increased morbidity and mortality.
- **Prevention of hypothermia:** Depending on the size of injury, hypothermia can develop quickly. During initial evaluation all efforts should be made to prevent hypothermia.
  - Provide a warm surround environment in the emergency room.
  - Cover exposed surfaces with sterile clean dressings to prevent heat loss.
  - Prevent vascular compromise/compartment syndrome.
- **Prophylactic antibiotics are *not indicated*** in the initial management of thermal injury.

Secondary assessment

The secondary assessment of a thermal injured patient should follow a systematic approach similar to that of a trauma patient. The thermal injuries should be evaluated and classified based on degree and extent of injury. A Lund and Browder chart can assist in the establishment of the extent and depth of thermal injury based on the body part affected.

First degree – superficial thermal injury
a. Extent of injury: one or more layers of the epidermis
b. Sensitivity: hyperalgesic
c. Appearance: erythema
d. Treatment: moisturizers and analgesics

Second degree – partial thickness thermal injury
a. Extent of injury: typically epidermis destroyed, dermis involved
b. Sensitivity: hyperalgesic
c. Appearance: blisters, pink, moist
d. Treatment: topical antibiotics and analgesics
e. A deep dermal injury may require excision and grafting

Third degree – full thickness thermal injury
a. Extent of injury: epidermis and dermis destroyed
b. Sensitivity: insensate
c. Appearance: opaque, white, black, leathery
d. Treatment: early excision and autografting

Fourth degree
a. Extent of injury: extends to the subcutaneous tissue, muscle/bone
b. Sensitivity: insensate
c. Appearance: disfiguring, black, leathery
d. Treatment: debridement, reconstruction, amputation

Triage

The American Burn Association has determined criteria for patients who would benefit from transfer to a burn center. These criteria include:

1. Partial thickness burns greater than 10% total body surface area (TBSA).
2. Burns that involve the face, hands, feet, genitalia, perineum, or major joints.
3. Third-degree burns in any age group.
4. Electrical burns, including lightning injury.
5. Chemical burns.
6. Inhalation injury.
7. Burn injury in patients with preexisting medical disorders that could complicate management, prolong recovery, or affect mortality.
8. Any patient with burns and concomitant trauma (such as fractures) in which the burn injury poses the greatest risk of morbidity or mortality. In such cases, if the trauma poses the greater immediate risk, the patient may be initially stabilized in a trauma center before being transferred to a burns unit. Physician judgment will be necessary in such situations and should be in concert with the regional medical control plan and triage protocols.
9. Burned children in hospitals without qualified personnel or equipment for the care of children.
10. Burn injury in patients who will require special social, emotional, or rehabilitative intervention.

REFERENCES

American Burn Association. *Advanced Burn Life Support (ABLS) Provider Manual.* Chicago, IL: American Burn Association; 2011.

Herndon DL. *Total Burn Care*, 3rd edn. Philadelphia: Elsevier Saunders; 2007.

Klien MB, Hayden D, Constance E, *et al.* The association between fluid administration and outcome following major burn – a multicenter study. *Ann Surg.* 2007; **245**: 622–8.

Orgill DP, Piccolo N. Escharotomy and decompressive therapies in burns. *BCR.* 2009; **30**: 759–68.

Phillips BJ. *Pediatric Burns.* New York: Cambria Press; 2012.

Sheridan RL. *Burns: A Practical Approach to Immediate Treatment and Long-Term Care.* London, UK: Manson Publishing; 2012.

Neurological emergencies

16

Ischemic strokes

Joshua W. Joseph and Ashley L. Greiner

Introduction

- Cerebrovascular accident (CVA) or stroke is an interruption of the blood supply to the brain.
- Most commonly due to **thrombosis** or **embolization** resulting in cell hypoxia, subsequently leading to cell edema and death.
- Thrombosis is caused by an in-situ clot at a site of atherosclerotic plaque.
- Embolization is caused by an intravascular embolus. Sources include atrial fibrillation, ventricular aneurysm, hypokinetic ventricle, myocardial infarction, prosthetic valve, infective endocarditis, and proximal friable atherosclerotic plaques.

Presentation

Classic presentation

- Middle cerebral artery syndrome
  - **The most common** stroke syndrome
  - Contralateral hemiplegia of the upper extremity > the lower extremity
  - Facial hemiplegia
  - Dominant hemisphere: aphasia
  - Nondominant hemisphere: inattention, neglect, apraxia
  - Contralateral homonymous hemianopia – eyes point toward side of lesion.

Practical Emergency Resuscitation and Critical Care, ed. Kaushal Shah, Jarone Lee, Kamal Medlej, and Scott D. Weingart. Published by Cambridge University Press. © Kaushal Shah, Jarone Lee, Kamal Medlej, and Scott D. Weingart 2013.

- Anterior cerebral artery syndrome
  - Contralateral hemiplegia and sensory neglect of the lower extremity > the upper extremity
  - Apraxia
  - Mutism and/or aphasia
- Posterior cerebral artery syndrome
  - Unilateral headache
  - Homonymous hemianopia
  - Patient unaware of defect (visual agnosia)
  - Third nerve palsy
  - Sensation deficits (pinprick, light touch)
- Vertebrobasilar artery syndrome
  - Ipsilateral cranial nerve palsy and contralateral hemiplegia
  - Ipsilateral facial parasthesia, vertigo, Horner syndrome, dysphagia, and dysphonia
  - Contralateral sensory deficits (pain and temperature)
  - Abnormal gait and cerebellar coordination testing
- Basilar artery occlusion
  - Quadriplegia
  - Coma
  - Locked-in syndrome
- Cerebellar infarction
  - The most common symptom is ataxia.
  - Can have headache, central vertigo, nausea and vomiting.
  - Can have herniation from edema manifest as decreased level of consciousness, abnormal respiratory pattern, and pupillary dilation
- Lacunar syndromes
  - Pure motor stroke (most common)
  - Pure sensory stroke
  - Clumsy hand-dysarthria syndrome

Critical presentation

- Patients may present with altered mental status or airway compromise requiring immediate treatment.

Diagnosis and evaluation

- **History** is important in identifying:
  - Time last *witnessed* "normal", establishing time of onset of CVA.
    - Patients waking from sleep with stroke symptoms are considered "normal" when last witnessed at their baseline while awake.
- Possible exclusion criteria for thrombolytics (Table 16.1).

Table 16.1. Indications for thrombolytics (tPA)

These statements must be true in order to consider tPA administration:
1. Ischemic stroke onset within 3 hours, or in certain causes within 4.5 hours.
2. Measurable deficit on NIH Stroke Scale examination.
3. Patient's computed tomography (CT) does not show hemorrhage or nonstroke cause of deficit.
4. Patient's age is >18 years.

Contraindications to thrombolytics (tPA)

Do NOT administer tPA if any of these statements are true:
1. Patient's symptoms are minor or rapidly improving.
2. Patient had seizure at onset of stroke.
3. Patient has had another stroke or serious head trauma within the past 3 months.
4. Patient had major surgery within the last 14 days.
5. Patient has known history of intracranial hemorrhage.
6. Patient has sustained systolic blood pressure >185 mmHg.
7. Patient has sustained diastolic blood pressure >110 mmHg.
8. Aggressive treatment is necessary to lower the patient's blood pressure.
9. Patient has symptoms suggestive of subarachnoid hemorrhage.
10. Patient has had gastrointestinal or urinary tract hemorrhage within the last 21 days.
11. Patient has had arterial puncture at noncompressible site within the last 7 days.
12. Patient has received heparin within the last 48 hours and has elevated PTT.
13. Patient's prothrombin time (PT) is >15 seconds.
14. Patient's platelet count is <100 000/microliter.
15. Patient's serum glucose is <50 mg/dL or >400 mg/dL.

Relative contraindications to thrombolytics (tPA)

If either of the following statements is true, use tPA with caution:
1. Patient has a large stroke with NIH Stroke Scale score >22.
2. Patient's CT shows evidence of large middle cerebral artery (MCA) territory infarction (sulcal effacement or blurring of gray-white junction in greater than 1/3 of MCA territory).

Additional contraindications to thrombolytics (tPA) for 3–4.5 hours
1. Age >80 years
2. History of prior stroke *and* diabetes
3. Any anticoagulant use prior to admission (even if INR <1.7)
4. NIHSS >25
5. CT findings involving more than 1/3 of the MCA territory (as evidenced by hypodensity, sulcal effacement or mass effect estimated by visual inspection or ABC/2 >100 mL)

Table 16.2. NIH Stroke Scale

1a. Level of consciousness: Alertness and response to stimuli	1. **Alert**; keenly responsive. 2. **Not alert**; but arousable by minor stimulation to obey, answer, or respond. 3. **Not alert**; requires repeated stimulation to attend, or is obtunded and requires strong or painful stimulation to make movements (not stereotyped). 4. Responds only with reflex motor or autonomic effects or totally unresponsive, flaccid, and areflexic.
1b. LOC questions: The month and patient's age	1. **Answers** both questions correctly. 2. **Answers** one question correctly. 3. **Answers** neither question correctly.
1c. LOC commands: Opening and closing eyes, opening and closing non-paretic hand	1. **Performs** both tasks correctly. 2. **Performs** one task correctly. 3. **Performs** neither task correctly.
2. Best gaze: Horizontal eye movements	1. Normal. 2. **Partial gaze palsy**; gaze is abnormal in one or both eyes, but forced deviation or total gaze paresis is not present. 3. **Forced deviation**, or total gaze paresis not overcome by the oculocephalic maneuver.
3. Visual: Test visual fields to confrontation	1. **No visual loss.** 2. **Partial hemianopia.** 3. **Complete hemianopia.** 4. **Bilateral hemianopia** (blind including cortical blindness).
4. Facial Palsy: Ask patient to show teeth, open/close eyes	1. **Normal** symmetrical movements. 2. **Minor paralysis** (flattened nasolabial fold, asymmetry on smiling). 3. **Partial paralysis** (total or near-total paralysis of lower face). 4. **Complete paralysis** of one or both sides (absence of facial movement in the upper and lower face).
5. Motor Arm: Extend arm, test for drift **5a.** Left Arm **5b.** Right Arm	1. **No drift**; limb holds 90 (or 45) degrees for full 10 seconds. 2. **Drift**; limb holds 90 (or 45) degrees, but drifts down before full 10 seconds; does not hit bed or other support. 3. **Some effort against gravity**; limb cannot get to or maintain (if cued) 90 (or 45) degrees, drifts down to bed, but has some effort against gravity. 4. **No effort against gravity**; limb falls. 5. **No movement.** UN = Amputation or joint fusion.

6. Motor Leg:
Extend leg, test for drift
6a. Left Leg
6b. Right Leg

1. **No drift**; leg holds 30-degree position for full 5 seconds.
2. **Drift**; leg falls by the end of the 5-second period but does not hit bed.
3. **Some effort against gravity**; leg falls to bed by 5 seconds, but has some effort against gravity.
4. **No effort against gravity**; leg falls to bed immediately.
5. **No movement.**
UN = Amputation or joint fusion.

7. Limb Ataxia:
Finger-nose and heel-shin tests

1. Absent.
2. Present in one limb.
3. Present in two limbs.
UN = Amputation or joint fusion.

8. Sensory:
Sensation to pinprick, withdrawal to noxious stimuli

1. **Normal**; no sensory loss.
2. **Mild-to-moderate sensory loss**; patient feels pinprick is less sharp or is dull on the affected side; or there is a loss of superficial pain with pinprick, but patient is aware of being touched.
3. **Severe to total sensory loss**; patient is not aware of being touched in the face, arm, and leg.

9. Best Language:
Patient is asked to describe a standard picture, name objects, read sentences

1. **No aphasia**; normal.
2. **Mild-to-moderate aphasia**; some obvious loss of fluency or facility of comprehension, without significant limitation on ideas expressed or form of expression. Examiner can identify picture or naming card content from patient's response.
3. **Severe aphasia**; all communication is through fragmentary expression; great need for inference, questioning, and guessing by the listener. Examiner cannot identify materials provided from patient response.
4. **Mute, global aphasia**; no usable speech or auditory comprehension.

10. Dysarthria:
Patient reads/repeats words

1. Normal.
2. **Mild-to-moderate dysarthria**; patient slurs at least some words and, at worst, can be understood with some difficulty.
3. **Severe dysarthria;** patient's speech is so slurred as to be unintelligible in the absence of or out of proportion to any dysphasia, or is mute/anarthric.
UN = Intubated or other physical barrier.

11. Extinction and inattention:
Extinction to bilateral visual/sensory stimuli

1. **No abnormality.**
2. **Visual, tactile, auditory, spatial, or personal inattention** or extinction to bilateral simultaneous stimulation in one of the sensory modalities.
3. **Profound hemi-inattention or extinction** to more than one modality; does not recognize own hand or orients to only one side of space.

Table 16.2. (*cont.*)

Sentences for Best Language Task:	Words for Dysarthria Task:
You know how.	MAMA
Down to earth.	TIP-TOP
I got home from work.	FIFTY-FIFTY
Near the table in the	THANKS
dining room.	HUCKLEBERRY
They heard him speak	BASEBALL PLAYER
on the radio last night.	

- **Physical examination**
  - National Institutes of Health Stroke Scale (NIHSS) (Table 16.2).
- **Ancillary testing**
  - Bedside glucose
  - Complete blood count, electrolyte panel and coagulation profile
  - ECG, as cardiac abnormalities are prevalent in stroke patients
  - Serial cardiac enzymes (i.e., troponin).
- **Imaging**
  - Noncontrast head CT: can be normal in the first 24 hours, especially in the first 3 hours from presentation.
  - MRI: more sensitive than CT during the immediate period, but is more time consuming to obtain and less available emergently at most institutions.

Critical management

Airway management as needed
Oxygen
IV access
Cardiac monitors
Fingerstick blood glucose test
Noncontrast head CT
Neurology consultation
Thrombolytics (if meet all criteria)
Blood pressure control
Glucose control
Temperature control

- If the patient is not protecting his/her airway due to neurological deficits or level of consciousness, **intubation** will be required. If possible, try to assess the neurological examination prior to intubation.

- Supplemental **oxygen** is only necessary in patients with oxygen saturation ≤92%.
- Patient should be placed on a **cardiac monitor** for evaluation of atrial fibrillation or other cardiac arrhythmias.
- After **fingerstick blood glucose** (to assess for hypoglycemia), obtain a STAT **noncontrast head CT**. Head CT will exclude intracranial hemorrhage as the etiology of the patient's presentation and is essential before consideration of intravenous thrombolytic therapy.
- **Neurology consultation** should be obtained early in the patient's presentation.
- Although controversial, consider **systemic thrombolysis** for those patients meeting criteria for tissue plasminogen activator (tPA) and presenting within 3–4.5 hours of symptom onset (Table 16.1).
  - Dose 0.9 mg/kg, maximum 90 mg:
    - 10% of the dose is given as an initial bolus over 1 minute.
    - Remainder of the dose is infused over 60 minutes.
  - Defer Foley placement, arterial lines, or nasogastric tubes until after infusion starts.
  - Admit the patient to an intensive care unit setting.
- **Blood pressure monitoring** is essential for maintaining brain perfusion and decreasing the risk of conversion to hemorrhagic stroke.
  - *For tPA candidates*
    - Begin treatment at systolic BP ≥185 mmHg and/or diastolic BP ≥110 mmHg. Consider labetalol IV push or nicardipine infusion.
    - If blood pressure does not decline and remains ≥185/110 mmHg, do not administer tPA.
    - During infusion, monitor blood pressure every 15 minutes, more frequently if the blood pressure is ≥185/110.
  - *For those excluded from tPA administration*, permissive hypertension is allowed.
    - Begin hypertensive treatment at systolic BP ≥220 mmHg and/or diastolic BP ≥120 mmHg.
    - Consider nicardipine, labetalol, esmolol, or enalaprilat for BP control.
    - The goal is BP reduction of ~15% during the first 24 hours after onset.
- **Blood glucose control** is controversial as there is no definitive evidence regarding the ideal glucose goal. Previous guidelines for tight control may precipitate hypoglycemia and worse outcomes. Current recommendations are to begin **insulin** therapy only at a threshold of **140–180 mg/dL**.
- Patients with **fever** should be given antipyretics. The role of induced hypothermia is still under investigation.

Sudden deterioration

- The most likely cause of sudden decompensation is **intracranial hemorrhage** during tPA administration or increased **intracranial pressure** due to cerebral edema.

- Signs and symptoms include new/worsening neurological deficits, nausea/vomiting, severe headache, acute hypertension, or decreased level of consciousness.
- If any of these develop during infusion, immediately stop the infusion. Check pupillary response and obtain a repeat noncontrast head CT.
- If there is concern for increased intracranial pressure:
  - Begin medical management with osmotic diuretics, elevating the head of the bed to 30°, keep the jugular neck veins straight, as well as by treating fever, pain, and agitation.
  - Hyperventilation is not recommended, as it reduces ICP by reducing cerebral blood flow, which can worsen infarction.
  - The goal should be to maintain normocarbia while minimizing positive end-expiratory pressure (PEEP). Increased PEEP can lower venous return to the heart, leading to reduced cardiac output and worsening cerebral perfusion.
  - Consult **neurosurgery** for consideration of cerebral fluid drainage or decompressive surgery. This can be pivotal during cerebellar infarcts or massive hemispheric infarcts.

REFERENCES

Adams HP Jr, del Zoppo G, Alberts MJ, *et al.* Guidelines for the early management of adults with ischemic stroke: a guideline from the American Heart Association/American Stroke Association Stroke Council, Clinical Cardiology Council, Cardiovascular Radiology and Intervention Council, and the Atherosclerotic Peripheral Vascular Disease and Quality of Care Outcomes in Research Interdisciplinary Working Groups: the American Academy of Neurology affirms the value of this guideline as an educational tool for neurologists. *Stroke.* 2007; **38**: 1655.

Hacke W, Kaste M, Bluhmki E, *et al.* Thrombolysis with alteplase 3 to 4.5 hours after acute ischemic stroke. *N Engl J Med.* 2008; **359**: 1317–29.

Heitsch L, Jauch EC. Management of hypertension in the setting of acute ischemic stroke. *Curr Hypertens Rep.* 2007; **9**: 506–11.

Kimberly WT, Sheth KN. Approach to severe hemispheric stroke. *Neurology.* 2011; **76**; S50.

Lukovits TG, Goddeau RP. Critical care of patients with acute ischemic and hemorrhagic stroke: update on recent evidence and international guidelines. *Chest.* 2011; **139**; 694–700.

National Institutes of Health. NIH Stroke Scale. Bethesda, MD: National Institutes of Health, National Institute of Neurological Disorders and Stroke; 2013. Available from: http://stroke.nih.gov/documents/NIH_Stroke_Scale.pdf (accessed April 30, 2013).

17

Intracranial hemorrhage

Jonathan C. Roberts and Timothy C. Peck

Introduction

- Intracranial hemorrhage is a devastating neurological emergency that demands prompt, thoughtful decision making in the emergency department.
- In intracranial hemorrhage, blood occupies space within the calvarium, irritates brain parenchyma and impairs outflow of cerebral spinal fluid (CSF) from the dural sinus venous network, which raises intracranial pressure (ICP) with a resultant decrease in cerebral perfusion.
- The clinical condition of these patients can change quickly and dramatically.
- Regardless of its source, when blood accumulates within a fixed volume space, pressure within that container increases. A healthy brain regulates cerebral blood flow by titrating vascular resistance. These mechanisms are disrupted in an injured brain and blood flow depends on cerebral perfusion pressure (CPP) which is the difference between mean arterial pressure (MAP) and ICP.

$$CPP = MAP - ICP \quad (\text{normal CPP} = 50-70\text{mmHg})$$

- In addition to occupying space, blood has several effects on surrounding tissues. It triggers an inflammatory cascade with capillary leak that promotes worsening edema. It irritates surrounding neurovascular bundles causing vasospasm, thrombosis, and seizure activity. Intraventricular extension of hemorrhage may block CSF and venous drainage resulting in acute noncommunicating hydrocephalus.
- There are several types of intracranial hemorrhage, and diagnostic and therapeutic approaches differ (Table 17.1).

Practical Emergency Resuscitation and Critical Care, ed. Kaushal Shah, Jarone Lee, Kamal Medlej, and Scott D. Weingart. Published by Cambridge University Press. © Kaushal Shah, Jarone Lee, Kamal Medlej, and Scott D. Weingart 2013.

Table 17.1. Type of intracranial hemorrhage categorized by location

Type	Location
Subarachnoid hemorrhage	Bleeding into the potential space between the arachnoid and pia mater
Subdural hematoma	Bleeding into the potential space between dura and arachnoid membrane
Epidural hematoma	Bleeding into the space between skull and the dura
Intracerebral hemorrhage	Bleeding into the space within the brain parenchyma

- *Subarachnoid hemorrhage (SAH)*
  - SAH accounts for 5% of all strokes, affecting 30 000 patients in the United States annually with a mortality rate approaching 45%.
  - SAH occurs when blood enters the potential space between the arachnoid and pia mater. The most common cause of SAH is spontaneous rupture of a cerebral aneurysm.
- *Subdural hemorrhage (SDH)*
  - SDH is classically from shearing of the bridging veins that drain the arachnoid to the dural sinuses and extravasate into the space between arachnoid and dura.
  - The majority of SDHs are acute in nature and from trauma.
  - SDH is a common injury of the elderly with even minor head injuries.
  - SDH can also be caused by low CSF pressure (CSF leak after lumbar puncture [LP]) or can be spontaneous in those with significant brain atrophy (the elderly and alcoholics).
  - Chronic SDHs are slow-forming hematomas that usually present insidiously.
- *Epidural hemorrhage (EDH)*
  - Epidural hematomas arise in the potential space between the dura and the skull, most often from injury to the meningeal arteries.
  - Most patients with EDH also have a skull fracture.
  - Nontraumatic causes include hemodialysis, pregnancy, abscess, and sickle cell disease.
  - EDH is rare in the elderly.
  - If recognized and treated early, the prognosis is excellent.
  - About 50% of patients have a "lucid interval," which is a window of consciousness that occurs between the initial transient loss of consciousness and eventual coma. During the lucid interval, the hematoma expands and causes increased intracranial pressure.
- *Intracerebral hemorrhage (ICH)*
  - Intracerebral hemorrhage accounts for 10–15% of first-time strokes, with a mortality rate ranging between 35% and 52%.

- ICH occurs when blood accumulates within the brain parenchyma itself. The most common cause of ICH is chronic hypertension with progressive cerebrovascular disease leading to degenerative changes of cerebral arterioles. Other etiologies include bleeding from amyloid angiopathy or tumor.

Presentation

Classic and critical presentation

- Patient presentation varies widely depending on location and extent of the hemorrhage and can include:
  - Altered mental status
  - Headache
  - Nausea/vomiting
  - Focal neurological deficits
  - Coma
  - Seizure
  - Brief loss of consciousness followed by lucid interval.
- The classic presentation of SAH is the *sudden onset of 'the worst headache of one's life.'* SAH accounts for 1% of all patients presenting to the ED with the complaint of "the worst headache of my life."
- The most common features of SAH include headache (74%), nausea or vomiting (77%), loss of consciousness (53%), nuchal rigidity (35%), and focal neurological deficits.

Diagnosis and evaluation

- **Radiology**
  - Emergent noncontrast head CT is the cornerstone for detection of intracranial hemorrhage. MRI is equally effective in identifying intracranial hemorrhage and better at detecting predisposing underlying parenchymal or vascular anomalies. However, for many emergent clinical scenarios, MRI is not practical.
  - For SAH, the most current AHA guidelines recommend lumbar puncture for detection of potential SAH if noncontrast head CT is negative; more recent literature suggests that the newer, multidetector CT scanners can safely rule out SAH if obtained within 6 hours of headache onset, thereby eliminating the need for LP.
  - The presence of red blood cells or xanthochromia in the CSF sample suggests possible SAH and warrants further evaluation and neurosurgical consultation. Current evidence suggests that it takes approximately 12 hours for xanthochromia to develop.

- In patients with confirmed SAH, immediate CTA of the head and neck should be obtained to evaluate for cerebral aneurysm as prompt intervention via clipping or coiling may improve patient outcomes.
- If trauma suspected, consider CT cervical spine as well.
- **Laboratory tests**
  - Check serum electrolytes as derangements can worsen brain function.
  - Check serum glucose as hypoglycemia can mimic the signs and symptoms of intracranial hemorrhage.
  - Check coagulation studies (PT/PTT) to identify coagulopathy.
  - Type and screen/cross-match blood products.
  - Consider toxicology screens.
  - Pregnancy test as needed.

Critical management

- Emergency department management focuses on protecting cerebral perfusion by balancing the forces of MAP and ICP.
- Patients should be positioned with the head of the bed elevated to 30 degrees to support cerebral venous drainage to reduce ICP.
- **Securing the airway**
  - Laryngeal manipulation transiently increases ICP. If anticipating endotracheal intubation, premedication with lidocaine 3–5 minutes prior to laryngoscopy may blunt this effect on ICP.
  - Induction agents for rapid sequence intubation should support MAP. Etomidate is an effective, fast-acting induction agent, which is hemodynamically neutral. Other potential induction agents include benzodiazepines, ketamine and propofol.
  - Depolarizing neuromuscular blockers such as succinylcholine produce diffuse muscle fasciculations that can raise ICP. Nondepolarizing neuromuscular blockers do not cause muscle contraction and have no effect on ICP. Consider one of the nondepolarizing neuromuscular blockers such as rocuronium.
  - Adequate sedation prevents agitation and subsequent elevations in ICP. Propofol is a rapid-onset sedative, which is cleared quickly once discontinued, thereby facilitating frequent monitoring of the neurological examination. Propofol can precipitate hypotension and should be used with caution as secondary insults to the brain are known to produce worse outcomes.
  - Respiratory rates should be titrated to a goal $PaCO_2$ of 35–40 mmHg to prevent cerebral vasodilation.
- **Blood pressure control**
  - *Hypertension*
    - Extremely elevated blood pressures in patients with intracranial hemorrhage may be associated with hematoma expansion and poor clinical outcomes.

- Current 2010 AHA guidelines recommend aggressive blood pressure reduction in hypertensive patients with intracranial hemorrhage. While current evidence is limited, a target of 160/90 is probably reasonable as long as CPP is preserved, but further study is warranted. This target may be lowered in patients with unsecured cerebral aneurysms, and discussion with a neurosurgeon for these patients is critical.
  - The INTERACT trial (published in *Lancet* in 2008) suggested that tight blood pressure control SBP <140 mmHg is safe and decreases hematoma expansion.
  - The ATACH trial (published in *Neuro Critical Care* in 2007) suggested that aggressive blood pressure reduction with nicardipine is not associated with neurological deterioration.
- Consider nicardipine, labetalol, and nitroprusside. Do not use hydralazine, as it causes cerebral vasodilatation and increased ICP.
- *Hypotension*
  - Injured brains depend on the balance between MAP and ICP for perfusion. MAP should be maintained >60 mmHg by vasoactive agents if necessary to protect cerebral perfusion pressure.
  - Consider arterial line insertion to help monitor all patients requiring antihypertensive drips or pressors for MAP management.
- **Anticoagulation reversal** (Table 17.2)
  - Immediate review of the patient's medications is crucial to identify potential underlying medication-induced coagulopathy. Rapid, aggressive reversal of anticoagulation can prevent hematoma expansion and improve clinical outcomes (see Table 17.2).
- **ICP management**
  - **Elevate the head of the bed to 30 degrees** to promote venous drainage from the head to reduce ICP. Be sure to maintain the head in a midline position to ensure drainage of the neck veins.
  - **Empiric treatment** for presumed herniation includes use of osmotic agents to reduce cerebral edema. These are purely temporizing measures until invasive ICP monitoring is established to guide therapy, or until surgical interventions become available.
    - *Mannitol* is a sugar alcohol used as an osmotic diuretic to draw hypotonic fluid (edema) into the hypertonic intravascular space. Mannitol can precipitate hypotension and should be used with caution in patients with low MAP and renal failure.
    - *Hypertonic saline* is an alternative osmotic agent that is effective in lowering ICP and improving CPP. It is generally not associated with hypotension unless infused rapidly. There are various concentrations of hypertonic saline with various dosing regimens that may be chosen based on the clinical scenario. Ultimately, close monitoring of serum sodium levels and serum osmolarity dictates infusion volume.

Table 17.2. Reversal of anticoagulation

Medication	Reversal agent
Coumadin	Vitamin K
	Fresh frozen plasma
	Prothrombin complex concentrates
Aspirin/Plavix	Platelets
	DDAVP
Heparin/Lovenox	Protamine

- **Invasive ICP monitoring** is crucial for aggressive management of patients with presumed ICP elevations.
  - Extraventricular drains allow real-time ICP monitoring while allowing drainage of CSF to help lower ICP.
  - Other devices including Camino bolts and intraparenchymal pressure catheters can also be used for ICP monitoring but do not offer the option of draining CSF to lower ICP.
- **Surgical intervention**
  - The majority of these patients will require a **neurosurgical consultation**.
  - **Timely consultation or transfer to a tertiary care center** for neurosurgical evaluation is an essential component of emergency medicine management. Continued management should be in a critical care setting as soon as feasible.
  - Various surgical procedures including craniotomy, craniectomy, stereotactic aspiration, and hematoma drainage may be used by neurosurgery to further lower ICP.
  - Various interventional and surgical techniques including clipping and coiling are crucial for management of spontaneous SAH from aneurysmal rupture.

Sudden deterioration

- The sudden deterioration of a previously stable patient may represent a critical increase in ICP and shift of intracranial structures that further compromises the CPP. This may manifest clinically as change in alertness, new neurological deficits, vomiting, or vital sign derangements including hypertension coupled with bradycardia (Cushing's response).
- The airway should be immediately secured and osmotic agents including mannitol or hypertonic saline can be used empirically to temporize impending herniation. Other quick measures to reduce ICP include adequate sedation, neuromuscular blockade, elevating the head of bed to 30 degrees, and adjusting the respiratory rate to achieve a goal $PaCO_2$ of 35 mmHg. Any potential coagulopathy should be fully and aggressively reversed if present.

- Emergent neurosurgical consultation should be initiated while immediate non-contrast head CT is performed to evaluate for interval change. If the emergency physician is practicing in a setting without neurosurgical services, arrangements should be made for emergent transfer to a tertiary care center. The main goal of emergency management is temporize ICP changes, avoid secondary insults (e.g., hypoxia and hypotension) and protect CPP while expediting neurosurgical evaluation for possible life-saving surgical intervention.

Vasopressor of choice: norepinephrine.

REFERENCES

Bederson JB, Connolly ES, Batjer HH, *et al.* Guidelines for the Management of Aneurysmal Subarachnoid Hemorrhage: A Statement for Healthcare Professionals from a Special Writing Group of the Stroke Council, American Heart Association/American Stroke Association. *Stroke.* 2009; **40**: 994–1025.

Birenbaum DS. Intracerebral hemorrhage. In: Winters ME, DeBlieux P, Marcolini EG, Bond MC, Woolridge DP, eds. *Emergency Department Resuscitation of the Critically Ill.* Dallas, TX: ACEP; 2011.

Broderick J, Connolly S, Feldmann E, *et al.* Guidelines for the Management of Spontaneous Intracerebral Hemorrhage in Adults from the Special Writing Group of the Stroke Council, American Heart Association/American Stroke Association. *Stroke.* 2007; **38**: 2001–23.

Davis SM, Broderick J, Hennerici M, *et al.* Hematoma growth is a determinant of mortality and poor outcome after intracerebral hemorrhage. *Neurology.* 2006; **66**: 1175–81.

Gijn JV, Rinkel GJ. Subarachnoid hemorrhage: diagnosis, causes and management. *Brain.* 2001; **124**: 249–78.

18

Status epilepticus

Matthew L. Wong and John W. Hardin

Introduction

- Seizures are caused by erratic electrical discharges in the brain.
- *Generalized convulsive status epilepticus* (GCSE) is defined as either continuous seizure activity lasting more than 30 minutes, or two or more seizures of any length without complete recovery of mental status between them.
- Seizures fatigue muscles, so twitching may decrease without termination of neurological activity.
- Status epilepticus can present with purely neurological symptoms without muscle involvement in nonconvulsive status epilepticus (NCSE).
- Seizures have many etiologies; therefore, treatment and diagnosis should be made in parallel.
- See Table 18.1 for a list of causes of seizures.

Presentation

Classic presentation

- Unresponsive with rhythmic movement of one or more body parts, or tonic eye deviation; of note, myotonic movements and incontinence may be seen in syncope as well as seizure.
- Less commonly, patients with altered mental status may actually be in NCSE.
- There is an association with seizures and posterior shoulder dislocations.
- Seizures are followed by a postictal state – defined as an altered mental status of variable duration.

Practical Emergency Resuscitation and Critical Care, ed. Kaushal Shah, Jarone Lee, Kamal Medlej, and Scott D. Weingart. Published by Cambridge University Press. © Kaushal Shah, Jarone Lee, Kamal Medlej, and Scott D. Weingart 2013.

Table 18.1. Causes of seizures

Metabolic	Primary central nervous system	Toxidromes/toxins
• Hypoxia • Hypoglycemia • Hyponatremia • Hypocalcemia • Hypomagnesemia • Inborn errors of metabolism	• Trauma • Infections • Cerebral vascular accident • Hemorrhage • Vasculitis • Seizure disorder with other medical condition • Seizure disorder medication abstinence • Seizure disorder with recent medication change • Pre- or postpartum eclampsia • Tumors	• Anticholinergic • Sympathomimetic • Ethanol withdrawal • Serotonin syndrome • Tricyclic antidepressant • Salicylate • Isoniazid • Tramadol • Bupropion • Venlafaxine • Strychnine

- A postictal state may include a Todd's paralysis in which focal neurological deficits may mimic a stroke.

Critical presentation

- Seizures, which may be the result of CNS infection, require **early and empiric** antibiotics, antivirals, and possibly steroids, ideally **before** lumbar puncture is performed. Do not delay administration of these medications while awaiting lumbar puncture.
- Seizures may require additional treatment and can be **refractory** to first-line agents (i.e., benzodiazepines) and second-line agents (i.e., phenytoin, phenobarbital, and valproate).
- Be aware that patients could be seizing with **little or no muscle twitching** or because of concomitant administration of neuromuscular blockade medications.

Diagnosis and evaluation

- **Immediate bedside tests**
  - Bedside **glucose** level to rapidly evaluate for hypoglycemia.
  - **Electrocardiogram** to screen for hyperkalemia or toxidrome.
- **Laboratory tests**
  - Obtain basic serum electrolytes, calcium, magnesium, phosphorus, and glucose.

- Lactate will be very elevated if blood is drawn during or immediately after tonic-clonic activity. Recheck the lactate level after seizures have successfully been aborted.
- Get total creatine phosphokinase (CK/CPK) to assess for associated rhabdomyolysis.
- Consider drug levels such as antiepileptic drug levels, ethanol, salicylate, acetaminophen, and tricyclic level.
- Urine toxicology test to screen for cocaine or other ingestions.
- Urine/serum pregnancy test to screen for **pregnancy**.
- **Imaging studies**
  - Consider **noncontrast head CT** to evaluate for structural cause for the seizure such as hemorrhage, or mass, particularly for first-time seizures.
- **Further testing**
  - Consider **lumbar puncture** and empiric administration of antibiotics/antiviral medications if an infectious etiology is suspected.
  - Consider **STAT bedside EEG** if concerned about NCSE.

Critical management

- Assess **airway** security. Patients unable to protect the airway may require rapid sequence intubation (RSI).
- Rapidly identify and correct hypoglycemia and hypoxia with dextrose and high-flow oxygen.
- Administer **benzodiazepines** as first-line therapy:
  - Typically lorazepam IV/IM (0.1 mg/kg every 5–10 minutes), diazepam IV/PR (0.2 mg/kg every 5 minutes), or midazolam IV/IM (0.2 mg/kg every 5 minutes).
  - Do not give diazepam IM because it is erratically absorbed.
- Administer **second-line agents** if necessary:
  - Phenytoin (20 mg/kg at 50 mg/minute) or fosphenytoin (20 mg/kg at 150 mg/minute).
  - If still seizing then consider
    - Propofol
    - Phenobarbital
    - Pentobarbital.
- If seizures are refractory to first- and second-line agents, consider levetiracetam or lacosamide, or induction with general anesthesia by inhalational anesthetics.
- **Treat the underlying cause**
  - *Infectious:* Early administration of antibiotics, antivirals, and steroids before lumbar puncture if infectious etiology is suspected.
  - *Hyponatremia:* If seizures are from hyponatremia, administer **hypertonic saline** (3% NS) 1–2 mL/kg over 10 minutes until seizures stop. Then recheck

sodium level hourly and correct by 1 mEq/L per hour to prevent **osmotic demyelination syndrome**.

- *Eclampsia:* If seizures are from **eclampsia** or hypomagnesemia, administer magnesium (4–6 g over 15–20 minutes then 2 g/hour).
- *Toxic ingestion:* Consider antidotes if isoniazid, tricyclic antidepressant, salicylate, or organophosphate overdose is suspected – contact local poison control center or toxicology consultants.
- Monitor and treat expectantly for hyperthermia, rhabdomyolysis, hyperkalemia, and acute kidney injury.
- Patients with status epilepticus should be admitted to an intensive care unit (ICU) setting.

Sudden deterioration

- The most likely causes for sudden decompensation are airway compromise/respiratory failure, sepsis/septic shock, and recurrent seizure activity.
- Patients requiring multiple boluses of medications or continuous infusions should be considered for intubation for airway protection.
- Patients with an infectious etiology may rapidly progress to sepsis and require additional hemodynamic support.
- Prolonged seizure activity with or without overt muscle twitching is associated with increased mortality.

Vasopressor of choice (if necessary): norepinephrine, but may depend on underlying etiology.

REFERENCES

Holtkamp M. Treatment strategies for refractory status epilepticus. *Curr Opin Crit Care.* 2011; **17**: 94–100.

Shearer P, Riviello J. Generalized convulsive status epilepticus in adults and children: treatment guidelines and protocols. *Emerg Med Clin North Am.* 2011; **29**: 51–64.

Silbergleit R, Durkalski V, Lowenstein D, *et al.* Intramuscular versus intravenous therapy for prehospital status epilepticus. *N Engl J Med.* 2012; **366**: 591–600.

Treiman DM, Meyers PD, Walton NY, *et al.* A comparison of four treatments for generalized convulsive status epilepticus. Veterans Affairs Status Epilepticus Cooperative Study Group. *N Engl J Med.* 1998; **339**: 792–8.

Zehtabchi S, Abdel Baki SG, Malhotra S, Grant AC. Nonconvulsive seizures in patients presenting with altered mental status: an evidence-based review. *Epilepsy Behav.* 2011; **22**: 139–43.

19

Acute spinal cord compression

Cristal Cristia and Timothy C. Peck

Introduction

- Acute spinal cord compression results from impingement on the spinal cord due to a variety of etiologies, including neoplasm, hemorrhage, infection, or structural impingement on the cord and spinal nerves at any vertebral level (Table 19.1).
- Spinal cord compression is a true surgical emergency, which may lead to permanent neurological deficits such as paralysis and death.
- **Time is critical**: the longer the patient has neurological deficit, the more likely it will become permanent, even with surgical intervention.
- Any patient who presents with a history of trauma, intravenous drug use (IVDU), or immunocompromised state with associated neurological deficits and/or back pain should be evaluated for acute cord compression.
- Neoplastic disease is rarely confined to a single location; therefore, the entire spine should be evaluated when metastatic disease is suspected.
- Cervical spine injury accounts for 50% of traumatic spinal cord injury, while thoracolumbar injuries comprise the remaining 50%.

Presentation

Classic presentation

- **Neck or back pain**
  - May be acute, subacute, or chronic in development.
  - May be associated with symptoms of the underlying disease process (e.g., fever).

Practical Emergency Resuscitation and Critical Care, ed. Kaushal Shah, Jarone Lee, Kamal Medlej, and Scott D. Weingart. Published by Cambridge University Press. © Kaushal Shah, Jarone Lee, Kamal Medlej, and Scott D. Weingart 2013.

Table 19.1. Etiologies of acute spinal cord compression

Neoplastic disease
- Most common presentation is metastatic lesion
  (lung/prostate/breast > renal/gastrointestinal/lymphoma)

Mechanical/structural abnormalities
- Traumatic/bony injury
- Osteoporosis/pathological fracture
- Degenerative joint disease
- Postsurgical complication

Infectious causes
- Extradural spinal abscess (IVDU, HIV, tuberculosis, immunosuppression)
- Diskitis/osteomyelitis

Vascular causes
- Ischemic
- Hemorrhagic (anticoagulation)

Inflammatory disease
- Rheumatoid arthritis (C1/2 dislocation)

- **Neurological signs and symptoms**
  - Associated with limb weakness/paresthesias in more advanced cases.
  - Neurogenic bladder and/or bowel.
  - Autonomic dysfunction is expected if the lesion is cervical/thoracic in origin.
  - Gait abnormality.

Critical presentation

- **Spinal shock**
  - Characterized by a loss of spinal cord function below the level of the lesion.
  - Cervical and thoracic level lesions may be associated with respiratory compromise.
  - Results in a disruption of sympathetic innervation causing unopposed para-sympathetic tone, which may also cause hypotension and bradyarrhythmias (neurogenic shock).
  - Flaccid paralysis, anesthesia distal to the lesion, and loss of bladder/bowel control are characteristic.
  - Priapism may also be present, caused by loss of sympathetic innervation below the level of the lesion.

Diagnosis and evaluation

- The diagnosis of acute spinal cord compression is suggested by history and physical examination, and confirmed by radiography or surgical intervention. Clinical presentations may vary depending on the level of neurological injury.

- CBC, ESR, CRP, chemistries, venous lactate.
- Coagulation studies, liver function tests.
- Urinalysis, ± beta-hCG.
- ECG, chest radiography.
- Spinal imaging:
  - Plain radiographic films may show bony destruction in the case of infectious or metastatic disease, or fracture in the setting of trauma. However, plain films may be falsely negative in up to 20% of cases.
  - CT scan of the spine provides improved delineation of bony structures.
  - Emergent spine MRI: MRI is preferred over CT because it can better evaluate soft tissue structures such as the spinal cord and ligamentous pathology.
  - CT myelography is useful for identifying spinal canal compromise in those patients unable to undergo MRI. However, it does not provide distinction between the various soft tissue lesions such as hematoma, epidural abscess, etc.

Critical management

Airway management as needed
Maintain spinal precautions, especially in the setting of trauma
Narcotic analgesia
NPO, IV fluids
Emergent MRI spine
± Vasopressor therapy
± Antibiotics
Neurosurgery consultation and admission

- **Manage ABCs**
  - Immediately place the patient on cardiac monitors and pulse oximetry.
  - Patients with a cervical lesion may require *intubation* for definitive airway control and to assist with ventilation and oxygenation.
  - If the patient is breathing spontaneously, obtain an FVC (forced vital capacity) to assess for impending airway compromise. Serial measurements should be obtained to monitor for progression of respiratory fatigue.
  - Respiratory muscle weakness and paralysis as evidenced by poor FVC or concerning clinical signs such as shallow rapid breathing should be managed immediately with endotracheal intubation.
  - Manual cervical in-line spinal stabilization should be maintained during intubation if a direct laryngoscopy approach is used, particularly in the setting of trauma. Fiberoptic intubation may be necessary.
- **Strict spinal precautions** (e.g., cervical collar, backboard) should be continued until imaging has been obtained to prevent further neurological injury.

- **IV narcotic analgesia** will likely be necessary. In those patients with a subacute onset of disease, such as with neoplastic disease, pain may have been present for day to weeks prior to presentation.
- Maintain **NPO** status – the patient with spinal cord compromise may require an operative intervention.
- If an infectious process is suspected, blood cultures should be drawn and broad-spectrum **IV antibiotic coverage** should be administered. Prompt recognition of possible infection based on history and physical examination, or indicators such as the presence of SIRS criteria or elevated ESR/CRP, is important to minimize delays in antibiotics.
- **Check a post-void residual** with a bladder ultrasound or catheterization, as **urinary retention** is very sensitive for spinal cord injury and cauda equina syndrome.
- **Steroid treatment** for spinal cord injury is controversial, especially in the setting of trauma, and is beyond the scope of this discussion. In contrast, administration of corticosteroids (most commonly dexamethasone) is an important component in the treatment of spinal cord compression secondary to metastatic disease. In this population, steroids have been shown to improve clinical outcomes and may also alleviate pain related to bony metastases and compression of neural structures.
- **Surgical consultation** should be considered for all patients with acute cord compression. Radiation therapy may have a role in relieving cord compression caused by malignancy. Continued management should occur in an intensive care setting.

Sudden deterioration

- The mostly likely causes for sudden decompensation include expansion of the offending lesion causing worsening neurological compromise or a high cervical/thoracic lesion, resulting in respiratory or hemodynamic compromise. Both scenarios require urgent surgical consultation, ± surgical decompression. Endotracheal intubation may also be required.
- Risk factors for sudden deterioration include weakened diaphragmatic function (poor FVC), advanced age, history of cardiopulmonary disease, tachypnea at presentation, etc.
- **Respiratory compromise** occurs with spinal cord lesions above the high thoracic level. Monitor for diaphragmatic and respiratory muscle weakness with forced vital capacity and provide intubation as needed.
- **Cardiopulmonary collapse** may occur with spinal shock. Hypotension and bradycardia are hallmarks. Keep in mind that neurogenic shock does not always present with bradycardia and depends on the level of the lesion.
  - Provide IV fluids and vasopressor therapy as needed to maintain adequate perfusion.

- Symptomatic or unstable bradycardia may require administration of atropine or cardiac pacing.
- Vasopressors with chronotropic properties, such as dopamine and norepinephrine, may be of particular advantage in those patients with persistent bradycardia.
- Adequate perfusion may be measured by standard resuscitation parameters, such as appropriate urine output and resolution of systemic acidosis.

Special circumstances

- **Cauda equina syndrome** is not a compression of the spinal cord but rather a syndrome whereby compression occurs at the spinal nerve roots below the level of the spinal cord.
  - A clinical diagnosis that classically presents with bilateral lumbosacral back pain with radiation to the legs, subjective urinary retention or overflow incontinence, bowel incontinence, and saddle anesthesia.
  - Presentation may be subtle: a high index of suspicion is required to prevent delay in diagnosis.
  - Examination should include a rectal examination and evaluation of sensory function in the perineal area.
  - Urinary retention (at least 500 mL) is a concerning late finding.
- Emergent MRI should be obtained in all patients in whom the diagnosis is being considered to evaluate for the number of etiologies that may cause this syndrome including neoplasm, inflammatory conditions, etc.
- Urgent surgical consultation should be obtained in parallel with imaging.

Vasopressor of choice: norepinephrine.

REFERENCES

Fehlings MG, Cadotte DW, Fehlings LN. A series of systematic reviews on the treatment of acute spinal cord injury: a foundation for best medical practice. *J Neurotrauma.* 2011; **28**: 1329–33.

George R, Jeba J, Ramkumar G, *et al.* Interventions for the treatment of metastatic extradural spinal cord compression in adults. *Cochrane Database of Syst Rev.* 2008; (4): CD006716.

Markandaya M, Stein DM, Menaker J. Acute treatment options for spinal cord injury. *Curr Treat Options Neurol.* 2011; **14**: 175–187.

Radcliff KE, Kepler CK, Delasotta LA, *et al.* Current management review of thoracolumbar cord syndromes. *Spine J.* 2011; **11**: 884–92.

Schiff D. Spinal cord compression. *Neurol Clin N Am.* 2003; **21**: 67–86.

Cardiovascular emergencies

20

Acute coronary syndrome

Steven C. Rougas

Introduction

- Ischemic heart disease is the leading cause of death in adults in the United States.
- Acute coronary syndrome (ACS) refers to symptoms attributable to atherosclerotic disease of the epicardial coronary arteries, usually caused by a fixed atherosclerotic lesion.
- ACS is a spectrum of disease and can present as acute myocardial infarction (AMI) or unstable angina (UA).
  - AMI: myocardial ischemia *with* necrosis; can occur with or without ST segment elevation. The latter is referred to as non-ST-segment elevation myocardial infarction (NSTEMI).
  - UA: reversible myocardial ischemia *without* necrosis.
- The etiologies for ACS can be divided into primary and secondary (see Table 20.1).

Table 20.1. Etiologies of ACS

Primary etiologies	Secondary etiologies
Coronary artery spasm	Increased myocardial oxygen demand
Disruption or erosion of atherosclerotic plaques	Reduced myocardial blood flow
Platelet aggregation or thrombus formation at the site of an atherosclerotic lesion	Reduced myocardial oxygen delivery

Practical Emergency Resuscitation and Critical Care, ed. Kaushal Shah, Jarone Lee, Kamal Medlej, and Scott D. Weingart. Published by Cambridge University Press. © Kaushal Shah, Jarone Lee, Kamal Medlej, and Scott D. Weingart 2013.

Presentation

Classic presentation

- **General signs and symptoms:**
  - Substernal or left-sided chest discomfort (heaviness, pressure, tightness, or squeezing).
  - Radiation to the arms, jaw, or neck.
  - Nausea, vomiting.
  - Diaphoresis.
  - Dyspnea.
- **Stable angina:**
  - Transient, episodic chest pain.
  - Exercise or stress may induce symptoms.
  - Episodes usually last <10 minutes.
  - Usually resolves with rest or glyceryl nitrate.
- **Unstable angina:**
  - Occurs with minimal exertion or at rest.
  - Episodes usually last >20 minutes despite glyceryl trinitrate or cessation of activity.
- **Acute myocardial infarction:**
  - Prolonged, continuous, severe chest discomfort at rest.
  - May not respond to immediate symptomatic management.

Critical presentation

- Patients may present with cardiogenic shock:
  - Hypotension
  - Pallor
  - Diaphoresis
  - Cardiac arrhythmias (ventricular fibrillation [VF] or ventricular tachycardia [VT])
  - Variations in systolic blood pressure
  - Bradycardia or heart block
  - New murmur secondary to papillary muscle rupture
  - Pulmonary edema manifested by shortness of breath and rales on auscultation
- Patients in extremis may also present in cardiac arrest.

Diagnosis and evaluation

- There are four main elements in the diagnosis of ACS:
  - Clinical history
  - Physical examination

- Electrocardiogram (ECG) findings:
  - In addition to interpretation of an initial ECG, it is imperative that any patient with a concerning story have a **repeat ECG within 10–15 minutes** to assess for evolution of ischemia or myocardial injury.
  - Myocardial distress is manifest in the ST segments of the ECG; ST segment depression indicates myocardial ischemia whereas ST segment elevation (STE) indicates acute myocardial infarction (>1 mm in two contiguous standard limb leads or >2 mm in two contiguous precordial leads).
  - ECG changes occur in patterns on the ECG and may be suggestive of the location of the culprit lesion (Table 20.2).
- Cardiac biomarkers:
  - Troponin:
    - Myocardial troponin I (TnI) and troponin T (TnT) are elevated as early as 3 hours, but may stay elevated for up to 7 days.
  - Creatine kinase (CK):
    - CK-MB is myocardial specific, usually elevated as early as 3 hours and peaking within 24 hours; it normalizes 2–3 days after injury.
  - Myoglobin:
    - Myocardial myoglobin is not distinguishable from skeletal muscle myoglobin and thus is not a useful marker in ACS.
    - Initially rises 1–2 hours post event, peaks at 5–7 hours, and normalizes by 24 hours.

Table 20.2. ECG findings in ACS

Common infarct locations	Corresponding electrocardiographic ST changes	Suggested potential lesion location
Anterior wall	V3, V4	Left anterior descending artery (LAD)
Anteroseptal wall	V1–V4, aVR	LAD, STE in aVR suggests left main coronary
Anterolateral wall	V3–V6, I, aVL	LAD, left circumflex artery (LCX)
Lateral wall	V5, V6, I, aVL	LAD and branches including perforators and obtuse marginals
Inferior wall	II, III, aVF	Right coronary artery (RCA), LCX
Right ventricle (often associated with inferior MI)	V1, V2, II, III, aVF, V3R–V6R	Proximal RCA
Posterior wall	V7–V9 (with ST depression in V1–V3)	RCA, LCX

Critical management of STEMI

- Any patient with STEMI (ST-segment elevation myocardial infarction) should undergo reperfusion with percutaneous coronary intervention (PCI) within 90 minutes of presentation.
- Fibrinolytics should be used for patients unable to undergo PCI within the recommended timeframe.
  - Initiation of therapy should occur as soon as possible after the diagnosis of STEMI is made.
  - Alteplase, tenecteplase and reteplase are all possible therapies.
  - Inclusion criteria:
    - Patients presenting with STEMI.
    - Survival benefit is greatest for patients presenting within 12 hours of symptoms.
    - ST segment elevations >1 mm in two contiguous standard limb leads or ST segment elevation >2 mm in two contiguous precordial leads.
  - Exclusion criteria:
    - Absolute contraindications:
      - Prior intracranial hemorrhage or known arteriovenous malformation (AVM).
      - Known intracranial mass.
      - Ischemic stroke within 3 months of presentation.
      - Active internal bleeding from other source.
      - Suspected aortic dissection.
    - Relative contraindications:
      - BP >180/100.
      - Elevated INR.
      - Trauma or major surgical procedure within the past 3 months.
      - Pregnancy.
- Other pharmacological agents include antiplatelets, antithrombins, beta-antagonists, nitrates, and morphine (see Table 20.3).
  - Antiplatelets such as aspirin have been linked to improved outcomes and should be uniformly used. The number needed to treat (NNT) to save 1 life is approximately 42.
  - Anticoagulants such as heparin should also be considered.
    - Either unfractionated (UF) or low–molecular weight (LMW) heparin can be used; no specific data supports one over the other.
  - Beta-blockers reduce myocardial oxygen demand and decrease the potential of arrhythmia. It is not necessary to give them in the emergency department (ED).
    - Contraindications to beta-blockade include hypotension, cardiogenic shock, or congestive heart failure.
  - Nitrates are used to decrease pain and increase myocardial blood flow.
    - They can be administered sublingually.
    - Intravenous (IV) infusions should be considered if the pain persists after repeated sublingual doses.

Table 20.3. Pharmacological agents in the treatment of ACS

Pharmacological agent	Example	Mechanism of action
Antiplatelets	Aspirin	Irreversibly acetylates platelet cyclooxygenase
Antithrombin	Heparin	Inhibits conversion of fibrinogen to fibrin
Beta-antagonists[a]	Metoprolol	Prevent tachycardia and increased inotropy
ACE inhibitors[b]	Lisinopril	Possibly cause a reduction in plaque rupture secondary to decreased shear force
Nitrates	Glyceryl trinitrate	Decrease myocardial preload and afterload
GP IIb/IIIa receptor inhibitors	Eptifibatide	Inhibit the glycoprotein IIb/IIIa receptor
Thienopyridine antiplatelets	Clopidogrel	Inhibit transformation of the glycoprotein IIb/IIIa receptor
Opioid analgesics	Morphine	Reduce pain/anxiety, leading to decreased myocardial oxygen consumption
Fibrinolytics	Alteplase	Bind to fibrin and convert plasminogen to plasmin.

[a] Beta-antagonists have been shown to benefit post-MI patients within 24 hours of the initial event when administered orally; early administration of IV doses does not appear to be beneficial.
[b] ACE inhibitors are also recommended within 24 hours post event, but not in the immediate treatment of ACS.

- In patients with a right ventricular infarction (a preload-dependent condition), the use of nitrates can cause severe hypotension and should be avoided.
- Morphine can be used to decrease pain and anxiety.

Critical management of NSTEMI and UA

- Therapy generally parallels that of STEMI.
- Immediate reperfusion is not indicated, though serial ECGs should be performed in patients with persistent symptoms to detect potential disease evolution.
- Aspirin (182 mg or 325 mg) should uniformly be administered.
- Beta-blockers can also be considered barring any contraindications.
- Pain control can be achieved with nitrates and opioids.

Sudden deterioration

The three most common reasons for decompensation of the ACS patient include cardiac arrhythmias, cardiogenic shock with congestive heart failure, and mechanical complications. Critical disruptions in the anatomy and function of the heart will often cause dyspnea, new murmurs, and potential hemodynamic compromise. A general approach to these patients should include simultaneous diagnostic and supportive efforts. Immediate ECG and bedside ultrasound may be helpful, and preparations for airway and hemodynamic support should be made.

- **Cardiac arrhythmias:**
  - These most commonly include sinus bradycardia, sinus tachycardia, atrial and ventricular premature complexes, and nonsustained ventricular tachycardia (VT).
  - Less common but more dangerous arrhythmias include second and third-degree heart blocks, sustained VT, ventricular fibrillation (VF), and asystole.
  - Antiarrhythmics including amiodarone, procainamide, lidocaine, propranolol, or diltiazem may be required for class-specific dysrhythmias.
  - Electrolyte repletion is also important in the treatment of certain dysrhythmias.
  - Temporary pacing may be required for symptomatic bradycardia or recurrent sinus pauses.
- **Cardiogenic shock:**
  - This is caused by a decrease in ventricular function secondary to acute infarction, and exacerbated by the concomitant increased myocardial oxygen demands as the pump fails.
  - Poor systolic function leads to hypotension, systemic hypoperfusion, and pulmonary congestion.
  - This condition may be complicated by simultaneous valvular disease.
  - It is the leading cause of death in patients with acute myocardial infarction. The in-hospital mortality rate approaches 50%.
  - The definitive intervention is emergent revascularization. Fibrinolysis is not usually effective in these patients.
  - Resuscitative efforts may be required in the ED prior to transport and must balance competing physiological priorities.
    - If severe **respiratory compromise** is present, orotracheal intubation may be required.
    - Managing hypotension in this setting can be challenging as both inotropic support and volume loading increase ventricular strain.
    - American Heart Association (AHA) guidelines suggest that dopamine is the agent of choice in this setting. Norepinephrine can also be used. Dobutamine is contraindicated in patients with a systolic blood pressure less than 80 mmHg.
    - Intra-aortic balloon counterpulsation may be used for patients with refractory hypotension.
- **Mechanical complications:**
  - Papillary muscle rupture:
    - Usually occurs 3–5 days post inferior myocardial infarction.

- Hypotension, pulmonary edema, and a new systolic murmur (indicative of mitral valve incompetence) are hallmarks of this condition.
- The diagnosis is confirmed by echocardiography.
- Medical management includes afterload reduction if possible.
- The definitive management is surgical repair.
- Patients with hypotension may require an intra-aortic balloon pump for stabilization.
  - Ventricular free wall rupture:
    - Rupture may occur anytime between day 1 and day 5 post MI.
    - Usually presents with sudden-onset chest pain with resultant hypotension, tachycardia, and signs of cardiac tamponade.
    - It is diagnosed by echocardiography and requires immediate surgical treatment.
  - Intraventricular septum rupture:
    - Usually occurs several days after acute infarction.
    - Associated with large anterior MI.
    - Patients present with chest pain, dyspnea, and a new systolic murmur as well as potential hemodynamic compromise.
    - Rupture causes left-to-right shunt.
    - It is diagnosed by color-Doppler flow echocardiography and requires surgical treatment.

Vasopressor of choice: Patients in cardiogenic shock post AMI suffer from a decrease in cardiac output associated with left ventricular dysfunction. The choice of inotrope and/or vasopressor will depend on the patient's systolic blood pressure (SBP):
- SBP ≥80 mmHg: dobutamine
- SBP <80 mmHg: dopamine
- SBP <70 mmHg: norepinephrine

REFERENCES

Brady WJ, Harrigan RA, Chan TC. Acute coronary syndrome. In: Marx JA, Hockberger RS, Walls RM, Adams J, Rosen P, eds. *Rosen's Emergency Medicine: Concepts and Clinical Practice*. 7th edn. Philadelphia, PA: Mosby Elsevier; 2010.

Hollander JE, Diercks DB. Acute coronary syndromes: acute myocardial infarction and unstable angina. In: Tintinalli JE, Stapczynski JS, Ma OJ, *et al.*, eds. *Tintinalli's Emergency Medicine: A Comprehensive Study Guide*. 7th edn. New York: McGraw-Hill; 2011.

Hollenberg SM, Parrillo JE. Myocardial ischemia. In: Hall JB, Schmidt GA, Wood LD, eds. *Principles of Critical Care*. 3rd edn. New York: McGraw-Hill; 2005.

21

Tachyarrhythmias

Joshua Jauregui

Introduction

- In adults, tachycardia is defined as a ventricular rate greater than 100 beats per minute (bpm).
- Tachyarrhythmias are rapid, abnormal heart rhythms that are broadly divided based upon the width of the QRS complex and whether the rhythm is regular or irregular (Table 21.1).
- The width of the QRS complex can be helpful in determining the origin of the arrhythmogenic impulse.
  - A narrow QRS complex is defined as a QRS with a duration < 0.12 seconds.
    - In narrow complex rhythms, the activation of the ventricles occurs via the normal His–Purkinje system, suggesting that the source of the arrhythmia originates above or within the atrioventricular (AV) node.
  - A wide QRS complex is defined as a QRS with a duration ≥ 0.12 seconds.
    - A wide complex rhythm suggests an aberrancy in the normal conduction system and is usually the result of one of the following:
      - A preexisting or rate-related abnormality within the normal conduction system (e.g., bundle branch block).
      - An accessory pathway (e.g., Wolff–Parkinson–White syndrome [WPW]).

Practical Emergency Resuscitation and Critical Care, ed. Kaushal Shah, Jarone Lee, Kamal Medlej, and Scott D. Weingart. Published by Cambridge University Press. © Kaushal Shah, Jarone Lee, Kamal Medlej, and Scott D. Weingart 2013.

Table 21.1. Classification of common tachyarrhythmias

Narrow-complex regular	Narrow-complex irregular	Wide-complex regular	Wide-complex irregular
Sinus tachycardia	Atrial fibrillation	Sinus tachycardia with aberrancy	Atrial fibrillation with aberrancy
Supraventricular tachycardia (SVT)	Atrial flutter with variable block	SVT with aberrancy	Atrial flutter with variable block and aberrancy
Atrial flutter	Multifocal atrial tachycardia (MAT)	Atrial flutter with aberrancy	MAT with aberrancy
		Ventricular tachycardia (VT)	Polymorphic ventricular tachycardia (torsades de point)
			Atrial fibrillation with Wolff–Parkinson–White syndrome (WPW)
			Ventricular fibrillation (VF)

Presentation

Classic presentation

- Ironically, the "classic presentation" mostly consists of nonspecific symptoms. Patients may complain of palpitations, chest pain, lightheadedness, dyspnea, or nonspecific weakness.
- Further evaluation will reveal a rapid heart rate on physical examination or on the electrocardiogram (ECG).

Critical presentation

- Patients with unstable tachyarrhythmias present with signs and symptoms of hypoperfusion and hemodynamic compromise while still maintaining a palpable pulse:
  - Hypotension
  - Altered mentation
  - Ischemic chest pain
  - Pulmonary edema.
- Patients who do not have a palpable pulse are deemed to be in cardiac arrest and are treated according to Advanced Cardiovascular Life Support (ACLS) guidelines.

Diagnosis and evaluation

- Primary evaluation consists of performing an ECG with a rhythm strip.
- Once tachyarrhythmia is confirmed, consideration should be given to whether the arrhythmia has an underlying noncardiac etiology such as a toxic ingestion or a metabolic disturbance.
  - Clinical history is useful and important. Attention should be paid to the patient's medical history and potential use of QT-prolonging medications.
  - A chest radiograph and basic blood work may be helpful in identifying a metabolic or infectious etiology of the arrhythmia.
- The type of arrhythmia can be determined on the basis of the ECG:
  - Sinus tachycardia:
    - Narrow-complex tachycardia.
    - Regular rate greater than 100 bpm.
    - Rates >160 bpm are not typically attributable to sinus tachycardia.
    - Each P wave is associated with a QRS complex.
    - There is a fixed P-R interval.
  - Supraventricular tachycardia (SVT):
    - Narrow-complex tachycardia.
    - Regular rate between 140 and 250 bpm.
    - P waves may be present but difficult to see due to the rate.
    - The most common cause of SVT is atrioventricular nodal reentrant tachycardia (AVNRT).
    - SVT may also present as a wide-complex tachycardia if it is associated with a rate-related or preexisting bundle branch block. This is often referred to as "SVT with aberrant conduction" and may mimic VT.
  - Atrial fibrillation:
    - Atrial fibrillation is the most common cardiac arrhythmia.
    - Usually narrow complex, but can present with a wide QRS in the presence of underlying disease of the conduction system.
    - Irregularly irregular rhythm with absent P waves and atrial rates varying from 400 to 700 bpm.
    - Ventricular response is usually 120–180 bpm.
    - Irregularly irregular rate distinguishes AF from other arrhythmias, even when the complex is wide.
  - Atrial flutter:
    - On a spectrum of sinus node dysfunction with atrial fibrillation.
    - Usually narrow complex.
    - Presents with a classic "sawtooth" pattern of P waves.
    - The atrial rate ranges between 250 and 350 bpm.
    - Atrial flutter is associated with varying degrees of AV block and can present as a regular or regularly irregular rhythm.
    - Most often, the atrial rate is regular at 300 bpm with a 2:1 block, producing a regular ventricular rate of 150 bpm.

- Multifocal atrial tachycardia:
  - Irregularly irregular tachyarrhythmia.
  - Diagnosed by the presence of at least three different P wave morphologies with varying P-R intervals.
  - MAT is almost always seen in the elderly and those with pulmonary disease. It is also associated with hypomagnesemia, hypokalemia, and coronary artery disease.
- Ventricular tachycardia:
  - Wide complex regular tachyarrhythmia.
  - Ventricular rate is greater than 120 bpm.
  - VT can be monomorphic or polymorphic:
    - Monomorphic VT usually presents with rates between 120 and 300 bpm.
    - Polymorphic VT usually has rates >200 bpm.
    - Torsades de pointes is a polymorphic VT with a prolonged QT. On the ECG, the QRS complex appears to be twisting around an axis. It is a subtype, not a synonym, of polymorphic VT.
  - All wide-complex regular tachycardias are potentially life threatening and should be considered VT until proven otherwise.
- Ventricular fibrillation:
  - Wide complex irregular tachyarrhythmia.
  - Always associated with unstable or pulseless patient.

Critical management

- In patients with tachyarrhythmias, critical management actions include
  - Assessment of overall stability with ABCs
  - ECG and continuous telemetry
  - Intravenous access
  - Placement of pacer/defibrillation pads on the patient in anticipation of potential deterioration
- Definitive therapy will vary depending on the underlying rhythm.
- Commonly used medications as well as their dosage are presented in Table 21.2.
  - **Sinus tachycardia**
    - The primary goal with a patient in sinus tachycardia (ST) is to treat the underlying condition rather than the tachycardia itself.
    - The primary indication for rate control in ST is during acute myocardial infarction, where tachycardia is associated with worse outcomes. Nodal agents, particularly beta-blockers, are useful in this setting.
  - **Paroxysmal supraventricular tachycardia**
    - Generally unrelated to an underlying cause.
    - Rhythm control is the primary intervention.
    - Vagal maneuvers can be attempted prior to pharmacological therapy.

- Adenosine is the medication of choice as it is both diagnostic and therapeutic.
  - Adenosine is metabolized quickly by nonspecific esterases in the plasma and therefore should be pushed quickly via the intravenous access closest to the heart.
  - If adenosine fails, consider synchronized cardioversion or rate control with agents that slow conduction through the AV node.
- **Atrial fibrillation and atrial flutter**
  - These rhythms are modulated by sinus automaticity and, like sinus tachycardia, can be driven by underlying etiologies.
  - Rate control is the primary treatment modality
    - Nodal blockers and digoxin are reasonable options.
    - Amiodarone is an appropriate alternative.
    - Of note, rapid atrial fibrillation with a wide QRS complex suggestive of WPW should not be treated with AV nodal blocking agents. In this setting, procainamide or synchronized cardioversion should be used.
- **Multifocal atrial tachycardia**
  - Initial therapy for MAT should be aimed at treating the underlying cause such as hypomagnesemia, hypokalemia, pulmonary, or cardiac disease.
  - Pharmacological therapy is indicated if the arrhythmia is causing significant symptoms such as ischemia, hypoxia, heart failure, or shock.
  - Nodal blockers can be used, though their efficacy is limited.
- **Ventricular tachycardia**
  - In stable patients with monomorphic VT, procainamide or amiodarone can be used.
  - Polymorphic VT is often caused by myocardial ischemia. Diagnosis and treatment of potential myocardial infarction should be pursued.
  - Treatment of torsades de pointes is aimed at decreasing the QT interval.
    - Intravenous magnesium sulfate is the first-line treatment.
    - Overdrive pacing also shortens the QT interval and can be used if magnesium therapy is ineffective. It can be achieved by transcutaneous pacing or with pharmacological agents such as isoproterenol.
- **Ventricular fibrillation:**
  - VF is an unstable rhythm that should be primarily managed by defibrillation.
  - ACLS should be initiated promptly in all patients exhibiting this rhythm.

Sudden deterioration

- Electrical cardioversion should be applied to all patients with a tachyarrhythmia who become hemodynamically unstable.
- Confirmation of a pulse is mandatory prior to performing cardioversion as it will determine whether the electrical charge should be synchronized or not.

Table 21.2. Common medications for the treatment of tachyarrhythmias

Medication	Initial dose	Repeat dose	Drip
Adenosine	6 mg fast IVP followed by saline bolus	12 mg after 2 minutes (may repeat the 12 mg dose once)	
Diltiazem	0.25 mg/kg IV over 2 minutes	0.35 mg/kg after 15 minutes	5–15 mg/hour
Verapamil	2.5–5 mg IV over 2 minutes	2.5–10 mg every 15 minutes (up to a total of 20 mg)	
Metoprolol	5 mg slow IV	5 mg every 5 minutes (up to a total of 15 mg)	
Esmolol			300–500 micrograms/kg bolus over 1 minute followed by 50 micrograms/kg per minute infusion (max infusion rate is 300 micrograms/kg per min)
Digoxin	0.5 mg IV	0.25 mg every 2 hours (up to a total of 1.5 mg)	
Amiodarone	150 mg IV bolus over 10 minutes		IV bolus is followed by infusion at 1 mg/minute IV for 6 hours then 0.5 mg/minute IV for 18 hours mixed in D5W
Procainamide	20 mg/minute until: QRS widens >50% Arrhythmia is suppressed Hypotension ensues Total of 17 mg/kg given		
Magnesium	2 g IV over 2 minutes	Repeat 2 g IV dose after 15 minutes if necessary	3–20 mg/minute
Isoproterenol			2–10 micrograms/minute titrated to a heart rate of 100 bpm

IVP, intravenous push; D5W, 5% dextrose in water.

Table 21.3. Guidelines for biphasic cardioversion

Rhythm	Energy (joules)
Atrial fibrillation	120–200
Atrial flutter and SVT	50–100
Ventricular tachycardia	100
Ventricular fibrillation/pulseless VT	120–200

- Preparations should be made for ACLS in the event that the cardiac rhythm deteriorates further.
- The minimum amount of energy required for successful cardioversion is rhythm-dependent. If the initial attempt fails, the amount of energy should be increased in a stepwise fashion (Table 21.3).

REFERENCES

Borloz MP, Mark DG, Pines JM, Brady WJ. Electrocardiographic differential diagnosis of narrow QRS complex tachycardia: an ED-oriented algorithmic approach. *Am J Emerg Med.* 2010; **28**: 378–81.

Fuster V, Rydé LE, Cannom DS, *et al.* ACC/AHA/ESC 2006 Guidelines for the Management of Patients with Atrial Fibrillation: A Report of the American College of Cardiology/ American Heart Association Task Force on Practice Guidelines and the European Society of Cardiology Committee for Practice Guidelines (Writing Committee to Revise the 2001 Guidelines for the Management of Patients with Atrial Fibrillation). *J Am Coll Cardiol.* 2006; **48**: 854–906.

International Liaison Committee on Resuscitation. 2005 International Consensus on Cardiopulmonary Resuscitation and Emergency Cardiovascular Care Science with Treatment Recommendations. Part 1: Introduction. *Resuscitation.* 2005; **67**: 181–6.

Neumar RW, Otto CW, Link MS, *et al.* Part 8: adult advanced cardiovascular life support: 2010 American Heart Association Guidelines for Cardiopulmonary Resuscitation and Emergency Cardiovascular Care. *Circulation.* 2010; **122**(18 Suppl 3): S729–67.

Sinz E, Navarro K. *Advanced Cardiovascular Life Support Provider Manual.* Dallas, TX: American Heart Association; 2011.

22

Bradyarrhythmias

Chad Van Ginkel

Introduction

- Bradycardia is defined as a heart rate of less than 60 beats per minute.
- The etiologies of bradyarrhythmias are varied and can be either physiological (e.g., sinus bradycardia) or pathological (Table 22.1).
- A pathological bradycardia can sometimes be caused by a dysfunction along the conduction system. This usually happens at the sinoatrial (SA) node, or the atrioventricular (AV) node.
- Noncardiac causes of bradycardia involve drug overdoses (e.g., calcium channel blockers), endocrine issues (e.g., hypothyroidism), and electrolyte imbalances (e.g., hyperkalemia).

Presentation

Classic presentation

- Although the symptoms are nonspecific, many will be related to inadequate cardiac output secondary to the low heart rate:
  - Orthostatic hypotension
  - Dizziness
  - Syncope
  - Generalized fatigue or malaise
  - Chest pain
  - Shortness of breath

Practical Emergency Resuscitation and Critical Care, ed. Kaushal Shah, Jarone Lee, Kamal Medlej, and Scott D. Weingart. Published by Cambridge University Press. © Kaushal Shah, Jarone Lee, Kamal Medlej, and Scott D. Weingart 2013.

Table 22.1. Causes of bradycardia

Sick sinus syndrome
Infiltrative diseases (e.g., sarcoidosis)
Collagen vascular diseases (e.g., scleroderma)
Atrioventricular conduction block
Acute or chronic ischemic heart disease
Increased vagal tone (e.g., Valsalva maneuver)
Drugs (e.g., digoxin, beta-blockers)
Obstructive sleep apnea
Hypothyroidism
Hypothermia
Vector-borne illness (e.g., Lyme disease)
Increased intracranial pressure (i.e., Cushing reflex)
Electrolyte disturbances (e.g., hypo/hyperkalemia)

Critical presentation

- Sinus bradycardia occurs in 15–20% of patients with acute myocardial infarction secondary to ischemia of the SA node.
- Syncope may result from primary dysrhythmia or from reduced cardiac output.
- Hemodynamic instability:
  - Similarly to patients with rapid heart rates, instability is defined as the evidence of hemodynamic compromise with a discernible pulse.
  - Patients will present with hypotension, altered mental status, ischemic chest pain, or respiratory distress from congestive heart failure and pulmonary edema.
  - Patients who do not have a palpable pulse are in cardiac arrest and are treated according to ACLS guidelines.

Diagnosis and evaluation

- A 12-lead electrocardiogram (ECG) is essential for the diagnosis of bradycardia and to differentiate between the different types of bradyarrhythmias.
- History should focus particularly on symptoms of ischemic heart disease, and on medications such as nodal blockers.
- Some laboratory values may be helpful, depending on the suspected etiology:
  - Troponin to assess for myocardial injury
  - Electrolytes to rule out hyperkalemia from changes in renal function
  - Digoxin level if appropriate
  - Thyroid-stimulating hormone (TSH).
- A rectal temperature should be taken to rule out hypothermia as a possible etiology.

- Once the ECG is performed, further information about the location and severity of the conduction delay can be obtained.
  - SA node dysfunction:
    - Irregular or absent sinus node activity.
    - Most common reason for pacemakers in the United States.
    - "Sick sinus syndrome":
      - Caused by a worsening fibrosis of the SA node or diminished blood flow to the SA nodal artery.
      - Most often seen in patients older than 70 years old.
      - Characteristics include inappropriate bradycardia, alternating bradycardia and tachyarrhythmias, and/or sinus pauses or sinus arrest.
  - AV node dysfunction:
    - AV conduction blocks can be either transient or permanent and can result from numerous etiologies.
    - The most common cause of AV nodal dysfunction is ischemic disease (40%), though other etiologies are possible:
      - Idiopathic fibrosis of the conduction system
      - Bacterial endocarditis
      - Vector-borne disease
      - Medication overdose
- AV node dysfunction can be classified as first-degree, second-degree (types I and II) or third-degree (i.e., complete heart block).
  - First-degree AV block:
    - Defined as a PR interval of greater than 200 milliseconds.
    - Each P is associated with a QRS and both the P-P and R-R intervals remain constant.
    - It is generally considered to be benign.
  - Second-degree AV block: Mobitz type I (aka: Wenckebach (see Figure 22.1):
    - Defined as a rhythm with an increasingly prolonged PR interval that will eventually lead to a dropped beat.
    - This pattern can happen intermittently or persistently, and in a variety of groupings.
    - Like first-degree AV blocks it is generally considered to be benign and does not require intervention.

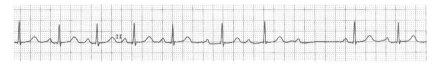

Figure 22.1. Second-degree AV block: Mobitz type I (Wenckebach).

  - Second-degree AV block: Mobitz type II (see Figure 22.2):
    - Defined as a consistent PR interval with intermittent failure of conduction through the AV node resulting in dropped beats.

- Can be seen in grouped beats as type I, but can also have varying degrees of block.
- Frequently progresses to complete heart block (third-degree heart block).
- Due to the potential for progression of the blockade, these patients require admission to the hospital and evaluation for a pacemaker.

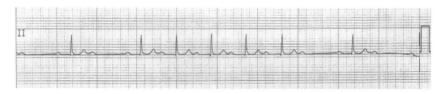

Figure 22.2. Second-degree AV block: Mobitz type II.

- Third-degree AV block (complete heart block) (see Figure 22.3):
  - Defined as a complete disassociation between atrial and ventricular activity.
  - No relationship exists between P-waves and the QRS complexes.
  - Ventricular escape beats can originate anywhere from the AV node (narrow complex) to the Purkinje system (wide QRS complex).
  - A permanent pacemaker is indicated in the setting of this rhythm.

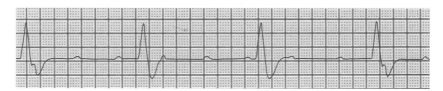

Figure 22.3. Third-degree AV block (complete heart block).

Critical management

- Asymptomatic patients only require admission and intervention if they are incidentally found to have a second-degree Mobitz type II or a third-degree AV block.
- First, look for a reversible cause for the bradyarrhythmia and treat the underlying etiology (i.e., myocardial ischemia, medication toxicity).
- In symptomatic bradycardic patients, a vagolytic drug such as atropine is the first-line therapy.
  - Administer 0.5 mg of atropine intravenously (IV) every 3–5 minutes until the patient is asymptomatic or you have reached a total dose of 3 mg.
  - Atropine is unlikely to be effective in Mobitz type II and in third-degree AV blocks. It can also lead to a slower ventricular rate in this setting and should therefore be used with caution.

- If atropine fails to relieve the bradycardia, positive inotropic agents, transcutaneous pacing, or transvenous pacing are recommended as second-line intervention:
  - Dopamine 2–10 micrograms/kg minute continuous infusion
  - Epinephrine 2–10 micrograms/minute continuous infusion
  - Isoproterenol 2–10 micrograms/minute continuous infusion
- In the setting of Mobitz type II and complete AV dissociation, external or transvenous pacing may be urgently indicated. Consultation for a permanent pacemaker placement will also be required.

Sudden deterioration

- As the bradycardia worsens, cardiac output will decrease as well. This will result in hypotension and hypoperfusion that will need to be corrected using medications or a pacemaker.
- In addition, a decrease in cardiac output can result in pulmonary edema.
- Even with the development of pulmonary edema, the bradycardia is the first thing that needs to be addressed. Treatment of the cardiogenic pulmonary edema can be instituted afterward.

Agent of choice: Atropine is the first-line agent for patients with symptomatic bradycardia although it should be used with caution in patients with Mobitz type II and complete heart block.

Isoproterenol has positive inotropic and chronotropic action and can be started on patients that require frequent doses of atropine.

REFERENCES

Epstein AE, DiMarco JP, Ellenbogen KA, *et al.* ACC/AHA/HRS 2008 Guidelines for Device-Based Therapy of Cardiac Rhythm Abnormalities: a report of the American College of Cardiology/American Heart Association Task Force on Practice Guidelines: developed in collaboration with the American Association for Thoracic Surgery and Society of Thoracic Surgeons. *Circulation*. 2008; **117**: e350–408.

Hartman D, Overton DT. Bradydysrhythmias. In: Wolfson AB, Hendey GW, Ling LJ, *et al.* eds. *Harwood-Nuss' Clinical Practice of Emergency Medicine*. 5th edn. Philadelphia: Lippincott Williams & Wilkins; 2009.

Morrison LJ, Deakin CD, Morley PT, *et al.* Part 8: Advanced life support: 2010 International Consensus on Cardiopulmonary Resuscitation and Emergency Cardiovascular Care Science With Treatment Recommendations. *Circulation*. 2010; **122**(16 Suppl 2): S345–421.

Mottram AR, Svenson JE. Rhythm disturbances. *Emerg Med Clin North Am*. 2011; **29**: 729–46.

23

Post–cardiac arrest care

Stephen Hendriksen

Introduction

- Post–cardiac arrest care has the potential to increase survival and improve quality of life by optimizing early hemodynamic function, addressing metabolic abnormalities, and preserving neurological function.
- After advanced life support has been provided and the return of spontaneous circulation (ROSC) has been achieved, a comprehensive approach to post–cardiac arrest care can minimize brain injury and multi-organ failure.
- Patient care after cardiac arrest is determined primarily by the etiology of the cardiac arrest (Table 23.1).

Table 23.1. Cardiac arrest etiologies

Cardiovascular disease
Arrhythmia
Electrolyte abnormality
Pulmonary embolus
Hypoxic arrest
Tension pneumothorax
Trauma
Cardiac tamponade
Hemorrhage/hypovolemia
Medication or drug overdose
Acidosis
Hypothermia

Practical Emergency Resuscitation and Critical Care, ed. Kaushal Shah, Jarone Lee, Kamal Medlej, and Scott D. Weingart. Published by Cambridge University Press. © Kaushal Shah, Jarone Lee, Kamal Medlej, and Scott D. Weingart 2013.

Diagnosis and evaluation

- An immediate assessment of a patient after the return of spontaneous circulation should include a focused history (usually obtained from bystanders or emergency medical services personnel), physical examination, diagnostic testing, and imaging studies.
- The physical examination should follow the ABCs, checking (1) the airway for appropriate endotracheal tube (ETT) placement, (2) the presence of bilateral breath sounds, (3) circulatory status and blood pressure, (4) heart rate and rhythm, (5) disability with neurological response and Glasgow coma scale, and (6) exposure to fully expose the patient and complete the examination.
- **Electrocardiogram (ECG)**
  - Cardiovascular disease is the most common cause of cardiac arrest; therefore, an ECG should be performed as soon as possible after ROSC to look for evidence of myocardial infarction.
  - If acute myocardial infarction is thought to have occurred, an emergency cardiac catheterization should be performed.
  - Other abnormalities on the ECG such as T-wave changes suggesting electrolyte abnormalities or ischemia, interval changes concerning for complete heart block, or prolonged QTc should also be promptly addressed.
- **Imaging studies**
  - Chest radiography: A chest radiograph (CXR) is taken to determine ETT position and to assess for potential etiologies of cardiac arrest such as congestive heart failure (CHF), chronic obstructive pulmonary disease (COPD), cardiac tamponade, aortic dissection, or tension pneumothorax. Certain complications of cardiac arrest such as aspiration or the acute respiratory distress syndrome (ARDS) can also appear on the initial CXR.
  - Echocardiography: When the diagnosis of cardiac disease is uncertain, a bedside echocardiogram may help detect wall motion abnormalities, assess left ventricular (LV) function, and rule out cardiac tamponade.
  - CT scan: A CT scan can be performed to exclude a primary intracranial process, or to evaluate the chest, abdomen, and pelvis.
- **Laboratory studies**
  - Basic serum electrolytes, complete blood count, arterial blood gas, serum troponin, serum lactate, and specific toxicological studies should be drawn as part of the patient workup.

Critical management

- The extent of brain injury and cardiovascular instability are the major determinants of mortality after cardiac arrest.
- Brain injury is responsible for mortality in 68% of out-of-hospital arrests and 23% of in-hospital arrests.
- Perfusion should be optimized early and aggressively.

- Therapeutic hypothermia should then be considered in comatose patients who do not have contraindications for its initiation.
- **Hemodynamic optimization**
  - The systolic blood pressure (SBP) should be kept above 90 mmHg or the mean arterial pressure (MAP) above 65 mmHg.
  - Treat hypotension with intravenous fluid (IVF) boluses.
  - Inotropic and vasopressor agents such as dopamine and norepinephrine may be used through a central access if the patient is refractory to IVF.
  - If ventricular fibrillation (VF) or ventricular tachycardia (VT) preceded the cardiac arrest, an antiarrhythmic agent such as amiodarone may be started.
  - Patients should be placed on continuous telemetry with serial 12-lead ECGs performed.
- **Pulmonary optimization**
  - An endotracheal tube should be placed in unconscious patients to protect the airway. If cardiopulmonary resuscitation is ongoing, care should be taken to avoid interruption of quality chest compressions for the purpose of endotracheal tube placement. A temporary device such as an extraglottic airway may be temporarily placed until ROSC is achieved.
  - Titrate the minute ventilation on the ventilator to keep the end-tidal carbon dioxide ($PetCO_2$) at 35–40 mmHg, or the partial pressure of carbon dioxide ($PaCO_2$) at 40–45 mmHg.
  - Hypocarbia can potentially cause cerebral vasoconstriction leading to decreased cerebral perfusion and neurological injury.
  - FiO_2 should also be titrated down to keep the oxygen saturation (SpO_2) at 94% or above in order to reduce the potential for oxygen toxicity.
- **Neurological protection**
  - Hypothermia has been shown to significantly improve meaningful neurological outcomes for patients who remain comatose after cardiac arrest from shockable rhythms (VF and VT).
  - "Comatose" has been generally defined as a lack of meaningful response to verbal commands.
  - Patients who remain comatose after ROSC should be cooled to 32–34°C (89.6–93.2°F) for 12–24 hours.
  - Hyperpyrexia should be avoided in these patients as it has been shown to exacerbate the extent of brain damage.

Hypothermia after cardiac arrest

- **Contraindications to cooling**
  - The only absolute contraindications for therapeutic hypothermia in comatose patients are a do not resuscitate (DNR) order or arrest secondary to traumatic injury.

- Relative contraindications include active bleeding, pregnancy, and septic shock as a cause of the arrest.
- Induction of therapeutic hypothermia can begin before cardiac catheterization and safely be continued throughout the procedure.
- **Cooling methods and monitoring**
  - There are multiple methods of cooling and none have been proven to be superior.
  - Internal systems using intravascular catheters and surface cooling devices are common.
  - Cooling blankets and ice bags can be used but patients should be monitored closely as the rate of cooling and the goal temperature cannot be programmed.
  - Intravascular cooling with cool IVF is an easy way to initiate cooling in the prehospital setting or in the emergency department: 30 mL/kg of 4°C (39°F) isotonic saline is administered through peripheral access.
  - A patient's core temperature should always be monitored through an esophageal thermometer, pulmonary artery catheter, or bladder catheter.
  - The goal temperature should ideally be reached within 6 hours and maintained for 12 to 24 hours.
- **Sedation and paralytics**
  - Sedation and paralytics are used to prevent shivering and decrease agitation, pain, and anxiety, during therapeutic hypothermia.
  - Shivering can increase temperature and delay reaching the hypothermia goal.
  - Sedation is most commonly provided with propofol or midazolam infusions.
  - Midazolam may cause less hypotension than propofol but its effects are longer lasting, which can affect neurological examinations.
- **Rewarming**
  - During the rewarming phase, the core temperature should be raised gradually by 0.2 to 0.5°C an hour until the goal of 37°C is reached.
  - Rapid rewarming can cause electrolyte abnormalities, cerebral edema, and seizures.

Common complications from cooling

- **Seizures**
  - Continuous electroencephalogram (EEG) monitoring should be used on all patients requiring neuromuscular blockade in order to monitor for seizures.
  - If seizures occur, propofol, midazolam, phenytoin, and phenobarbital can be used and are similarly effective. Multiple medications may be required.
- **Coagulopathy**
  - Hypothermia impairs coagulation and therefore any active bleeding should be controlled before the initiation of cooling.

- In the event of significant bleeding; a significant drop in hemoglobin, hemo-dynamic instability, intracranial hemorrhage, or noncompressive bleeding, therapeutic hypothermia should be stopped and the patient rewarmed to at least 35°C.
- **Increased risk of infection**
  - When hypothermia is continued for longer than 24 hours, it has been shown to increase the risk of infection due to decreased leukocyte function.
  - Concern for sepsis and septic shock as the cause of arrest is a relative contra-indication to the initiation of hypothermia.
- **Arrhythmias**
  - Hypothermia can lead to arrhythmias such as bradycardia and QT interval prolongation.
  - If the blood pressure remains adequate then the bradycardia does not need to be addressed.
- **Hyperglycemia**
  - Hyperglycemia due to insulin resistance has been shown to result in worse neurological outcomes and increased mortality in post–cardiac arrest patients. However, intense glucose control can also lead to episodes of hypoglycemia and adverse outcomes.
  - Glucose control should therefore aim to maintain glucose between 140 and 180 mg/dL (7.77–9.99 mmol/L).
- **Electrolyte abnormalities**
  - Hypothermia can lead to increased urine output, a condition known as "cold diuresis," which in turn can lead to hypovolemia and electrolyte abnormalities.
  - Fluid balance should be continuously monitored in all patients and electro-lytes measured every 3–4 hours and replaced as needed.

Special circumstances

- In post–cardiac arrest patients with arrest secondary to known or suspected pul-monary embolism, fibrinolytics should be considered.
- If adequate hemodynamic stability cannot be achieved through IVF and inotro-pic support, placement of an intra-aortic balloon pump may be necessary.
- If these therapies fail, a left ventricular assist device, or extracorporeal mem-brane oxygenation (ECMO), may be considered.

Critical care considerations

Vasopressor of choice: Patients who are hypotensive post cardiac arrest from a shockable rhythm (VT or VF) are likely suffering from a degree of cardiogenic shock. The choice of inotrope and/or vasopressor will depend on the patient's systolic blood pressure (SBP):

- SBP ≥80 mmHg: dobutamine
- SBP <80 mmHg: dopamine
- SBP <70 mmHg: norepinephrine.

In patients with ROSC post cardiac arrest with pulseless electrical activity (PEA), the choice of inotrope and/or pressor will depend on the etiology of the arrest.

REFERENCES

Arrich J, Holzer M, Havel C, *et al.* Hypothermia for neuroprotection in adults after cardiopulmonary resuscitation. *Cochrane Database Syst Rev.* 2012 Sep 12; **9**: CD004128.

Nolan JP, Neumar RW, Adrie C, *et al.* Post-cardiac arrest syndrome: epidemiology, pathophysiology, treatment, and prognostication. A Scientific Statement from the International Liaison Committee on Resuscitation; the American Heart Association Emergency Cardiovascular Care Committee; the Council on Cardiovascular Surgery and Anesthesia; the Council on Cardiopulmonary, Perioperative, and Critical Care; the Council on Clinical Cardiology; the Council on Stroke. *Resuscitation.* 2008; **79**: 350–79.

Peberdy MA, Callaway CW, Neumar RW, *et al.* Part 9: Post–cardiac arrest care: 2010 American Heart Association Guidelines for Cardiopulmonary Resuscitation and Emergency Cardiovascular Care. *Circulation.* 2010; **122**(18 Suppl 3): S768–86.

Reynolds JC, Lawner BJ. Management of the post–cardiac arrest syndrome. *J Emerg Med.* 2012; **42**: 440–9.

Stub D, Bernard S, Duffy SJ *et al.* Post cardiac arrest syndrome: a review of therapeutic strategies. *Circulation.* 2011; **123**: 1428–35.

24

Acute decompensated heart failure

Brandon Maughan

Introduction

- Acute decompensated heart failure (ADHF) describes a set of clinical syndromes characterized by reduced cardiac output secondary to impaired ventricular function.
- Impaired ventricular function can be caused by new pathology (i.e. as myocardial infarction), or exacerbation of an underlying chronic process (Table 24.1).
- Heart failure can generally be classified on the basis of the cardiac cycle (systolic or diastolic heart failure), or by which ventricle is predominantly impaired (left- or right-sided heart failure).
  - In systolic heart failure, patients develop an elevated systemic vascular resistance due to poor cardiac output from a decrease in systolic pump function.
    - This results in decreased renal perfusion and increased fluid accumulation through the renin–angiotensin–aldosterone axis.
    - In addition, this increase in intravascular volume leads to an elevated hydrostatic pressure and leakage of fluid from the capillaries into nearby tissues.
  - Diastolic heart failure is characterized by low cardiac output secondary to poor ventricular filling during diastole. This typically occurs as a result of impaired ventricular wall relaxation.
- Less frequently, patients may develop high-output heart failure which is associated with low systemic vascular resistance and above-normal cardiac index.
  - Acute anemia is a common cause of high-output failure.

Practical Emergency Resuscitation and Critical Care, ed. Kaushal Shah, Jarone Lee, Kamal Medlej, and Scott D. Weingart. Published by Cambridge University Press. © Kaushal Shah, Jarone Lee, Kamal Medlej, and Scott D. Weingart 2013.

Table 24.1. Etiologies of decompensated heart failure

Systolic dysfunction	Diastolic dysfunction
Impaired contractility	*Structural abnormality*
Myocardial infarction	Ventricular hypertrophy (often related to
Dilated cardiomyopathy, including	hypertension)
peripartum cardiomyopathy	Hypertrophic or constrictive
Myocarditis	cardiomyopathy
Alcohol abuse	Constrictive pericarditis
Papillary muscle rupture	Infiltrative disease such as sarcoidosis
Increased afterload	*Impaired myocyte relaxation*
Systemic hypertension, including	Myocardial ischemia or hypoxia
hypertensive crisis caused by underlying	Medications (e.g., digitalis)
disease (e.g., pregnancy or thyrotoxicosis)	Hypercalcemia
Pulmonary hypertension, including	
pulmonary embolism	
Aortic stenosis	
Cocaine abuse	
Medication noncompliance	
Dietary intake	

Presentation

Classic presentation

- Left-sided heart failure classically presents with dyspnea, usually related to pulmonary vascular congestion.
  - The symptoms may be acute or subacute in onset.
  - The duration of symptoms may be helpful in identifying the etiology of the decompensation.
- Orthopnea and paroxysmal nocturnal dyspnea may be noted in the history.
- On examination, the lungs may reveal crackles or wheezing.
- Right-sided heart failure presents with jugular venous distension (JVD), hepatic congestion, and dependent edema.
- Patients may report significant weight gain due to increased fluid retention.
- Many cases of ADHF will present with a mixed clinical picture that includes signs and symptoms of both left- and right-sided heart failure.
- The differential diagnosis of ADHF includes other etiologies of poor cardiac output and dyspnea such as
  - Acute coronary syndromes (ACS)
  - Chronic obstructive pulmonary disease (COPD) exacerbation
  - Pulmonary embolism

- Pneumonia (including severe sepsis and septic shock)
- Pneumothorax
- Pericardial tamponade
- Hypertensive crisis
- Noncardiogenic pulmonary edema (including acute respiratory distress syndrome)
- Papillary muscle rupture.

Critical presentation

- Patients with severe ADHF will present with respiratory distress and impending respiratory failure.
- Associated symptoms may include frothy oral secretions, diaphoresis, and hypoxia.
- Patients may also have other symptoms related to poor cardiac output and poor perfusion such as chest pain and altered mental status.
- Patients may be hypertensive or hypotensive depending on the etiology of symptoms.
  - Hypotension can be indicative of cardiogenic shock and is particularly concerning.

Diagnosis and evaluation

- **History**
  - Important elements of history will include past history of cardiac dysfunction and potential causes of new cardiac dysfunction:
    - Prior history of heart disease
    - Recent weight gain or increasing edema
    - Dietary or medication noncompliance
    - Alcohol or cocaine abuse
    - Recent use of negative inotropic agents (e.g., calcium channel blockers)
    - Medication changes
    - Duration of symptoms.
- **Physical examination**
  - Vital signs:
    - Typically, patients with ADHF have abnormal vital signs. Tachypnea, hypertension, and tachycardia are common given the pathophysiology of the disease.
    - Hypoxia is also possible, and may indicate impending respiratory failure.
    - Hypotension is particularly concerning, and may indicate that the patient is in cardiogenic shock.
      - Hypotension should prompt further evaluation into other etiologies of shock that may have exacerbated any underlying cardiac pathology.

- These patients will usually be euthermic.
- On examination, patients will exhibit signs of poor cardiac output and pulmonary congestion:
  - General: respiratory distress, diaphoresis
  - HEENT: cyanosis, frothy oral secretions
  - Cardiac: S3, murmurs corresponding to valvular lesions, JVD
  - Pulmonary: crackles in lower lung fields, wheezing, diminished breath sounds
  - Extremities: edema, cyanosis, mottled or diaphoretic skin. Patients in cardiogenic shock will have cool and clammy extremities because of the increased systemic vascular resistance.
- **Laboratory tests**
  - A complete blood count with differential is obtained to assess for anemia or elevated white count.
  - Electrolytes are useful to evaluate for any disturbances associated with ADHF or cardiac rhythm (e.g., hyponatremia, hypokalemia, hyperkalemia, or hypomagnesemia).
  - An elevated troponin level may reflect a recent myocardial infarction (MI) causing acute heart failure, or may be caused by myocardial ischemia from ventricular strain.
  - Brain (or B-type) natriuretic peptide (BNP) can aid clinical decision-making in patients with undifferentiated dyspnea and an intermediate risk of heart failure. A BNP >500 pg/mL suggests heart failure while levels <100 pg/mL decrease the likelihood of heart failure. BNP levels may be difficult to interpret in the setting of atrial fibrillation or renal failure.
  - An alcohol level or urine toxicology panel for common drugs of abuse (e.g., cocaine, amphetamines) can be sent based on clinical suspicion.
  - A TSH level can be requested to rule out thyrotoxicosis.
  - Blood cultures, urine cultures, and lactic acid should be ordered if sepsis is suspected.
- **Imaging and ancillary tests**
  - Chest radiography:
    - Look for signs of pulmonary edema (increased interstitial markings, Kerley B lines, widened pulmonary fissures, cephalization of pulmonary vessels).
    - Rule out other causes of respiratory distress (e.g., pneumothorax).
    - Evaluate for focal infiltrate suggestive of pneumonia.
  - ECG:
    - Evaluate for ischemia, dysrhythmias, or signs of pericardial effusion (e.g., electrical alternans).
    - The ECG can also be useful to evaluate underlying cardiac disease or electrolyte abnormalities.
  - Echocardiography:

- Should be obtained emergently in an unstable patient if there is a concern for cardiac tamponade physiology. It can also detect wall motion abnormalities if there is a concern for ischemia.

Critical management

- When approaching a patient with ADHF, one must be sure to address any underlying cause while simultaneously managing the physiological derangements.
- Optimize oxygenation:
  - Sitting patients upright will improve oxygenation. Avoid recumbent or supine positioning as this will exacerbate respiratory distress.
  - Provide suctioning for frothy oral secretions.
  - Supplement oxygen as needed to maintain a saturation of ≥90%.
- Consider supportive respiratory adjuncts and prepare for potential respiratory deterioration:
  - For patients with moderate to severe respiratory distress who are able to maintain their airway, consider immediate noninvasive positive-pressure ventilation (NPPV).
  - NPPV reduces both preload and afterload, thereby relieving heart failure symptoms. Anticipate and prepare for relative hypotension after starting NPPV.
  - Both continuous positive airway pressure (CPAP) and bi-level positive airway pressure (Bi-PAP) have demonstrated efficacy in patients with ADHF, particularly if initiated early.
    - Begin with a PEEP of 5 cmH$_2$O and increase incrementally until an improvement in oxygenation is seen.
    - If Bi-PAP is used, the initial inspiratory pressure can be set at 10–12 cmH$_2$O and incrementally increased. The inspiratory pressure should not exceed 20 cmH$_2$O.
- Modulation of preload and afterload are the primary components of therapy for ADHF.
  - Nitrate therapy is among the mainstays of treatment for ADHF.
    - Glyceryl trinitrate causes venodilation, thereby decreasing preload.
    - It can be administered as sublingual tablets (0.4 mg/tablet) while intravenous (IV) access is obtained.
    - Nitrate therapy can also be given as a continuous infusion.
      - Start with 20–50 micrograms/minute and titrate by 20 micrograms/minute every 3–5 minutes until a maximum of 200 micrograms/minute or a MAP ≤65 mmHg.
  - Angiotensin-converting enzyme (ACE) inhibitors work by decreasing afterload and, in the long term, preventing ventricular remodeling.
    - Though not always given during initial assessment and stabilization, captopril can be used sublingually for immediate afterload reduction.

- IV enalaprilat (5–10 mg) can also be used as primary or adjunctive therapy.
- Avoid giving these drugs to patients with potential hyperkalemia, or during pregnancy.
- Diuretics, and particularly loop diuretics, can be used to combat the renin-angiotensin mediated increases in circulating blood volume.
  - It is important to realize that not all patients with pulmonary edema are volume overloaded.
  - In the absence of evidence of chronic volume overload, diuresis should only be initiated after other modalities of treatment including NPPV and nitrate therapy have been attempted. Inappropriate diuresis can lead to hypotension and acute kidney injury.
  - Furosemide (40–80 mg IV), torsemide (10–20 mg IV), or bumetanide (0.5–1 mg IV) can be used as initial therapy.
  - If the patient is on home diuretics, give a bolus dose equal to 100–200% of the home dose.
    - Diuretics can be used as a continuous infusion, but this will likely not be required in the immediate stabilization.
- Hypotension will limit the use of any of the above therapies and should prompt consideration for vasopressors or inotropes (see below).

Sudden deterioration

- Patients who become hypoxic, lethargic, or more confused despite NPPV should be intubated.
- Patients who are hypotensive, especially those requiring intubation, may require cautious use of inotropes or vasopressors to enhance cardiac output and maintain their coronary filling pressure. Titrate these agents to a MAP >60 mmHg, or less if limited by signs or symptoms of cardiac ischemia.
  - Dobutamine: start IV infusion at 5–10 micrograms/kg/minute.
  - Milrinone: load 50 micrograms/kg IV over 10 minutes, then infuse 0.375–0.75 micrograms/kg/minute.
  - Dopamine: start IV infusion at 5–10 micrograms/kg/minute.
- Some patients may need specialized interventions based on their underlying disease:
  - Cardiac catheterization for ongoing ischemia.
  - Intra-arterial balloon pump for cases of severe cardiogenic shock.
  - Implantable cardioverter-defibrillators (ICDs) may be indicated for patients with ischemic or dilated cardiomyopathy and impaired systolic function (left ventricular ejection fraction <30%).
  - Cardiac resynchronization therapy (CRT) may be appropriate for patients with severe systolic heart failure and QRS interval prolongation (>120 milliseconds).

- Patients with severe end-stage systolic heart failure may be considered for a left ventricular assist device (LVAD) as a bridge to heart transplant.

Vasopressor of choice: Patients with ADHF who are hypotensive can be suffering from low-output heart failure or cardiogenic shock. Inotropes and/or vasopressors should be used judiciously in order to avoid exacerbating the condition:
- SBP ≥80 mmHg: dobutamine
- SBP <80 mmHg: dopamine
- SBP <70 mmHg: norepinephrine.

REFERENCES

Heart Failure Society of America, Lindenfeld J, Albert NM, Boehmer JP, *et al.* HFSA 2010 Comprehensive Heart Failure Practice Guideline. *J Card Fail.* 2010; **16**: e1–194.

Hunt SA, Abraham WT, Chin MH, *et al.* 2005 Guideline Update for the Diagnosis and Management of Chronic Heart Failure in the Adult: a report of the American College of Cardiology/American Heart Association Task Force on Practice Guidelines (Writing Committee to Update the 2001 Guidelines for the Evaluation and Management of Heart Failure): developed in collaboration with the American College of Chest Physicians and the International Society for Heart and Lung Transplantation: endorsed by the Heart Rhythm Society. *Circulation.* 2005; **112**: e154–235.

Jessup M, Abraham WT, Casey DE, *et al.* 2009 focused update: ACCF/AHA Guidelines for the Diagnosis and Management of Heart Failure in Adults: a report of the American College of Cardiology Foundation/American Heart Association Task Force on Practice Guidelines: developed in collaboration with the International Society for Heart and Lung Transplantation. *Circulation.* 2009; **119**: 1977–2016.

O'Connor CM, Starling RC, Hernandez AF, *et al.* Effect of nesiritide in patients with acute decompensated heart failure. *N Engl J Med.* 2011; **365**: 32–43.

Vital FM, Saconato H, Ladeira MT, *et al.* Noninvasive positive pressure ventilation (CPAP or bilevel NPPV) for cardiogenic pulmonary edema. *Cochrane Database Syst Rev.* 2008; (3): CD005351.

25

Aortic dissection

Gregory Hayward

Introduction

- Aortic dissection represents the most frequent aortic catastrophe with approximately 10 000 cases annually in the United States.
- Dissection occurs with a primary tear of the aortic intima layer and subsequent infiltration of the media layer, creating a false lumen which may extend the entire length of the aorta.
- Propagation of the false lumen may result in obstruction of any vascular branches of the aorta, leading to acute hypoperfusion of the brain, heart, kidneys, spine, or extremities.
- The location of injury (i.e., ascending versus descending aorta) predicts mortality and guides management decisions.

Presentation

Classic presentation

- Over 90% of patients report chest or back pain, often of sudden onset, and described as tearing, ripping, or sharp. Patients may describe symptoms as most severe at onset.
- While uncommon, pulse deficits or blood pressure differentials when comparing upper extremities may be present.
- A number of well-established risk factors exist:
  - Hypertension
  - Genetic syndromes such as Marfan, Turner, and Ehlers–Danlos

Practical Emergency Resuscitation and Critical Care, ed. Kaushal Shah, Jarone Lee, Kamal Medlej, and Scott D. Weingart. Published by Cambridge University Press. © Kaushal Shah, Jarone Lee, Kamal Medlej, and Scott D. Weingart 2013.

- Structural abnormalities such as coarctation of the aorta or a bicuspid aortic valve
- Traumatic injuries from motor vehicle accidents, coronary catheterization, coronary stenting, aortic balloon pump placement, vascular surgery, or valve replacement
- Inflammatory diseases such as giant cell or Takayasu's arteritis
- Infections such as syphilis
- Cocaine use
- Third-trimester pregnancy

Critical presentation

- In addition to chest pain, patients may present with focal neurological deficits secondary to the physical obstruction of either one of the carotid arteries by an intimal flap, or false lumen propagation.
- Vascular obstruction and ischemia may occur at any level, leading to syncope, stroke symptoms, acute myocardial infarction (frequently from right coronary artery compromise), mesenteric ischemia, paraplegia (from hypoperfusion of the spinal arteries), or limb ischemia.
- Patients often present hypertensive, although proximal dissection may cause aortic root dilatation and severe aortic regurgitation (resulting in a new diastolic murmur) with ensuing heart failure and hypotension.
- Cardiogenic shock may also arise as a complication of dissection into the pericardium resulting in cardiac tamponade. Beck's triad of hypotension, muffled heart sounds, and jugular venous distension can sometimes be found.
- A hemothorax may develop in the setting of a ruptured or leaking descending aorta.

Diagnosis and evaluation

- **Electrocardiogram (ECG)** findings rarely aid in the diagnosis, though ST elevations may be present in as many as 20% of patients due to ostial coronary involvement.
  - Myocardial infarctions resulting from acute aortic dissection versus thrombosis or embolization of the coronaries may not be immediately discernible.
  - Because both conditions are time-sensitive, patients should be managed in the most expeditious manner.
  - ST elevations should prompt immediate consideration of cardiac catheterization and involvement of interventional cardiology, even if a CT angiogram has not been completed.
  - Myocardial infarction (MI) from aortic and coronary artery dissection has a much lower incidence than from coronary thrombosis or embolization, and can be detected during the catheterization.

- In 60–90% of patients, a **chest radiograph** will demonstrate one or more abnormalities including a widened mediastinum, an irregular aortic knob, an apical cap, or a pleural effusion.
- Early definitive imaging will confirm the diagnosis. A **helical computed tomography (CT)** with intravenous (IV) contrast is the most commonly used study (Figure 25.1).
- **Magnetic resonance imaging (MRI)** is highly sensitive and specific though it may be impractical in the emergency setting.
- **Transesophageal ultrasonography** can be performed at bedside, providing useful dynamic information. **Transthoracic ultrasonography** may be utilized, though it has low sensitivity for an acute dissection.
- Studies have demonstrated a high sensitivity of **D-dimer** to rule out an aortic dissection, though the specificity was low. The clinical role of D-dimer in the evaluation of aortic dissection has not been well established, however.
- Aortic dissections are generally classified depending on whether or not they involve the ascending aorta or aortic arch (Table 25.1).

Table 25.1. Aortic dissection classification systems

Stanford classification	
Type A	Dissection involving the ascending aorta, as defined as proximal to the brachiocephalic artery, with or without involvement of the descending aorta
Type B	Dissection of the descending aorta alone, defined as distal to the left subclavian artery
DeBakey classification	
Type 1	Dissection of the entire aorta
Type 2	Dissection of the ascending aorta alone
Type 3	Dissection of the descending aorta alone

Critical management

- Place two large-bore IVs in preparation for potential massive resuscitation with fluids and blood products.
- Connect the patient to a monitor with continuous blood pressure monitoring and electrocardiogram.
- Obtain a 12-lead ECG to rule out cardiac ischemia or infarction.
- In the hemodynamically unstable patient with suspected acute aortic dissection, a transesophageal ultrasound is the confirmatory test of choice as it can be done at bedside and does not require for the patient to be taken out of the emergency department.
- Provide pain relief with opiates (morphine, fentanyl, or hydromorphone).

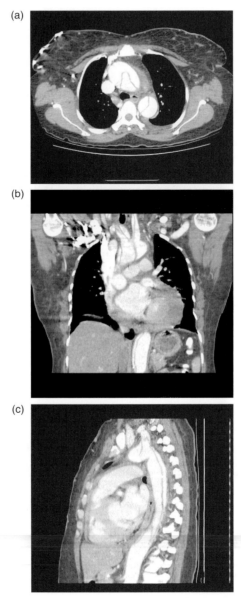

Figure 25.1. Aortic dissection diagnosed on CT angiography is visible in transverse (a), coronal (b) and sagittal (c) views. (Images courtesy of Amanda Holland Yang, MD.)

- Aggressive early blood pressure control serves as the critical intervention in acute dissection.
- The blood pressure should be dropped rapidly to a goal of 100–120 mmHg systolic, and the heart rate to 60–80 bpm.

- Beta-blockers are the initial agents of choice. They should be administered prior to vasodilators in order to prevent reflex tachycardia that may exacerbate shear forces.
  - **Labetalol:** Bolus 10–20 mg IV, double the dose every 10 minutes to a maximum of 80 mg/dose, *or* start a continuous infusion starting at 2–10 mg/minute IV and increase by 1 mg/minute every 10 minutes until the desired blood pressure is achieved.
  - **Esmolol:** Bolus 500 micrograms/kg IV followed by a continuous infusion starting at 25–300 micrograms/kg/minute. Titrate by 50 micrograms/kg/minute every 4 minutes.
- If necessary, vasodilators can be added after initiation of the beta-blockers.
  - **Sodium nitroprusside:** Start a continuous infusion at 1–4 micrograms/kg/minute and titrate by 0.25–0.5 microgram/kg/minute every 2–3 minutes.
  - **Glyceryl trinitrate:** Start a continuous infusion at 10–200 micrograms/minute and titrate by 5–10 micrograms/minute every 5–10 minutes.
  - **Nicardipine:** Start a continuous infusion at 2.5–15 mg/hour and titrate by 2.5 mg/hour every 5–10 minutes.
- Monitor for signs of oliguria or neurological dysfunction.
- Early surgical consultation should be obtained for patients with Stanford type A dissections.
- Stanford type B dissections are frequently treated with medical therapy alone.

Sudden deterioration

- Sudden decompensation will most likely result from cardiovascular catastrophe.
- Maintain a low threshold for intubation and ventilation in cases of hemodynamic instability or neurological deficit leading to airway compromise.
- In cases of hypotensive shock, consider acute myocardial infarction, aortic rupture, and hemopericardium.
- Pericardiocentesis should be considered but only be aimed at removing enough pericardial fluid to raise the blood pressure to an acceptable level.
- In the presence of acute myocardial infarction or stroke, aortic dissection is a contraindication to thrombolytic therapy.
- Indications for surgical management of type B dissections include persistent pain, rapid expansion on serial imaging, evidence of organ or peripheral ischemia, or acute rupture.
- Active hemorrhagic stroke is a relative contraindication to surgery.

Critical care considerations

Vasopressor of choice: Patients with acute aortic dissection usually present with hypertension but can become hypotensive with progression of the condition. These patients will need to be aggressively resuscitated with blood products. Infusion of crystalloids and use of vasopressors such as phenylephrine and norepinephrine can be initiated as a temporizing measure.

REFERENCES

Braverman AC. Aortic dissection: prompt diagnosis and emergency treatment are critical. *Cleve Clin J Med*. 2011; **78**: 685–96.

Golledge J, Eagle KA. Acute aortic dissection. *Lancet*. 2008; **372**(9632): 55–66.

Hagan PG, Nienaber CA, Isselbacher EM, *et al*. The International Registry of Acute Aortic Dissection (IRAD): new insights into an old disease. *JAMA*. 2000; **283**(7): 897–903.

Hines G, Dracea C, Katz DS. Diagnosis and management of acute type A aortic dissection. *Cardiol Rev*. 2011; **19**: 226–32.

Klompas M. Does this patient have an acute thoracic aortic dissection? *JAMA*. 2002; **287**: 2262–72.

26

Pericarditis and myocarditis

Jennifer L. Carey

Introduction

Pericarditis

- Pericarditis is an inflammatory disorder of the pericardial sac.
- It is most commonly idiopathic (75–80% of cases).
- In the United States, up to 10% of cases are attributed to viral infections such as coxsackievirus, parvovirus, and the human immunodeficiency virus (HIV).
- A number of other conditions can result in pericarditis and myocarditis (see Table 26.1).
- Patients classically present with chest pain, electrocardiogram (ECG) changes, and a friction rub.
- Patients may also have a pericardial effusion that, if large enough, may result in cardiac tamponade.

Myocarditis

- Myocarditis is an inflammatory disorder of the cardiac muscle characterized by infiltration of the myocardium by immune cells, and myocyte necrosis.
- The inflammation may be focal or diffuse.
  - Any or all cardiac chambers may be involved.
  - It may result in regional or global contractile impairment, chamber stiffening, or conduction system disease.
  - Clinical manifestation are highly variable depending upon the region of involvement, and include chest pain, acute heart failure, or cardiac arrhythmias.

Practical Emergency Resuscitation and Critical Care, ed. Kaushal Shah, Jarone Lee, Kamal Medlej, and Scott D. Weingart. Published by Cambridge University Press. © Kaushal Shah, Jarone Lee, Kamal Medlej, and Scott D. Weingart 2013.

Table 26.1. Etiologies of pericardial and myocardial disease

Viral
Bacterial
Fungal
Parasitic
Radiation induced
Drug induced
Neoplastic
Systemic inflammatory disease
Myocardial infarction/Dressler syndrome (pericarditis)
Traumatic (pericarditis)
Metabolic (pericarditis)
Peripartum (myocarditis)

- Viral illnesses (coxsackievirus, parvovirus, and human herpes virus 6) are the most common causes of myocarditis in the United States.
- Diphtheria is the most common bacterial cause worldwide.

Presentation

Pericarditis

Classic presentation
- Chest pain: sharp, pleuritic, and worse with recumbency (95%).
- Pericardial friction rub heard over the left sternal border (15–30%).
- ECG changes: diffuse ST elevations, PR depression in the lateral leads.
- Pericardial effusion.

Critical presentation
- Hemodynamic instability secondary to cardiac tamponade.
- Patients may complain of chest pain and dyspnea.
- Heart sounds may be muffled.
- Jugular venous distension.
- ECG demonstrating electrical alternans.
- Large effusion with diastolic right ventricular collapse on bedside echocardiogram.

Myocarditis

Classic presentation
- Chest pain that may mimic cardiac ischemia.
- Heart failure: dyspnea, fatigue, orthopnea, exercise intolerance.

Critical presentation
- Fulminant decompensated heart failure.
- Dysrhythmias, including complete heart block.
- Syncope and sudden cardiac death.

Diagnosis and evaluation

Pericarditis

- Acute pericarditis is largely a clinical diagnosis.
- Two of the following four criteria should be met:
  - Classic chest pain (sharp, pleuritic, and worse with recumbency).
  - Pericardial friction rub.
  - ECG changes with new diffuse ST elevation or PR depression in the lateral leads (Table 26.2; Figure 26.1).
    - The ST elevations associated with pericarditis can be differentiated from those seen with ST elevation myocardial infarction.
      - ST elevations in pericarditis rarely exceed 5 mm.
      - ST elevations are diffuse rather than in a vascular distribution.
      - Reciprocal ST depression and PR elevation should only be seen in leads aVR and V1.
      - Associated temporal changes, such as hyperacute T-waves or Q-waves, are not typically seen in pericarditis.
  - Pericardial effusion (Figure 26.2):
    - Presence of effusion confirms the diagnosis, though absence does not exclude it.
- Chest radiograph: enlarged cardiac silhouette if effusion is present.
- Inflammatory markers: leukocytes may be normal or elevated, ESR is usually elevated although it is not specific.
- Cardiac markers: may be elevated in myocarditis or postinfarction pericarditis.
- Echocardiogram:
  - Normal wall motion.
  - Evaluate for coexisting effusion; effusion size can be estimated by the distance between the epicardium and the pericardium (<0.5 cm = small effusion; 0.5–2 cm = moderate effusion; >2 cm = large effusion).
  - Presence of a large effusion on a bedside echocardiogram with RV collapse during diastole should prompt consideration of impending tamponade.

Myocarditis

- The diagnosis of myocarditis is nearly entirely clinical but is supported by noninvasive diagnostic methods such as cardiovascular magnetic resonance imaging.
- Cardiac biomarkers such as troponin and CK-MB may be elevated.

Table 26.2. ECG manifestations of acute pericarditis

Stage 1 (hours to days)	Concave upward ST segment elevation PR segment depression
Stage 2 (first week)	ST segments returns to baseline T wave amplitude decreases PR segments may be depressed
Stage 3 (weeks 2–3)	T wave flattening T wave inversion in leads with previous ST segment elevation
Stage 4 (months later)	Normalization of all segments

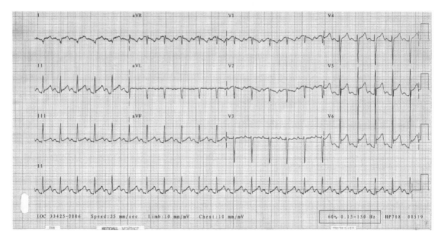

Figure 26.1. Electrocardiogram showing PR and ST segment changes consistent with acute pericarditis.

- Inflammatory markers such as ESR, CRP, and leukocytes may be elevated although they are not specific.
- ECG findings:
  - Nonspecific T-wave changes
  - Nonspecific ST abnormalities
  - Atrial or ventricular ectopic beats
  - Ventricular arrhythmias
  - Atrial tachycardia or atrial fibrillation
  - Diffuse or regional ST elevations and Q waves
- Chest radiograph: may be normal or show cardiomegaly with or without pulmonary vascular congestion or pleural effusions.
- Echocardiography:
  - There are no specific echocardiographic features of myocarditis.

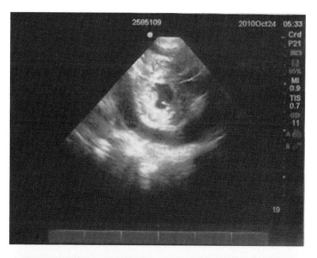

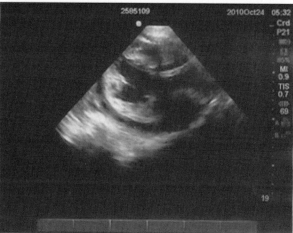

Figure 26.2. Echocardiogram showing a pericardial effusion in two different windows.

- Echocardiography is used to exclude other causes of heart failure and identify ventricular thrombi.
- It may show new regional or global wall motion abnormalities that are not associated with a coronary distribution.
- Impaired right ventricular function is a strong predictor of death or need for transplantation.
- Cardiac MRI is a sensitive and noninvasive test to diagnose acute myocarditis.
- Cardiac biopsy is the gold standard for diagnosis of myocarditis and provides immunohistological evidence of an inflammatory cell infiltrate with or without myocyte damage.

Critical management

Pericarditis

- The management of pericarditis is based on providing symptom relief and reducing the inflammation. The treatment should be for 7–14 days.
  - Aspirin 2–4 g/day.
  - Ibuprofen 1200–1800 mg/day.
  - Indomethacin 75–150 mg/day.
  - Colchicine can be considered for the initial treatment in combination with an NSAID.
  - Systemic corticosteroids are not recommended, except in some cases of pericarditis associated with connective tissue disease, uremia, or immune-mediated diseases.
- If identified, the underlying cause of the pericarditis should be treated as well (e.g., uremia).
- Viral studies are not warranted as they will not alter management or disease course.
- ST elevations in the presence of chest pain must be carefully considered; immediate treatment for myocardial infarction, including cardiac catheterization, should be considered if the ECG findings are equivocal.
- Consider admission in high-risk patients:
  - Fever >38°C
  - Subacute onset
  - Immunosuppression
  - Trauma
  - Anticoagulation therapy
  - Myopericarditis
  - Large effusion

Myocarditis

- Treatment is mostly symptomatic and targeted at the underlying cause.
- It largely parallels the treatment of pericarditis, unless ventricular function or the conduction system is impaired.
- Patients with acutely decreased ventricular function should be admitted to the hospital for further evaluation. Emergent management may include therapies used for the treatment of acute decompensate heart failure.
- Physical activity should be limited in the acute phase of myocarditis.

Sudden deterioration

Pericarditis

- The most likely cause for sudden deterioration is pericardial effusion with cardiac tamponade (occurs in 3% of cases).
  - This may be the initial presentation of the disease.
  - Symptoms include: chest pain, dyspnea, and orthopnea.
  - Tachycardia is particularly concerning as it can be a sign of compensation for decreased cardiac filling.
- The ECG can show low voltage (<0.5 mV in the limb leads, or <1 mV in the precordial leads), or electrical alternans.
- Echocardiography findings in cardiac tamponade:
  - Heart-swinging within the fluid-filled pericardial sac.
  - Collapse of the right atrium (RA) during systole.
  - Right ventricular (RV) collapse may be seen during diastole.
- Immediate measures to support hemodynamics should be initiated.
  - Volume expansion and increased preload may transiently temporize the hypotension.
  - In patients requiring intubation for airway protection, it should be recognized that positive-pressure ventilation will further impede venous return and may worsen the hypotension.
- A pericardiocentesis should be urgently performed in patients with decompensated cardiac tamponade.
- Surgical intervention for pericardial window and potential pericardial drain may be required, and surgical consultation should be sought early on.

Myocarditis

- Critical presentations of myocarditis include arrhythmias and decompensated heart failure.
- In the event of high degree heart blocks with hypotension, temporary transcutaneous or transvenous pacing should be initiated.
- Medical management for heart failure, including afterload reduction and inotropic agents, should be started as needed.
- In the case of cardiogenic shock:
  - Inotropic and/or vasopressor support can be initiated in the emergency department.
  - Invasive therapy may be required, including:
    - Intra-aortic balloon pump
    - Left ventricular assist device
    - Extracorporeal membrane oxygenation (ECMO)
    - Cardiac transplant

Critical care considerations

Vasopressor of choice: Patients presenting with hypotension associated with cardiac tamponade should undergo emergent pericardiocentesis. Patients with myocarditis can present in cardiogenic shock. The choice of inotrope and/or vasopressor will depend on the patient's systolic blood pressure (SBP):

- SBP ≥80 mmHg: dobutamine
- SBP <80 mmHg: dopamine
- SBP <70 mmHg: norepinephrine.

REFERENCES

Kindermann I, Barth C, Mahfoud F, *et al.* Update on myocarditis. *J Am Coll Cardiol.* 2012; **59**: 779–92.

Sagar S, Liu PP, Cooper LT Jr. Myocarditis. *Lancet.* 2012; **379**(9817): 738–47.

Schultheiss HP, Kühl U, Cooper LT. The management of myocarditis. *Eur Heart J.* 2011; **32**: 2616–25.

Seferović PM, Ristić AD, Imazio M, *et al.* Management strategies in pericardial emergencies. *Herz.* 2006; **31**: 891–900.

Sparano DM, Ward RP. Pericarditis and pericardial effusion: management update. *Curr Treat Options Cardiovasc Med.* 2011; **13**: 543–55.

27

Hypertensive emergencies

Nadine Himelfarb

Introduction

- Hypertension is defined as a systolic blood pressure (SBP) higher than 140 mmHg, or a diastolic blood pressure (DBP) higher than 90 mmHg.
- Hypertension may be essential (primary), meaning that it is not linked to an obvious underlying cause, or it may be secondary to a known etiology such as a disorder of the endocrine system.
- Of people with known hypertension 1–2% will present with an acutely elevated blood pressure referred to as a "hypertensive crisis." It is often due to factors that exacerbate a preexisting hypertension, such as medication noncompliance or substance abuse.
- Hypertensive crisis is defined as SBP >180 mmHg or DBP >120 mmHg.
- Increases in blood pressure cause mechanical stress and endothelial damage at the level of the arterioles and capillary beds, leading to microvascular derangements and ischemia. Ultimately, hypoperfusion of organs results, with manifestations of signs of end-organ damage.
- Hypertensive crisis without evidence of acute end-organ damage is termed "hypertensive urgency."
- Hypertensive crisis with evidence of acute end-organ damage is termed "hypertensive emergency."
- Clinical manifestations of hypertensive emergency are directly related to the specific organ affected, usually the brain, heart, or kidneys (Table 27.1).

Practical Emergency Resuscitation and Critical Care, ed. Kaushal Shah, Jarone Lee, Kamal Medlej, and Scott D. Weingart. Published by Cambridge University Press. © Kaushal Shah, Jarone Lee, Kamal Medlej, and Scott D. Weingart 2013.

Table 27.1. Clinical manifestations of hypertensive emergencies

Hypertensive encephalopathy
Acute ischemic stroke
Acute intracerebral hemorrhage
Aortic dissection
Unstable angina/acute myocardial infarction
Acute pulmonary edema
Preeclampsia/HELLP syndrome/eclampsia
Acute renal failure

Diagnosis and evaluation

- **History**
  - Ask for symptoms related to specific organ dysfunction:
    - Neurological symptoms: headache, altered mental status, visual changes.
    - Cardiovascular symptoms: chest pain, dyspnea.
    - Renal failure: oliguria, anuria, altered mental status, symptoms related to electrolyte abnormalities.
  - Elements of the past medical history, including coronary artery disease, prior cerebrovascular events, and renal disease should be obtained.
  - Patients should also be asked about current prescription medications for blood pressure control, as well as recent changes in their medications or dose.
  - Always consider pregnancy as a possible etiology for hypertensive symptoms in women of childbearing age.
  - Investigate potential use of recreational drugs such as cocaine, amphetamines, or phencyclidine.
- **Physical examination**
  - Confirm blood pressure measurement using an appropriately sized cuff.
  - If there is a concern for aortic dissection, the blood pressure should be taken in both upper extremities and compared for discrepancies.
  - An elevated temperature may suggest thyrotoxicosis or an underlying infection.
  - Tachypnea and hypoxia may suggest an underlying pulmonary dysfunction or acute pulmonary edema.
  - Clinical signs of congestive heart failure such as elevated jugular venous pressure, a third heart sound, or rales may be present as well.
  - The fundoscopic examination evaluating for arteriolar changes may reveal papilledema, retinal hemorrhage, and exudates.
  - A full neurological examination should be performed to assess for mental status changes, focal neurological deficits, and visual changes.
- **Laboratory tests and imaging**
  - Complete blood count and peripheral smear to assess for hemolysis and microangiopathic anemia.
  - Complete serum chemistry panel to assess for renal function and presence of electrolyte derangements.

- Liver panel, particularly in pregnant patients, to help rule out the HELLP syndrome (hemolysis, elevated liver enzymes, and low platelet count.)
- Urinalysis with microscopic examination of the urine for presence of proteinuria, red blood cells, and/or casts.
- Electrocardiogram (ECG) to look for signs of ischemia or left ventricular hypertrophy.
- For patients with dyspnea or chest pain, a chest radiograph (CXR) may demonstrate pulmonary edema or mediastinal widening.
- A computed tomography (CT) of the chest has higher sensitivity and specificity than CXR and may provide additional information if aortic dissection is suspected.
- For patients presenting with a headache, changes in mental status, or abnormal neurological findings, a non-contrast CT of the brain should be performed to rule out an acute intracerebral hemorrhage.
- An MRI may be needed to identify an ischemic stroke and should be ordered in consultation with a neurologist.

Critical management

- Critical management will depend on the presence of end-organ damage. Only patients with a diagnosis of hypertensive emergency will require immediate interventions in the emergency department for blood pressure lowering.
- Patients with chronically elevated blood pressure may suffer detrimental consequences if their blood pressure is lowered too quickly. Dramatic and rapid decreases in blood pressure can result in critical hypoperfusion of the brain, heart, and kidneys, resulting in ischemia or infarction.
- Patients with hypertensive urgency can be managed as outpatients as long as reliable follow-up can be arranged. They are usually started on oral antihypertensives with a goal of lowering their blood pressure to less than 160/100 mmHg over 12–48 hours.
- Admission may be considered for patients with multiple medical problems, or those without access to follow-up care.
- If there is evidence of end-organ dysfunction on history, physical examination, or laboratory evaluation, the diagnosis of hypertensive emergency is made.
- Correction of blood pressure in a hypertensive emergency should be via continuous infusion of medications that have a rapid onset and are both short-acting and titratable.
- The immediate goal is to reduce the mean arterial pressure (MAP) by no more than 20–25%, or to reduce the diastolic blood pressure to 100–110 mmHg within 2–6 hours. There are certain exceptions, however, and these are detailed in the "Special considerations" section below.
- Agents should be chosen based on the specific organ(s) being damaged (Tables 27.2 and 27.3).

Table 27.2. Parenteral drugs for the treatment of hypertensive emergencies

Drug	Mechanism	Initial dose	Time of onset	Duration
Nitroprusside	Arterial and venous dilator	0.5 mg/kg/minute drip	Immediate	1–2 minutes
Glyceryl trinitrate	Venous dilator	5 mg/minute drip	2–5 minutes	5–10 minutes
Labetalol	α and β adrenergic blocker	1 mg/minute drip	5–10 minutes	3–6 hours
Nicardipine	Calcium channel blocker	5 mg/hour drip	5–10 minutes	15–30 minutes
Clevidipine	Calcium channel blocker	1 mg/hour drip	1–2 minutes	5–15 minutes
Hydralazine	Arterial dilator	10 mg bolus	10–20 minutes	1–4 hours
Phentolamine	α adrenergic blocker	5 mg bolus	1–2 minutes	10–30 minutes

Table 27.3. Parenteral drugs for the management of specific complications of hypertensive emergency

Condition	Recommended	Contraindicated
Hypertensive encephalopathy	Labetalol, nicardipine, fenoldopam, clevidipine	Hydralazine, nitroprusside
Aortic dissection	Esmolol **and** nitroprusside, or nicardipine, or fenoldopam	Arterial and venodilators should be used in combination with a beta-blocker
Acute coronary syndrome	Labetalol, or esmolol **and** glyceryl trinitrate	Hydralazine
Acute pulmonary edema	Nitroprusside or glyceryl trinitrate	Hydralazine, labetalol
Preeclampsia/eclampsia	Labetalol, nicardipine	Nitroprusside, ACE inhibitors
Sympathetic crises (pheochromocytoma/cocaine use)	Phentolamine, nicardipine, fenoldopam (consider adding a benzodiazepine)	Beta-blockers should only be used in combination with an alpha-blocker
Acute renal failure	Fenoldopam, nicardipine	Nitroprusside

Special considerations

Aortic dissection

- Should always be a consideration in patients with high blood pressure and chest pain.
- Mortality is 75% if not treated during the initial presentation.
- Medical management involves reducing the shear stress on the artery. This is accomplished by regulating both vascular tone and heart rate.
  - Blood pressure control may result in a reflex tachycardia that may in turn increase shear stress. Therefore, heart rate should be controlled with a beta-blocker prior to the administration of vasodilators.
  - The goal is to rapidly reduce heart rate to less than 60 beats per minute (bpm), and the SBP to 100–120 mmHg (or MAP to <80 mmHg) within 5–10 minutes.
  - Agents of choice are usually a beta-adrenergic antagonist and a vasodilator. Calcium channel blockers may be used for rate control in situations where beta-blockers are contraindicated.
- Consultation for surgical management should be obtained on all patients with aortic dissection.

Acute ischemic stroke

- Blood pressure is commonly elevated after an ischemic cerebrovascular accident (CVA). This occurs physiologically in order to maintain cerebral perfusion pressure (CPP) in the ischemic areas of the brain.
- Lowering blood pressures during an acute CVA could cause further ischemia and damage to the brain by reducing the CPP.
- If tPA is to be administered, blood pressure should be lowered to an SBP <185 mmHg and a DBP <110 mmHg.
- If tPA is not a consideration, blood pressure should be lowered when the SBP >220 mmHg or the DBP >120 mmHg.

Acute intracerebral hemorrhage (ICH)

- Patients who are hypertensive in the context of ICH should have their blood pressure reduced rapidly with labetalol or nicardipine infusions.
- No evidence for a specific blood pressure target currently exists for ICH. However, some sources recommend targeting an SBP of less than 140 mmHg.
- Primary data suggests that patients with ICH are more tolerant of large drops in blood pressure due to differences in pathophysiology.
- Because cerebral perfusion is impacted by both systemic blood pressure and intracranial pressure (ICP), care should be taken to avoid dropping the MAP too much.

CPP = MAP − ICP

- Nitroprusside is contraindicated in these patients, as direct arterial vasodilation can increase the intracranial pressure.
- Both neurology and neurosurgical consultations should be initiated, and early invasive intracranial pressure monitoring should be considered.

Preeclampsia and eclampsia

- Delivery of the fetus is the definitive treatment.
- Obstetric consultation should be sought.
- Management involves the use of magnesium sulfate and blood pressure lowering agents.
- Blood pressure must be lowered cautiously to avoid decreasing uteroplacental blood flow.
- The goal is to maintain an SBP of 140 mmHg and a DBP of 90 mmHg.
  - Blood pressure management can be achieved using intravenous labetalol or nicardipine.
  - Hydralazine is no longer recommended due to unpredictable decreases in blood pressure, duration of effect, and side effects that can mimic worsening pre-eclampsia.

REFERENCES

Chobanian AV, Bakris GL, Black HR, *et al.* Seventh Report of the Joint National Committee on Prevention, Detection, Evaluation, and Treatment of High Blood Pressure. *Hypertension.* 2003; **42**: 1206–52.

Marik PE, Rivera R. Hypertensive emergencies: an update. *Curr Opin Crit Care.* 2011; **17(6)**: 569–80.

Marik PE, Varon J. Hypertensive crises: challenges and management. *Chest.* 2007; **131**: 1949–62.

Rodriguez MA, Kumar SK, De Caro M. Hypertensive crisis. *Cardiol Rev.* 2010; **18**: 102–7.

28

Valvular diseases

Elena Kapilevich

Introduction

- Valvular pathologies are common in emergency department patients and may be acute or chronic.
- Valvular dysfunction alters the basic physiology of the heart and impacts the management of hemodynamic compromise.
- Valvular diseases are classified depending on whether the valve is obstructing outflow (stenosis) or is not closing adequately (regurgitation).

Presentation

Classic presentation

- **Aortic stenosis (AS)**
  - Patients with AS have impaired left ventricular (LV) outflow due to a chronic valvular stenosis.
  - Subclinical AS is often asymptomatic.
  - Classic symptoms of advancing AS are exertional dyspnea, pre-syncope and angina with an associated harsh crescendo–decrescendo ejection murmur.
  - AS can mimic or exacerbate other types of cardiac disease, including acute coronary syndrome (ACS) and acute decompensated heart failure (ADHF).
- **Aortic regurgitation (AR)**
  - *Chronic AR:*
    - Patients with chronic AR have inadequate closure of the aortic valve at end-systole resulting in flow regurgitation back into the LV.

Practical Emergency Resuscitation and Critical Care, ed. Kaushal Shah, Jarone Lee, Kamal Medlej, and Scott D. Weingart. Published by Cambridge University Press. © Kaushal Shah, Jarone Lee, Kamal Medlej, and Scott D. Weingart 2013.

- This results in increased LV end-diastolic volume (LVEDV) and increase in LV size.
- AR is associated with a diastolic murmur best heard at the upper sternal border.
- It may be largely asymptomatic, depending on the function and compliance of the LV.
- Concomitant ventricular dysfunction can result in exertional dyspnea, ADHF, and conduction abnormalities.
- Angina is uncommon with isolated AR.
- *Acute AR* is a medical emergency and discussed in the "Critical presentation" section below.
- **Mitral stenosis (MS)**
  - Patients with MS have obstruction of flow between the left atrium (LA) and the LV.
    - This results in increased pressure in the LA, the pulmonary vasculature, and the right side of the heart.
    - LV function in isolated MS is largely unimpeded.
    - Symptoms of MS are related to the degree of pressure gradient across the valve.
      - Mild and moderate MS are generally asymptomatic.
      - Symptoms are exacerbated by tachycardia as diastolic filling time decreases.
      - MS is associated with a "low and rumbling" diastolic murmur best heard at the apex, as well as a classic "opening snap".
    - As the stenosis worsens, patients become symptomatic at rest.
      - Exertional dyspnea secondary to pulmonary congestion is the most common symptom of MS.
      - Hemoptysis.
      - Hoarseness or cough from the enlarged left atrium compressing the recurrent laryngeal nerve.
      - Dysphagia from the enlarged left atrium compressing the esophagus.
      - Malar flush or "mitral facies."
      - Progressive RV dilatation, right-sided heart failure and pulmonary hypertension.
      - Similar to AR, chest pain is uncommon with isolated MS.
- **Mitral regurgitation (MR)**
  - *Chronic MR:*
    - Patients with chronic MR have inadequate closure of the mitral valve at end-systole with resultant regurgitant flow back into the LA.
    - It can be caused by primary valvular problems, or as a result of a dilated LV.
    - This results in increased LA volume and subsequent LA dilation.
    - MR is associated with an early systolic or holosystolic murmur best heard at the upper sternal border.
    - Chronic mild MR may be largely asymptomatic.

- Symptoms from isolated, chronic MR are related to both LA overload and decreases in effective cardiac output.
  - Dyspnea
  - Atrial fibrillation (AF) due to LA enlargement
  - Progressive congestive heart failure (CHF) leading to right heart failure
  - Systemic emboli.
- *Acute MR* is a medical emergency and discussed in the "Critical presentation" section below.

Critical presentation

- **Aortic stenosis (AS)**
  - Aortic stenosis can exacerbate other cardiac pathologies including ACS and ADHF.
  - Patients with AS are particularly sensitive to changes in cardiac output due to the pressure gradient across the aortic valve.
    - Tachycardia decreases diastolic filling time and LVEDV, effectively decreasing stroke volume.
    - Intravascular volume depletion also decreases stroke volume.
    - Hemodynamics will deteriorate without appropriate preload, making AS a "preload-dependent" condition.
- **Aortic regurgitation (AR)**
  - Chronic aortic regurgitation is rarely a critical problem.
  - Acute AR is a medical emergency caused by sudden insufficiency of the aortic valve related to endocarditis, a perivalvular abscess, or acute aortic dissection.
  - In acute AR, the LV is unable to compensate for the dramatic and sudden increases in LVEDV.
  - Patients with acute AR will present with symptoms of acute volume overload, ADHF, or cardiogenic shock.
- **Mitral stenosis (MS)**
  - As MS worsens, clinical symptoms can become severe.
  - Atrial fibrillation (due to LA dilation) can cause tachycardia and hypotension.
  - Pulmonary vascular congestion can cause severe dyspnea.
  - Similarly to AS, symptoms of MS are exacerbated by tachycardia:
  - LVEDV decreases and cardiac output falls.
  - LA pressure increases, worsening pulmonary congestion.
  - Thromboembolic events increase with age and the degree of stenosis.
- **Mitral regurgitation (MR)**
  - *Chronic MR:*
    - Critical presentations of patients with chronic MR include rapid atrial fibrillation, dyspnea, and pulmonary edema.
    - Patients with chronic MR may also have a dilated LV, or decreased ventricular function which can lead to ADHF.

- *Acute MR* is a medical emergency caused by a flail leaflet or papillary muscle rupture.
  - These are often caused by endocarditis, trauma, or ACS.
  - Mitral valve failure leads to pulmonary edema and cardiogenic shock.
    - With ventricular contraction, reverse flow substantially decreases effective cardiac output while also causing acute overload of the LA.
    - Notably, due to the low pressure gradient between LV and LA in acute MR, a typical murmur will be difficult to discern. Up to 30–50% of patients with acute MR will have no murmur.

Diagnosis and evaluation

- Evaluation of any valvular pathology begins with the history and physical examination, paying particular attention to whether a valvular defect has been previously noted.
- Patients with acute valvular disease will require immediate stabilization as described below.
  - If a new acute AR is discovered, the diagnosis of aortic dissection should be ruled out with a CTA or a transthoracic or transesophageal echocardiogram.
  - If a new acute MR is discovered, ACS must be considered.
    - If the ECG is unrevealing, an echocardiogram may be useful to identify a flail leaflet, vegetations, ruptured chordae tendineae or papillary muscle rupture.
- Patients with known valvular disease should be evaluated based upon presenting symptoms.
  - The ECG may demonstrate findings of chronic structural changes from valvular dysfunction (Table 28.1).
  - A chest radiograph (CXR) is needed for patients presenting with dyspnea.
  - Basic laboratory studies including complete blood count, chemistry, cardiac enzymes, brain natriuretic peptide (BNP), and coagulation profiles may be helpful and should be ordered after a proper clinical assessment.
  - Blood culture and antibiotics may be indicated if endocarditis or a perivalvular abscess are suspected.
  - Characterization of valve dysfunction in the emergency department is not imperative if patients are hemodynamically stable.
  - Echocardiography should be considered in patients who are hemodynamically unstable.

Sudden deterioration and critical management

- **General principles**
  - Initial management should focus on acute stabilization:
    - Expectant airway management
    - Supplemental oxygen
    - Cardiac monitoring.

Table 28.1. Common findings of valvular pathology on ECG and CXR

Valvular lesion	Common ECG findings	Common CXR findings
Aortic stenosis	Left ventricular hypertrophy (LVH)	Enlarged cardiac silhouette, aortic calcifications, potential pulmonary edema
Aortic regurgitation (chronic)	LVH, left heart strain	May have no acute findings
Aortic regurgitation (acute)	May have no acute findings	Widened mediastinum, enlarged cardiac silhouette
Mitral stenosis	P mitrale due to LA enlargement, potential AF	May have no acute findings
Mitral regurgitation (chronic)	P mitrale due to LA enlargement, potential AF	Enlarged LA and LV
Mitral regurgitation (acute)	No specific changes related to valvular disease, though may indicate underlying etiology (e.g., STEMI)	Severe pulmonary edema

- Following stabilization, treatment should be symptom-focused.
- Acute valvular dysfunction is usually secondary to a precipitating critical problem. The latter will have to be addressed as well.
- **Lesion-specific issues**
  - *Aortic stenosis:*
    - Patients with AS are exquisitely sensitive to preload.
    - Exaggerated hypotension after intubation should be anticipated.
    - Depending on the underlying pathology, hemodynamics may be optimized by controlling the heart rate and increasing stroke volume.
    - In patients with acute CHF, afterload reduction will decrease the pressure gradient across the valve.
    - Loop diuretics should be used judiciously.
  - *Acute aortic regurgitation:*
    - Like acute MR, this is a true medical emergency and often presents with acute onset dyspnea from CHF.
    - Early medical management focuses on lowering LV end-diastolic pressure and increasing forward flow by reducing afterload.
    - IV nitroprusside or other vasodilators can be used for afterload reduction.
    - Cardiac inotropes such as dobutamine or dopamine can help increase contractility.
    - Avoid beta-blockers in the acute setting.
    - Unlike in MR, the use of intra-aortic balloon pumps is contraindicated since inflation of the balloon during diastole will worsen the severity of AR.

- Treat other causes of acute AR such as infective endocarditis or aortic dissection.
- The mainstay of treatment is early surgery to replace or repair the incompetent valve.
- *Mitral stenosis:*
  - Like AS, it may impact hemodynamics but does not often present critically.
  - Heart rate control may improve hemodynamics.
- *Acute mitral regurgitation:*
  - This is a medical emergency, as patients typically present in acute pulmonary edema and cardiogenic shock.
  - Early medical management focuses on the reduction of afterload to increase ventricular ejection fraction, and therefore reduce regurgitant volume.
  - If the patient is hypotensive, nitroprusside should be administered along with dobutamine.
  - Intra-aortic balloon pumps are often used to increase cardiac output.
  - Mild to moderate tachycardia may be beneficial as it limits the amount of regurgitation. Beta-blockers should therefore be avoided.
  - Surgical management is the mainstay of treatment in most cases of acute MR.
  - MR secondary to myocardial ischemia may be managed with early revascularization to restore blood flow to the papillary muscles.

Critical care considerations

Vasopressor of choice: while there is no good evidence on the use of pressors in patients presenting with hypotension and shock related to acute valvular emergency, vasopressors with primarily vasoconstrictive effects such as phenylephrine should be avoided as they increase afterload and decrease cardiac output. The following pressors and/or inotropes can be considered:

- SBP ≥80 mmHg: dobutamine
- SBP <80 mmHg: dopamine
- SBP <70 mmHg: norepinephrine.

REFERENCES

Carabello BA, Crawford FA. Valvular heart disease. *N Engl J Med.* 1997; **337**: 32–41.

Chandrashekhar Y, Westaby S, Narula J. Mitral stenosis. *Lancet.* 2009; **374**(9697): 1271–83.

Chen RS, Bivens MJ, Grossman SA. Diagnosis and management of valvular heart disease in emergency medicine. *Emerg Med Clin North Am.* 2011; **29**: 801–10, vii.

Mokadam NA, Stout KK, Verrier ED. Management of acute regurgitation in left-sided cardiac valves. *Tex Heart Inst J.* 2011; **38**: 9–19.

Stout KK, Verrier ED. Acute valvular regurgitation. *Circulation.* 2009; **119**: 3232–41.

29

Upper airway emergencies

Brian C. Geyer and Susan Wilcox

Introduction

- An upper airway emergency is the actual or impending loss of air movement through any of the structures cephalad to the mainstem bronchi.
- Representing a true life-threatening emergency, this process may be viewed as a common presentation from a diverse range of etiologies (Table 29.1).

Presentation

Classic presentation

- Patients with upper airway emergencies may have variable initial presentations, from presenting calmly and without distress, to presenting with cyanosis and obtundation.
- Patients may complain of airway symptoms such as hoarseness, shortness of breath, or speech changes. Patients may also complain of systemic symptoms such as an allergic reaction or fever.
- The wide variety of presentations mandates a high index of suspicion for potential airway compromise.

Critical presentation

- There is often rapid progression from benign to life-threatening symptoms, and one of the key challenges is to anticipate a patient's clinical course.

Practical Emergency Resuscitation and Critical Care, ed. Kaushal Shah, Jarone Lee, Kamal Medlej, and Scott D. Weingart. Published by Cambridge University Press. © Kaushal Shah, Jarone Lee, Kamal Medlej, and Scott D. Weingart 2013.

Table 29.1. Differential diagnosis for upper airway emergencies

Allergic
- Anaphylaxis
- Angioedema

Infectious
- Ludwig's angina
- Retropharyngeal abscess/other deep space infections of the neck
- Peritonsillar abscess
- Epiglottitis

Traumatic and caustic
- Thermal burn
- Traumatic hematoma
- Caustic ingestion
- Inhaled toxins

Anatomical and mechanical
- Tumor/postradiation therapy changes
- Postsurgical changes
- Muscle weakness
- Congenital
- Foreign body

- Key warning signs of impending airway collapse include
  - Signs of upper airway obstruction: stridor, muffled "hot potato" voice
  - Difficulty managing secretions: drooling, tripod position, pooled secretions in posterior pharynx
  - Signs of respiratory failure: dyspnea, tachypnea, accessory muscle recruitment, hypoxia.
- Patients may not demonstrate hypoxemia until late in their presentation.

Diagnosis and evaluation

- The first step in the evaluation of the patient with suspected upper airway emergency is to determine the need for emergent intubation or surgical airway.
- If possible, a brief history should be obtained focusing on history of cancer, allergies, exposure to medications including ACE inhibitors, a family history of C1 esterase inhibitor deficiency, trauma, and recent surgery.
- A targeted physical examination should include assessment for stridor, hoarseness, urticaria, edema of skin, lips, mouth, and throat.
  - Burns to facial skin or mouth, singed nose hairs, soot in airway should be considered high-risk features in burn patients.
  - Trauma patients should be evaluated for blood in airway, facial injuries, penetrating neck injuries, and neck hematomas or ecchymosis.

- Laboratory testing should be guided by the suspected underlying etiology.
- Imaging studies:
  - **Patients at risk for impending airway collapse should not be sent to radiology**
  - Lateral neck radiographs may demonstrate prevertebral swelling.
  - CT scan of the neck may provide better anatomical detail and define the amount and location of swelling or mass.

Critical management

Recognize the severity of the presentation
Evaluate for the need for immediate and definitive airway control
Consider the differential diagnosis of the underlying etiology
Secure the airway with simultaneous surgical airway setup
Provide medical therapies as indicated to treat the underlying process

- Given the high-risk, time-sensitive nature of these presentations, all practitioners should be familiar with their local resources, algorithms, and airway management options prior to seeing patients.
- **Risk stratification of the patient by expected clinical course**
  - *High-risk patients:*
    - For patients with severe anaphylaxis/angioedema, upper airway burns and signs of upper airway obstruction, consider intubation preemptively.
    - For trauma patients with any signs of airway involvement or "hard signs" of penetrating trauma to the neck, consider immediate intubation.
    - Video laryngoscopy with simultaneous surgical airway setup is recommended.
    - The high risk of airway collapse and decompensation during sedation and neuromuscular blockade must be considered in these patients.
    - The endotracheal tube should be at the smaller end of the acceptable range. A back-up tube of 5.5 or smaller should be immediately available.
  - *Moderate-risk patients:*
    - Patients with deep space infections and upper airway tumors have lower risk for rapid evolution and acute decompensation. However, these patients may present late in their course with an impending airway obstruction.
- **Awake visualization/intubation**
  - In patients with a rapidly evolving upper airway obstruction, awake evaluation can provide invaluable information about potential complications before paralytics are administered. Paralytics should never be administered if a "cannot intubate, cannot ventilate" situation is anticipated.

- Giving sedation carries the risk of airway collapse during most upper airway emergencies. Optimization of local anesthesia is recommended to minimize need for sedation and to preserve airway reflexes.
- The nasal route is usually preferred for cases mandating immediate visualization only. When planning intubation, the nasal route allows a direct passage to the vocal cords and may be easier for an awake patient to tolerate. Downsides to the nasal route include the need for greatly reduced tube diameter and the increased risk of inadvertent extubation due to a longer pathway for the tube. Therefore, the nasal route is primarily used in cases of angioedema or when an oral mass hinders oral visualization.
- If the patient requires immediate intubation, but not an immediate surgical airway, oral visualization/intubation is the preferred method. This may be accomplished with a flexible endoscope loaded with an endotracheal tube, or video/standard laryngoscope.
- Adequate preparation, including preoxygenation, gathering appropriate staff, having desired medications drawn up, and having a detailed algorithm including back-up and surgical options is critical prior to initiating any airway manipulation unless the patient is rapidly deteriorating.
- The major steps to awake visualization/intubation are
  - Pretreatment with glycopyrrolate, if time allows, to minimize secretions
  - Topical anesthesia with atomized 2–4% lidocaine
  - Sedation
  - Airway visualization
  - Intubation
  - Postintubation management.
- **Cricothyrotomy**
  - In many cases, cricothyrotomy is the definitive management technique for upper airway emergencies.
  - Patients with upper airway obstruction who are high risk for hypoxia should be prepared for cricothyrotomy while the endotracheal intubation is attempted ("double setup").
- **Medical therapy**
  - Once the airway is secured, or for patients of moderate risk not immediately requiring airway intervention, medical therapy should target the underlying etiology.
  - For anaphylaxis and angioedema, treat with IM epinephrine, IV H_2-blockers, diphenhydramine, IV methylprednisolone, and albuterol. In cases of angioedema with a known or suspected C1 esterase inhibitor deficiency, consider treatment with fresh frozen plasma.
  - For infections, treat with IV antibiotics as indicated by the underlying infection and dexamethasone.

Sudden deterioration

- Sudden deterioration is the hallmark of upper airway pathology and should be expected.
- For this reason, it is **generally inappropriate to transfer patients with risk of deterioration without a definitive airway** in place. This recommendation includes interfacility transfers, as well as intrafacility transfers to radiology or the intensive care unit. The sole exception is transport to the OR for definitive airway management, when the ED attending deems that the benefits of management in the OR outweigh the risks of transport.

Special circumstances

- **Foreign bodies in the airway** represent a special class of high-risk patients.
  - Need to rapidly distinguish complete from incomplete obstruction.
  - Liquid and semiliquid obstructions (blood, vomit, etc.) may be cleared with suction.
  - Solid and poorly visualized obstructions are higher risk for poor outcomes.
- In patients with incomplete obstruction from solid material, the goal is to temporize the patient and move to the operating room for definitive management.
  - Patients should be provided supplemental oxygen to prevent hypoxemia, but bag mask ventilation should be avoided as this may worsen the obstruction.
  - If the OR is not an option, the practitioner should be aware that topical anesthesia and sedation may facilitate laryngoscopy but may also result in complete obstruction.
- Complete obstructions require immediate action to relieve the obstruction.
  - In this case, basic life support techniques should be used on the conscious patient to expel the foreign body.
  - Subdiaphragmatic thrusts may be applied to both the semi-upright and supine patient.
- If the patient loses consciousness or arrives unconscious:
  - Immediate direct laryngoscopy should be performed to attempt removal of the obstruction using forceps.
  - Cricothyrotomy is indicated if the obstruction is above the vocal cords and cannot be removed.
  - If no obstruction is visible, endotracheal intubation should be performed immediately.
  - Inability to ventilate the patient with subglottic obstruction indicates a tracheal obstruction. In this case:
    - Stop ventilation, deflate the cuff, replace the stylet, and advance the endotracheal tube as far as possible in an attempt to displace the obstruction into one of the mainstem bronchi.

- Then retract the endotracheal tube to the proper position and ventilate utilizing the contralateral lung.
- Failure to ventilate at this point indicates either bilateral mainstem bronchial obstruction (which is not survivable without immediate extracorporeal membrane oxygenation) or unilateral obstruction with a contralateral pneumothorax. Thus bilateral needle thoracostomies should be considered as the final salvage maneuver.

Vasopressor of choice: none.

REFERENCES

Adams JG, Barton ED, Collings J, *et al.*, eds. *Emergency Medicine*. Philadelphia, PA: Saunders; 2008: 17–30.

American Society of Anesthesiologists Task Force on Management of the Difficult Airway. Practice guidelines for management of the difficult airway: an updated report by the American Society of Anesthesiologists Task Force on Management of the Difficult Airway. *Anesthesiology*. 2003; **98**: 1269–77.

Langeron O, Amour J, Vivien B, Aubrun F. Clinical review: management of difficult airways. *Crit Care*. 2006; **10**: 243.

Orebaugh SL. Difficult airway management in the emergency department. *J Emerg Med*. 2002; **22**: 31–48.

Walls RM, Murphy MF. *Manual of Emergency Airway Management*. 4th edn. Philadelphia, PA: Lippincott Williams & Wilkins; 2012: 266–74, 377–82.

30

Asthma

Andrew Eyre

Introduction

- Asthma is a chronic inflammatory disorder of the airways characterized by increased responsiveness and sensitivity to irritating stimuli.
- Inflammatory episodes create obstruction to airflow due to bronchospasm, airway edema, bronchial smooth muscle contraction, and mucous plugs, leading to recurrent episodes of wheezing, shortness of breath, chest tightness, and coughing.
- The inflammatory episodes also lead to lung hyperinflation, increased work of breathing, ventilation–perfusion mismatch.
- A hallmark of asthma is that the inflammatory episodes are reversible.
- Asthma is extremely common, under-diagnosed and undertreated, and leads to significant morbidity, mortality, and healthcare costs.

Presentation

Classic presentation

- Patients present with cough, wheezing, and dyspnea. Other signs and symptoms include: mucous production, acid reflux, tachypnea, chest tightness, diaphoresis, accessory muscle use, and a prolonged expiratory phase.
- Key questions help risk stratify and guide management:
  - Number of prior hospital visits and admissions for asthma?
  - History of requiring intubation or ICU-level treatment?
  - Current asthma regimen?
  - What rescue medications have been used so far?

Practical Emergency Resuscitation and Critical Care, ed. Kaushal Shah, Jarone Lee, Kamal Medlej, and Scott D. Weingart. Published by Cambridge University Press. © Kaushal Shah, Jarone Lee, Kamal Medlej, and Scott D. Weingart 2013.

- Known asthma trigger?
- Current or recent use of systemic corticosteroids?
- Baseline pulmonary function tests or spirometry values?

Critical presentation

- Airflow restriction may be severe, leading to patients presenting in an upright or tripod position, with cyanosis, altered mental status, and respiratory arrest.
- **Beware of patients with suspected asthma who are not wheezing but are dyspneic.** Patients with severe disease may not have enough airflow to create a wheeze, and instead present with a "silent chest."

Diagnosis and evaluation

- **Physical examination**
  - Carefully monitor heart rate, respiratory rate, blood pressure, temperature, pulse oximetry, and pain.
  - Monitor for signs of altered mental status that could indicate impending respiratory failure.
- **Capnography**
  - Asthma exacerbations initially produce tachypnea and a resultant low carbon dioxide level; a normal or elevated carbon dioxide level may indicate fatigue and impending respiratory failure.
- **Bedside spirometry**
  - Measure peak flow and/or FEV_1 (forced expiratory volume in one second) on initial assessment to evaluate severity and response to treatment. Requires patient cooperation. Record the best of three attempts.
  - Values can be compared to a patient's baseline and personal best.
  - Peak flow of under 200 L/minute usually represents severe exacerbation/disease.
- **Arterial blood gas**
  - Not routinely required or recommended. Consider when not able to accurately monitor pulse oximetry, capnography, or with severe or otherwise complicated patients. May be used to differentiate asthma from other etiologies.
- **Chest radiography**
  - Not routinely required.
  - Should be used to differentiate asthma from other etiologies or comorbid conditions including pneumothorax, congestive heart failure, and pneumonia.
- **Laboratory testing and ECG**
  - Laboratory testing and ECG should not be routinely undertaken for straightforward cases. Use them to differentiate asthma exacerbations from alternative etiologies or comorbid conditions.

Critical management

Oxygen
Inhaled beta-agonists
Inhaled anticholinergics
Corticosteroids
Adjunctive medications
Noninvasive ventilation
Intubation as needed
Ventilator management

- **Manage ABCs**
  - *Oxygen:* Patients should be placed on supplemental oxygen therapy as needed to maintain adequate oxygen saturations.
  - Patients must be monitored for signs of impending respiratory failure.
- **Medications** (see Table 30.1)
  - *Inhaled beta-agonists:*
    - Inhaled albuterol is the initial rescue medication of choice.
    - Side effects include tremor, nervousness, tachycardia, palpitations, headache, and hyperglycemia.
    - Delivered by nebulizer or metered-dose inhaler (MDI) with spacer device. In severe exacerbations, albuterol should be delivered as a continuous nebulized treatment.
  - *Inhaled anticholinergics:*
    - Ipratropium bromide is an effective adjunctive therapy by addressing airway smooth muscle constriction and airway secretions.
    - Should not be used alone, but has additive effect with inhaled beta-agonists.
  - *Corticosteroids:*
    - Address the inflammatory component of the disease.
    - Administer early in treatment, as they do not take effect for a few hours.
    - There is no difference in treatment effect between enteral (prednisone) and parenteral (methylprednisone) administration; use intravenous/intramuscular route when the patient is unable to take oral medications.
  - *Subcutaneous epinephrine:*
    - An effective adjunct for patients with severe disease or those unable to tolerate inhaled therapy.
    - May produce tachycardia, arrhythmia, vasoconstriction; use with caution in patients with heart disease.
  - *Subcutaneous terbutaline:*
    - Long-acting beta2-agonist.
    - Adjunct for patients with severe disease.

Table 30.1. Common medications in acute asthma management for adults

Medication	Dosing	Comments
Albuterol (nebulized)	2.5–5 mg every 20 minutes ×3 doses, then space as able	May provide continuous therapy for severe cases
Albuterol (MDI)	2–8 puffs every 20 minutes up to 4 hours, then space as able	Consider using spacer
Ipratropium bromide (nebulized)	0.5 mg every 30 minutes ×3 doses, then space as needed	May mix with albuterol
Ipratropium bromide (MDI)	4–8 puffs	
Epinephrine (1:1000)	0.3–0.5 mg subcutaneously, may repeat every 20 minutes ×3 doses as needed	
Terbutaline	0.25 mg subcutaneously every 20 minutes ×3 doses as needed	
Prednisone	40–80 mg/day	For steroid burst: 40–60 mg daily
Methylprednisolone	60–125 mg/day	
Magnesium sulfate	1–2 g over 20–30 minutes	

- May produce tremor or tachycardia.
- *Intravenous magnesium sulfate:*
  - An adjunctive medication indicated for patients with severe asthma that works by dilating airways and relaxing smooth muscle.
- *Heliox:*
  - An inhaled mixture of helium and oxygen that is indicated only in severe asthma exacerbations.
  - Works by decreasing the density of any inhaled gas thereby reducing the airflow resistance and work of breathing.
  - A temporary intervention intended to "buy time" while other therapies take effect.
- **Airway and ventilatory support**
  - *Noninvasive positive-pressure ventilation (NPPV):*
    - Constant positive airway pressure (CPAP) and bi-level positive airway pressure (Bi-PAP) may be considered for patients with severe asthma.
    - NPPV works by decreasing the work of breathing but requires a patient with a patent airway and who will be compliant with the therapy.
    - Patients receiving noninvasive positive-pressure ventilation must be carefully monitored for signs of decompensation including altered mental status, hemodynamic instability, hypercarbia, vomiting, and increased dyspnea.
    - If noninvasive methods fail, the patient will require intubation

- *Intubation:*
  - Patients with altered mental status, severe acidosis, or hemodynamic instability should not be given a trial of NPPV but should be immediately intubated.
  - Lidocaine pretreatment blunts the bronchospastic response from airway manipulation.
  - Consider ketamine for induction, as this may improve bronchodilation.
- *Ventilator management:*
  - The goal of ventilator management in the asthmatic is to oxygenate and ventilate without worsening hyperinflation, which causes barotrauma and hemodynamic instability.
  - Often requires low tidal volumes, low respiratory rates, long expiratory times, and high inspiratory flow rates.
  - Permissive hypercapnia may be required.
  - Aggressive pharmacological therapy should continue once the patient is intubated.

Sudden deterioration

- If patients acutely decompensate while receiving invasive or noninvasive positive pressure ventilation, consider the possibility of pneumothorax and intrinsic positive end-expiratory pressure (auto-PEEP). If concern is for auto-PEEP, disconnect the ventilator circuit to allow for full exhalation. If concern is for tension pneumothorax, proceed with needle decompression and tube thoracostomy.

REFERENCES

Fanta CH. Treatment of acute asthma exacerbations in adults. *UpToDate* (Online). Wolters Kluwer Health; 2011. Available from: www.uptodate.com/contents/treatment-of-acute-exacerbations-of-asthma-in-adults (accessed April 30, 2013).

Lugogo NL, MacIntyre NR. Life-threatening asthma: pathophysiology and management. *Respir Care.* 2008; **53**: 726–35.

31

Chronic obstructive pulmonary disease

Andrew Eyre

Introduction

- COPD is defined as "a treatable and preventable disease … characterized by airflow limitation that is not fully reversible" (Global Initiative for Chronic Obstructive Lung Disease [GOLD] guidelines definition).
- It includes chronic bronchitis and emphysema.
- Most COPD is caused by exposure to tobacco smoke or chemicals.
- It leads to alveolar damage, increased mucous production, air trapping, hyper-inflation and airflow obstruction.
- Acute COPD exacerbations are typically caused by exposure to infection (viral or bacterial) or chemical irritant.

Presentation

Classic presentation

- Patients present with coughing, wheezing, a prolonged expiratory phase, increased sputum production, and dyspnea. Other signs may include tachypnea, accessory muscle use, pursed lip breathing, retractions, tripod position, altered mental status, cor pulmonale, right ventricular hypertrophy, subxiphoid heave, S3 or S4 heart sound, rales, and rhonchi.
- Patients with COPD may exhibit long-term changes including barrel chest, weight loss, and muscle wasting.

Practical Emergency Resuscitation and Critical Care, ed. Kaushal Shah, Jarone Lee, Kamal Medlej, and Scott D. Weingart. Published by Cambridge University Press. © Kaushal Shah, Jarone Lee, Kamal Medlej, and Scott D. Weingart 2013.

Critical presentation

- Airflow restriction may be severe, leading to patients presenting in an upright or tripod position, with cyanosis, altered mental status, and respiratory arrest.

Diagnosis and evaluation

- **Physical examination**
  - Carefully monitor heart rate, respiratory rate, blood pressure, temperature, pulse oximetry, and pain.
  - Monitor for signs of altered mental status that could indicate impending respiratory failure.
  - Many other etiologies present with similar symptoms as a COPD exacerbation.
- **Continuous pulse oximetry and capnography**
  - Continuous pulse oximetry and waveform capnography allow therapy to be titrated and changes in clinical status to be assessed.
  - A goal SpO_2 of 92% is adequate in order to avoid over-oxygenation.
  - COPD patients tend to retain CO_2. On continuous waveform capnography, the plateau phase of the waveform will tend to have a sharper angle.
- **Arterial blood gas**
  - ABGs are recommended in moderate to severe exacerbations to monitor pH, $PaCO_2$ and PaO_2.
  - May be used to compare to a baseline or differentiate COPD from other etiologies.
- **Chest radiography**
  - Recommended to evaluate for underlying etiology of a COPD exacerbation or to differentiate from other disease processes such as pneumothorax, pneumonia, CHF, or pleural effusions.
- **ECG**
  - Consider obtaining ECGs in older patients, in patients with chest pain, and to differentiate from other etiologies.
  - In chronic or severe cases of COPD, may see evidence of cor pulmonale.
- **Laboratory testing**
  - Use laboratory tests to differentiate COPD exacerbations from alternative etiologies or comorbid conditions. Consider complete blood count, electrolytes, cardiac enzymes, brain natriuretic peptide, D-dimer, and medications levels.

Critical management

Oxygen
Inhaled beta-agonists
Inhaled anticholinergics
Corticosteroids
Antibiotics
Noninvasive ventilation
Intubation
Ventilator management

- **Manage ABCs**
  - Patients should be placed on supplemental oxygen therapy as needed to maintain adequate oxygen saturations of 88–92%.
  - Beware of over-oxygenating the COPD patient as this can lead to worsening ventilation–perfusion mismatch and apnea.
  - Patients must be monitored for signs of impending respiratory failure.
- **Medications** (Table 31.1)
  - *Inhaled beta-agonists:*
    - Inhaled albuterol is the initial rescue medication of choice.
    - Common side effects include tremor, nervousness, tachycardia, palpitations, headache, and hyperglycemia.
    - Delivered by nebulizer or metered-dose inhaler (MDI) with spacer device.
  - *Inhaled anticholinergics:*
    - Ipratropium bromide is an effective therapy and treats airway smooth muscle constriction and airway secretions.
    - Although previously suggested to be more effective than beta2-agonists in acute COPD, recent data suggests that anticholinergics should be used as adjuncts in most cases.
  - *Corticosteroids:*
    - Systemic corticosteroids are critical in COPD exacerbations to address the inflammatory component of the disease.
    - Administer early in treatment as they do not take effect for hours. There is no difference between enteral and parenteral administration.
    - There is no benefit to high-dose steroids.
  - *Antibiotics:*
    - For most moderate/severe COPD exacerbations, it is appropriate to start antibiotics with coverage for common respiratory pathogens. Mortality benefit has been demonstrated when antibiotics are given to all patients admitted to the hospital for COPD exacerbation.
    - Common classes include macrolides and fluoroquinolones.

Table 31.1. Common medications for acute COPD management in adults

Medication	Dosing	Comments
Albuterol (nebulized)	2.5–5 mg every 20 minutes ×3 doses, then space as able	May provide continuous therapy for severe cases
Albuterol (MDI)	2–8 puffs every 20 minutes up to 4 hours, then space as able	Consider using spacer
Ipratropium bromide (nebulized)	0.5 mg every 30 minutes ×3 doses, then space as needed	May mix with albuterol
Ipratropium bromide (MDI)	4–8 puffs	
Prednisone	40–80 mg/day	Followed by steroid taper
Methylprednisolone	60–125 mg/day	
Levofloxacin	500–750 mg PO or IV daily	
Ceftazidime	1 g IV every 8–12 hours	
Azithromycin	500 mg PO or IV, then 250 mg daily	

- **Airway and ventilatory support**
  - *Noninvasive positive pressure ventilation:*
    - CPAP and BiPAP may be considered for certain patients with moderate to severe COPD exacerbations.
    - NPPV decreases the work of breathing, but requires a patient to have a patent airway and be compliant with the therapy.
    - Patients receiving NPPV must be carefully monitored for signs of decompensation including altered mental status, hemodynamic instability, worsening hypercarbia, vomiting, and increased dyspnea.
    - If noninvasive methods fail, the patient will require intubation.
  - *Intubation:*
    - If intubation is required, use the largest tube possible that will not cause damage to decrease airway resistance during mechanical ventilation.
  - *Ventilator management:*
    - The goal of ventilator management in the COPD patient is to oxygenate and ventilate without causing barotrauma and hemodynamic instability.
    - May require low tidal volumes, low respiratory rates, long expiratory times, and high inspiratory flow rates.
    - Permissive hypercapnia may be required. Follow capnography or ABG values to adjust ventilator settings.
    - Pharmacological therapy should continue once the patient is intubated.

Sudden deterioration

- If patients acutely decompensate while receiving invasive or noninvasive positive pressure ventilation, consider the possibility of pneumothorax and intrinsic positive end-expiratory pressure (auto-PEEP). If concern is for auto-PEEP, disconnect the ventilator circuit to allow for full exhalation. If concern is for tension pneumothorax, proceed with needle decompression and tube thoracostomy.

REFERENCES

Brulotte CA, Lang ES. Acute exacerbations of chronic obstructive pulmonary disease in the emergency department. *Emerg Med Clin North Am.* 2012; **30**: 223–47, vii.

NHLBI/WHO Workshop Report: Global Initiative for Chronic Obstructive Lung Disease (GOLD): Global Strategy for the Diagnosis, Management and Prevention of Chronic Obstructive Pulmonary Disease. Bethesda, MD: National Institutes of Health, National Heart, Lung and Blood Institute, April 2001; updated 2005.

Stoller JK. Management of acute exacerbations of chronic obstructive pulmonary disease. *UpToDate*: Wolters Kluwer Health; 2012. Available from: www.uptodate.com/contents/management-of-acute-exacerbations-of-chronic-obstructive-pulmonary-disease (accessed April 30, 2013).

32

Acute respiratory distress syndrome

Elisabeth Lessenich

Introduction

- Acute respiratory distress syndrome (ARDS) is severe respiratory distress of an acute and persistent nature, caused by one or more predisposing conditions, and resulting in refractory arterial hypoxemia.
- Approximately 50% of cases are due to severe infection, either focal (such as pneumonia) or systemic (such as sepsis). Other etiologies are listed in Table 32.1.

Presentation

Classic presentation

- This condition typically manifests in one of two ways:
  - Shortly after the patient's initial presentation, as in someone who has just sustained a major insult – such as significant smoke inhalation in a fire or near-drowning
  - Several days after admission, in severely ill patients whose initial presentation was more indolent – such as a patient with urosepsis.
- In the acute, exudative phase of ARDS, damage to the lungs causes fluid to leak across the alveolar-capillary basement membrane, causing alveolar edema and subsequent hypoxemia.
  - As a result of alveolar edema, surfactant activity is significantly compromised and lung compliance decreases
- The acute phase of ARDS can progress to a fibrotic phase, in which case patients will exhibit continued hypoxemia, increasing dead space, pulmonary hypertension, and even greater loss of lung compliance.

Practical Emergency Resuscitation and Critical Care, ed. Kaushal Shah, Jarone Lee, Kamal Medlej, and Scott D. Weingart. Published by Cambridge University Press. © Kaushal Shah, Jarone Lee, Kamal Medlej, and Scott D. Weingart 2013.

Table 32.1. Etiologies of ARDS

Direct injuries to lungs	Indirect injuries
Pneumonia	Sepsis
Aspiration	Severe trauma
• Gastric contents	• Multiple fractures
• Near-drowning	• Head injury
• Hydrocarbons/solvents	• Burns
Smoke or toxic gas inhalation	Pancreatitis
Pulmonary contusion	Multiple blood transfusions
Embolism	Drug toxicity
• Thromboembolism	• Salicylates
• Fat embolism	• Hydrochlorothiazide
• Amniotic fluid embolism	• Opiates
Oxygen toxicity	• Amiodarone
Reperfusion pulmonary edema	• Cyclosporine
	• Tricyclic antidepressants
	• Chemotherapeutic agents
	Cardiopulmonary bypass
	High-altitude exposure

- Pulmonary edema in ARDS is heterogeneous and leads to atelectatic or consolidated areas of lung interspersed with relatively unaffected regions, creating areas of intrapulmonary shunt, which results in hypoxemia that does not improve with oxygen administration alone.

Critical presentation

- As pulmonary edema accumulates in the initial exudative phase of the disease, patients will become dyspneic and will demonstrate increased work of breathing.
- Due to worsening lung compliance, tidal volumes will decrease and respiratory rate will increase. Patients will become progressively hypoxemic due to both worsening V/Q mismatch and shunt physiology.
- As above, patients may present to the ED in hypoxemic respiratory failure due to a rapidly progressive etiology, or they may present late.
- Patients may deteriorate rapidly during their ED course despite appropriate therapy.

Diagnosis and evaluation

- The diagnosis of ARDS is made clinically based on a standardized definition:
  - The syndrome must develop within one week of a known clinical insult or worsening pulmonary symptoms.
  - Chest imaging demonstrates bilateral opacities not fully explained by lobar collapse, nodules, or effusions.
  - The respiratory failure is not fully explained by cardiac failure or volume overload. If a known risk factor for ARDS is not present, objective assessment such as echocardiography should be obtained to rule out hydrostatic edema.
  - The PaO_2/FiO_2 ratio is <300 on at least 5 cmH$_2$O of positive end-expiratory pressure (PEEP) or continuous positive airway pressure (CPAP).

ARDS degree	PaO$_2$/FiO$_2$ ratio
Mild	200–300
Moderate	100–200
Severe	<100

- **Imaging**
  - On a chest radiograph, ARDS looks essentially the same as cardiogenic pulmonary edema. The syndrome usually develops 4–24 hours after the appearance of radiographic abnormalities (Figure 32.1).
  - On CT, one sees alveolar filling and consolidation often in a heterogeneous pattern.

Critical management

Identification and treatment of underlying cause
Mechanical ventilation, with the following parameters/settings:
- Ventilator in volume-control mode
- Tidal volume of 4 to 8 mL/kg of predicted body weight
- PEEP in the range of 5 to 20 cmH$_2$O
- Plateau pressure not to exceed 30 cmH$_2$O
Ensure adequate systemic perfusion for optimal oxygen delivery
Provide neuromuscular blockade as needed
Consider rescue therapies
- Inhaled nitric oxide or prostacyclins
- Advanced ventilation strategies
- Prone positioning
- Extracorporeal membrane oxygenation (ECMO)

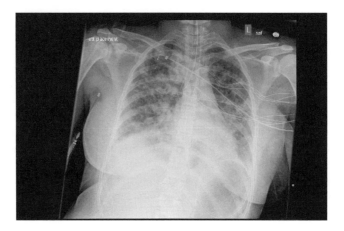

Figure 32.1. Chest radiograph of a 16-year-old girl who developed ARDS from aspiration of gastric contents, after having prolonged seizure activity with vomiting.

- Lung-protective ventilation is the mainstay of management in ARDS.
- The goal of this strategy is to support a patient's oxygenation until the inflammation and edema has cleared while minimizing further damage due to mechanical ventilation.
  - Specifically, lung-protective ventilation aims to obtain adequate gas exchange with the lowest possible tidal volumes, airway pressures, and oxygen concentrations.
- Plateau pressures, obtained via an inspiratory pause on the ventilator, represent the pressures seen by the alveoli. Elevated plateau pressures can over-distend undamaged alveoli.
  - The goal tidal volumes are 4–8 mL/kg of ideal body weight.
  - The goal plateau pressures are ≤30 cmH$_2$O.
- To protect the lungs with small tidal volumes and low pressures, many clinicians will allow for alveolar hypoventilation and subsequent respiratory acidosis, if necessary. This practice is known as "permissive hypercapnia."
- Positive end-expiratory pressure can stabilize damaged alveoli and increase their surface area by recruiting areas of atelectasis, resulting in:
  - Improved gas exchange
  - Smaller degree of hypoxic pulmonary vasoconstriction
  - Reduction in the amount of intrapulmonary shunt
  - Reduced damage from repetitive opening and closing of atelectatic alveoli.
- Goal oxygen saturation is set at 88–92% to minimize FiO$_2$ concentrations to reduce the risk of oxygen toxicity and worsening atelectasis.
- Early neuromuscular blockade with cisatracurium has been demonstrated to reduce 90-day mortality in patients with a PaO$_2$/FiO$_2$ ratio of less than 150. Once

patients are adequately sedated, cisatracurium infusions should be considered for severe hypoxemia.

- In patients with refractory hypoxemia, rescue therapies may be considered. Although these therapies may improve oxygenation in some patients, none have been conclusively shown to reduce mortality or long-term morbidity. There is not enough evidence to support use of these measures on a routine basis in ARDS.
  - Inhaled nitric oxide and prostacyclin may temporarily improve hypoxemia.
  - Airway pressure release ventilation (APRV) and high-frequency oscillatory ventilation (HFOV) are advanced ventilator modes designed to maximize oxygenation while minimizing further lung injury. These should only be initiated by an expert practitioner.
  - Prone positioning may improve oxygenation, but increases the risk of extubation.
  - Studies of steroids in ARDS have demonstrated mixed outcomes.
  - ECMO may be considered in intractable cases.

Sudden deterioration

- The most common causes for sudden decompensation are related to:
  - The respiratory system or mechanical ventilation from pneumothorax, bronchial plugging, or ET tube displacement
  - The overall state of critical illness, such as GI bleeding from a stress ulcer or septic shock from progression of the initial infection.
- Death in ARDS is most often caused by multiple organ failure rather than respiratory failure.

Vasopressor of choice: should be based on underlying etiology because isolated ARDS should not require vasopressor therapy.

REFERENCES

Esan A, Hess DR, Raoof S, *et al.* Severe hypoxemic respiratory failure: part 1 – ventilatory strategies. *Chest.* 2010; **137**: 1203–16.

Hemmila MR, Napolitano LM. Severe respiratory failure: advanced treatment options. *Crit Care Med.* 2006; **34**(9 Suppl): S278–90.

Papazian L, Forel JM, Gacouin A, *et al.* Neuromuscular blockers in early acute respiratory distress syndrome. *N Engl J Med.* 2010; **363**: 1107–16.

Piantadosi CA, Schwartz DA. The acute respiratory distress syndrome. *Ann Intern Med.* 2004; **141**: 460–70.

Ranieri VM, Rubenfeld GD, Thompson BT, *et al.* Acute respiratory distress syndrome: the Berlin Definition. *JAMA.* 2012; **307**: 2526–33.

33

Massive hemoptysis

Karen A. Kinnaman and Susan Wilcox

Introduction

- Hemoptysis is the expectoration of blood from the respiratory tract that originates from below the vocal cords.
- Massive hemoptysis is defined by the expectoration of a large amount of blood with or without a rapid rate of bleeding. The exact volume of blood has not been universally defined, but proposed volumes range anywhere from 200 to 1000 mL over 24 hours.
- Common etiologies of massive hemoptysis are listed in Table 33.1.
- Massive hemoptysis is a medical emergency, as patients can die from:
  - Asphyxiation due to flooding of the alveoli with blood (most common)
  - Intractable hypoxemia from ventilation–perfusion mismatch
  - Exsanguination from massive hemorrhage (least common).
- Less than 5% of hemoptysis cases are massive, but massive hemoptysis carries a mortality rate of 80%. Mortality correlates with amount of blood expectorated, rate of bleeding, and the underlying pulmonary reserve.
- **Anatomy**
  - Bronchial arteries branch from the thoracic aorta or intercostal arteries, and supply oxygenated blood to the lung parenchyma.
    - These arteries are at systemic pressure, may bleed profusely, and are the source of massive hemoptysis in >80% cases.
    - Vessel injury from inflammation (arteritis), trauma, bronchiectasis, or erosion from an adjacent malignancy can result in massive hemorrhage.
  - Pulmonary arteries carry large volumes of deoxygenated blood from the right ventricle across the pulmonary capillary bed and return oxygenated blood via the pulmonary veins.

Practical Emergency Resuscitation and Critical Care, ed. Kaushal Shah, Jarone Lee, Kamal Medlej, and Scott D. Weingart. Published by Cambridge University Press. © Kaushal Shah, Jarone Lee, Kamal Medlej, and Scott D. Weingart 2013.

Table 33.1. Common causes of massive hemoptysis

Bronchitis
Bronchiectasis
Aspergilloma
Tumor
Tuberculosis
Lung abscess
Emboli
Coagulopathy
Autoimmune disorders
Arterial venous malformation
Alveolar hemorrhage
Mitral stenosis
Pneumonia

- This is a low-pressure circuit and is less frequently the source of massive bleeding.

Presentation

Classic presentation

- Worldwide, tuberculosis (TB) is the most common cause of massive hemoptysis. In the United States, patients frequently have a history of pulmonary disease and/or smoking, cancer, prior hemoptysis, immunosuppression, cardiac disease, or coagulopathy/anticoagulant use.
- Patients may present with a sentinel bleed, with only a small amount of initial hemoptysis.

Critical presentation

- The clinical course of these patients can be difficult to predict, as small amounts of hemoptysis may suddenly become massive.
- Patients may present to the ED in extremis with active hemorrhage and respiratory failure.

Diagnosis and evaluation

- **Focused history and physical examination**
  - One must exclude bleeding from nonpulmonary source, such as a GI (hematemesis) or ENT (epistaxis) etiology. Expectorated material that has an alkaline

pH, is foamy, or contains purulence suggests lower respiratory source rather than GI source.
- One should inquire about prior episodes of hemoptysis, known etiology of hemoptysis, and the location of the lesion, if known.
- History of cancer, pulmonary disease, or smoking should be obtained. A history of anticoagulant use or other coagulation disorders should be determined.

- **Laboratory tests**
  - All patients should have complete blood count, prothrombin time and partial thromboplastin time, electrolytes, arterial blood gas, liver function tests.
  - Rapid type and cross-matching of blood should be performed.
  - If necessary, consider arterial blood gases to assess oxygenation status.
  - When obtainable, sputum samples should be sent for bacterial, fungal, and mycobacterial cultures.

- **Imaging studies**
  - Chest radiography may be helpful in identifying infiltrates, lymphadenopathy, or cavitary/mass lesions.
  - If the patient does not have active bleeding and is stable enough to go to radiology, chest CT may assist finding the etiology of hemoptysis. Bronchiectasis, lung abscess, pulmonary artery aneurysm, pulmonary embolism, and mass lesions are all abnormalities that are difficult to detect by bronchoscopy and angiography but can be identified by chest CT.

Critical management

Rapidly assess the patient's airway, breathing, and circulation
Establish and maintain airway patency
Transfuse blood products as needed for resuscitation and reversal of coagulopathy
Localize the source of bleeding
Position patient with suspected bleeding lung down
Early consultation with pulmonary, interventional radiology, and thoracic surgery services
  as indicated
Control the bleeding (i.e., bronchoscopy, angiography or surgery)
Definitive treatment of underlying source of bleeding

- **Prompt airway assessment and management**
  - If emergent intubation is indicated due to hypoxemia, poor gas exchange, hemodynamic instability, or ongoing hemoptysis, a large endotracheal tube of 8.0 mm or greater will allow for diagnostic and therapeutic bronchoscopy. Intubation should generally occur before bronchoscopy as bleeding may be accelerated or recur during the procedure.

- Unilateral lung ventilation by selective intubation into the mainstem bronchus of the nonbleeding lung can minimize spillage of blood to the unaffected lung.
- A double-lumen endotracheal tube may be used to isolate the lungs and provide selective ventilation in severe cases.
- An endobronchial blocker is a device placed bronchoscopically that may also be used to isolate the bleeding area from the rest of the lung parenchyma. Placement of these advanced tracheal and bronchial devices requires an experienced operator.
- **Resuscitation**
  - Large-bore IV access (18-gauge or larger) is imperative.
  - Blood product transfusion should be initiated for those who are coagulopathic, anemic, or bleeding rapidly.
- **Patient positioning**
  - If the bleeding site is known, immediately place the patient in lateral decubitus position with the affected lung in dependent position in order to protect the nonbleeding lung.
- **Localize source of bleeding**
  - Flexible bronchoscopy is the initial diagnostic and therapeutic procedure of choice and can easily be performed at the bedside. Localizing the bleeding requires visualization of active bleeding.
  - Rigid bronchoscopy provides benefits of greater suctioning and superior visualization but is used less often because it must be performed in the OR and it cannot visualize distal airways like flexible bronchoscopy.
  - When bronchoscopy is nondiagnostic or if bleeding continues, angiography is the next test of choice allowing for both localization and therapeutic embolization.
- **Control the bleeding**
  - *Bronchoscopic techniques:*
    - Techniques to control hemorrhage include irrigation with cold saline (causing local vasoconstriction); topical administration of vasoconstrictive agents (epinephrine or vasopressin) or topical coagulant; endobronchial balloon tamponade; laser therapy; electrocautery; and unilateral lung ventilation.
  - *Bronchial artery embolization:*
    - Embolization may be a first-line treatment in many cases.
    - This is often a definitive treatment and has replaced the need for emergent surgery in many patients. It is used primarily for hemorrhage involving bronchial circulation refractory to bronchoscopic interventions.
    - In patients requiring surgical treatment, embolization can stop or slow bleeding, which reduces operative risk.
  - *Surgical means:*
    - Uncontrollable, unilateral massive hemoptysis refractory to bronchoscopy or angiographic embolization should be evaluated promptly by a thoracic surgeon for potential lung resection.

- Relative contraindications to surgery include severe or diffuse underlying pulmonary disease and active TB. Every effort should be made to stabilize patient before surgery as perioperative mortality is much higher with active bleeding.
- Definitive therapy for massive hemoptysis includes treatment of the underlying cause.

Sudden deterioration

- If the patient has worsening respiratory distress, intubate the patient to protect the airway.
- If the patient becomes hemodynamically unstable due to exsanguination, transfuse blood products through a large-bore IV or central access, reverse any coagulopathy that exists, and initiate inotropic support as needed.

Vasopressor of choice: give blood products first then consider norepinephrine.

REFERENCES

Corder R. Hemoptysis. *Emerg Med Clin North Am*. 2003; **21**: 421–35.

Ingbar DH. Massive hemoptysis: Initial management. In: Wilson KC, ed. *UpToDate*. Waltham, MA: UpToDate; 2012.

Jean-Baptiste E. Clinical assessment and management of massive hemoptysis. *Crit Care Med*. 2000; **28**: 1642.

Sopko DR, Smith TP. Bronchial artery embolization for hemoptysis. *Semin Intervent Radiol*. 2011; **28**: 48–62.

Sukkar A. Hemoptysis. *Piccini & Nilsson: The Osler Medical Handbook*. Philadelphia: Saunders. 2006; 892–898.

34

Pulmonary embolism

Liza Gonen Smith

Introduction

- Acute pulmonary embolism (PE) carries a high risk of morbidity and mortality and has a wide spectrum of severity, from incidental diagnosis in an asymptomatic patient to sudden refractory shock and cardiovascular collapse.
- Although the exact incidence remains uncertain, it is estimated that approximately 600 000 patients are diagnosed with PE annually in the United States, with mortality rates as high as 30% for patients with hemodynamic instability at presentation.
- The diagnosis of PE is often complicated by presentations that can be subtle, atypical, or confounded by another coexisting disease.

Presentation

Classic presentation

- Suspect PE in any patient with new or worsening dyspnea, chest pain (particularly pleuritic or atypical chest pain), syncope, hypoxemia, or prolonged hypotension.
- Suspicion must be heightened in patients with a higher risk for venous thromboembolism (Table 34.1), as about 79% of patients diagnosed with acute PE have evidence of deep vein thrombosis (DVT), such as pain or swelling, in their legs.
- Fever, tachypnea, and tachycardia are common but nonspecific findings.

Practical Emergency Resuscitation and Critical Care, ed. Kaushal Shah, Jarone Lee, Kamal Medlej, and Scott D. Weingart. Published by Cambridge University Press. © Kaushal Shah, Jarone Lee, Kamal Medlej, and Scott D. Weingart 2013.

Table 34.1. Risk factors for venous thromboembolism

Age >40 years
History of venous thromboembolism
Prolonged immobilization, including long air or ground travel
Cancer
Trauma or major surgery
Obesity
Pregnancy
Hormonal contraceptives or hormonal replacement therapy
Acute illness or inflammatory diseases (such as inflammatory bowel disease)
Genetic or acquired thrombophilia
- Factor V Leiden
- Lupus anticoagulant
- Antiphospholipid antibody syndrome
- Antithrombin III deficiency
- Protein C or protein S deficiency

Critical presentation

- With significant clot burden, right heart strain can develop, with right ventricular dilation and hypokinesis and clinical signs of right heart failure.
- Decreased flow of blood through the right-heart system can lead to impaired left ventricular filling, causing tachycardia and systemic hypotension.
- Pulseless electrical activity (PEA) is the most common rhythm in cardiac arrest caused by obstructive PE.

Diagnosis and evaluation

- The evaluation for suspected PE is tailored to the level of the clinician's suspicion for this diagnosis based on the patient's history, physical examination, and risk factors.
- **ECG**
  - ECG changes in PE are usually the result of acute pulmonary hypertension, manifesting as tachycardia, symmetrical T wave inversion in the anterior leads (V_1–V_4), the nonspecific McGinn–White $S_1Q_3T_3$ pattern, P-wave pulmonale, and right bundle branch block.
- **Chest radiography and ultrasonography**
  - A chest radiograph is rarely diagnostic for PE, but can identify alternative diagnoses.
  - "Hampton's hump," a pleural-based, wedge-shaped area of infiltrate, can be seen in pulmonary infarction and is suggestive of PE.

Table 34.2. Clinical prediction score for suspected acute pulmonary embolism

---

Canadian (Wells) prediction score
  Symptoms of deep-venous thrombosis – 3.0
  PE as likely as or more likely than alternative diagnosis – 3.0
  Heart rate >100 beats/minute – 1.5
  Immobilization or surgery in previous 4 weeks – 1.5
  Previous DVT or PE – 1.5
  Hemoptysis – 1.0
  Cancer – 1.0
Total score
  <2 – low pretest probability
  2 to 6 – moderate pretest probability
  >6 – high pretest probability

- "Westermark's sign," unilateral lung oligemia, is a rare radiographic manifestation of a large PE.
- If DVT is identified on venous ultrasonography of the lower extremities in a hemodynamically stable patient with suspected PE, anticoagulant therapy can be initiated before further testing.
- **Laboratory tests**
  - The D-dimer assay, which detects the presence of fibrin degradation products, can be used as a screening test for the presence of thromboembolic disease.
  - Positive screens are nonspecific, as this test can become positive in many inflammatory states including trauma, infection, or other acute illness.
  - If a patient is deemed to have low-to-moderate clinical probability for PE estimated by clinical prediction rules (Table 34.2), a negative D-dimer test can preclude the need for further evaluation and imaging studies.
  - **Troponin** and **brain natriuretic peptide (BNP)** levels can risk-stratify patients with confirmed diagnosis of PE, but are not diagnostic tools.
  - Elevated BNP and troponin have independently been associated with increased risk of adverse outcome and death in acute PE.
- **Pulmonary imaging**
  - If the clinical probability for PE is high or the D-dimer screen is positive, perform CT angiography of the lungs (Figure 34.1) or ventilation–perfusion (VQ) scintigraphy if CT is contraindicated, such as in renal failure or allergy to intravenous contrast dye.
  - Magnetic resonance angiography has insufficient sensitivity for the diagnosis of PE.
  - Due to the accuracy of noninvasive imaging, use of conventional pulmonary angiography is rare.

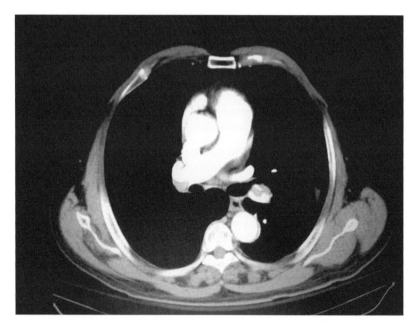

Figure 34.1. Computed tomography angiography of the chest showing a pulmonary embolism.

Critical management

Maintain a high index of suspicion for PE
Risk-stratify stable patients
Test with D-dimer, or CT scan as indicated
Promptly resuscitate hypoxemic or hemodynamically unstable patients
Consider lysis or thrombectomy in hemodynamically unstable patients
Evaluate for submassive PE with troponin, brain natriuretic peptide, and echo
Initiate anticoagulation

- **Manage ABCs**
  - Consider intubation for patients with refractory, severe hypoxemia.
  - Resuscitate hemodynamically unstable patients with volume to maintain pre-load. Also consider vasopressor and inotropic support for fluid unresponsive hypotension.
  - If a central line is indicated, this should be placed before starting anticoagulation or thrombolysis.

- **Risk-stratify massive and submassive PEs**
  - Massive PE is a PE leading to sustained hypotension (SBP <90 mmHg for 15 minutes), bradycardia, or pulselessness.
  - Submassive PE shows evidence of right heart dysfunction or myocardial necrosis:
    - Troponin I >0.4 ng/mL (or troponin T >0.1 ng/mL)
    - Brain natriuretic peptide (BNP) >90 pg/mL or N-terminal pro-BNP >500 pg/mL
    - ECG changes with a new right bundle-branch block, anteroseptal ST elevation or depression, or anteroseptal T-wave inversion
    - Echocardiography demonstrating right ventricular dilation or hypokinesis.
  - Intravenous thrombolysis has been associated with reduced mortality among hemodynamically unstable patients with PE and is typically reserved for patients with massive PEs as they have a high risk of circulatory collapse, respiratory failure, and death.
  - Patients in whom fibrinolysis is determined to be indicated should receive alteplase 15 mg bolus followed by 85 mg over 2 hours.
  - Data do not support routine thrombolysis of submassive PEs; these should be carefully assessed on an individual basis. Special consideration for thrombolysis should be given to patients with submassive PEs with RV strain by echo or who develop hypotension or respiratory failure. Consultation with Cardiology is recommended.
  - Surgical or percutaneous mechanical thrombectomy should be reserved for unstable patients with an absolute contraindication to thrombolytic treatment.
- **Anticoagulation**
  - Patients diagnosed with PE should be started on anticoagulation unless otherwise contraindicated to prevent clot propagation.
  - Patients with a high clinical probability of PE should be started on anticoagulation therapy while awaiting diagnostic confirmation.
  - Intravenous unfractionated heparin, subcutaneous low–molecular weight heparin, or fondaparinux should be initiated as bridging therapy to a vitamin-K antagonist:
    - Unfractionated heparin: Initial bolus dose of 80 IU/kg IV (up to 5000 IU) followed by continuous infusion of 18 IU/kg per hour to target activated thromboplastin time 1.5–2.5 times normal value
    - Enoxaparin: 1 mg/kg subcutaneously given twice daily
    - Fondaparinux: 5 mg subcutaneously once daily for patients weighing less than 50 kg; 7.5 mg once daily for patients weighing 50–100 kg; and 10 mg once daily for patients weighing >100 kg
    - Warfarin: daily oral dosing to achieve a target international normalized ratio (INR) of 2.0–3.0.

- Low–molecular weight heparin and fondaparinux are renally cleared and should not be used in patients with a creatinine clearance less than 30 mL/minute.
- Enoxaparin is the preferred anticoagulation regimen for pregnant women and patients with cancer.
- Oral direct thrombin inhibitors, such as dabigatran, and factor Xa inhibitors such as rivaroxaban, are not yet approved for anticoagulation therapy in pulmonary embolism.
- Patients diagnosed with PE in the setting of a major contraindication to anticoagulation should have an inferior vena caval filter (IVC filter) placed to prevent further embolic burden from reaching the lungs.
- Most hemodynamically stable patients with PE will recover completely with anticoagulation therapy.

Sudden deterioration

- The most common causes for sudden decompensation are respiratory and hemodynamic as the result of sudden shift or increase in clot burden.
- Intubation may be necessary to improve oxygenation/ventilation and establish control of the airway.
- If hypotension develops or remains refractory to resuscitation, consider inotropic support and thrombolysis.

Vasopressor of choice: norepinephrine.

REFERENCES

Agnelli G, Becattini C. Acute pulmonary embolism. *N Engl J Med*. 2010; **363**: 266–74.

Jaff MR, McMurtry MS, Archer SL, *et al.* American Heart Association Council on Cardiopulmonary, Critical Care, Perioperative and Resuscitation; American Heart Association Council on Peripheral Vascular Disease; American Heart Association Council on Arteriosclerosis, Thrombosis and Vascular Biology. Management of massive and submassive pulmonary embolism, iliofemoral deep vein thrombosis, and chronic thromboembolic pulmonary hypertension: a scientific statement from the American Heart Association. *Circulation*. 2011; **123**: 1788–830.

Marx JA, *et al. Rosen's Emergency Medicine: Concepts and Clinical Practice*, 6th edn. Vol. 2. Philadelphia, PA: Mosby Elsevier; 2006: 1368–82.

Piazza G, Goldhaber SZ. Acute pulmonary embolism. *Circulation*. 2006; **114**: e28–47.

Tapson VF. Acute pulmonary embolism. *N Engl J Med*. 2008; **358**: 1037–52.

35

Gastrointestinal bleeding

Bina Vasantharam and Joel Moll

Introduction

- **Upper gastrointestinal bleed (UGIB)**
  - UGIB is defined as bleeding proximal to the ligament of Treitz (esophageal, gastric, or duodenal source).
  - More common than lower gastrointestinal bleeding.
  - Most common cause is peptic ulcer disease.
  - Common etiologies are listed in Table 35.1 (in order of frequency).
  - Emergency management can be divided into variceal versus nonvariceal bleeding.
  - Esophageal varices result from increased portal resistance and blood flow. They can cause upper or lower GI bleeds, and have a higher mortality than nonvariceal bleeding, with an estimated 30–50% mortality during the first variceal bleed episode.
- **Lower gastrointestinal bleed (LGIB)**
  - LGIB is defined as bleeding distal to the ligament of Treitz.
  - Less common than UGIB, approximately one-fourth to one-third of patients with GIB.
  - LGIB generally has lower mortality rate than UGIB.
  - Most common cause is diverticular disease.
  - Often self-limited, although can be massive.
  - Common etiologies are listed in Table 35.2 (in order of frequency).
- **Differential diagnosis considerations**
  - Black stools: iron or bismuth (Pepto-Bismol), but will be guaiac negative.

Practical Emergency Resuscitation and Critical Care, ed. Kaushal Shah, Jarone Lee, Kamal Medlej, and Scott D. Weingart. Published by Cambridge University Press. © Kaushal Shah, Jarone Lee, Kamal Medlej, and Scott D. Weingart 2013.

Table 35.1. Common etiologies of UGIB

Adult patients
Peptic ulcer disease
Erosive gastritis, esophagitis, or duodenitis
Varices (esophageal and gastric)
Portal hypertensive gastropathy
Mallory Weiss tears
Malignancy
Aortoenteric fistula
Pediatric patients
Esophagitis
Gastritis
Peptic ulcer disease

Table 35.2. Common etiologies of LGIB

Adult patients
Diverticular disease
Vascular ectasia
Ischemic colitis
Hemorrhoids
Inflammatory bowel disease
Malignancy
Meckel's diverticulum
Pediatric patients
Infectious colitis
Inflammatory/infectious enteritis/colitis
If the patient is under 2 years old, consider Meckel's diverticulum or intussusception

- Bright red stools or emesis: red foods including wine, beets.
- Potential false-positive guaiac tests: certain fruits (cantaloupe, grapefruit, figs), uncooked vegetables, red meat, methylene blue, chlorophyll, iodide, cupric sulfate, bromides – however, **any positive test should not be second-guessed.**
- Potential false-negative guaiac test: dry stools, low pH, antacids, antioxidants (e.g., high-dose vitamin C); use of hemoccult developer and card on gastric contents will cause false-negative due to the pH (use separate gastroccult developer and card).
- Oropharyngeal or nasopharyngeal bleeding.

Presentation

Classic presentation

- **UGIB**
  - Patients typically present with hematemesis, coffee-ground emesis, and/or melena.
  - *Hematemesis:* more easily recognized as "coffee grounds," usually signifies higher risk of active bleeding.
  - *Melena:* dark, tarry stools. Usually suggests a minimum loss of 100–200 mL of blood from UGI tract. Dark color is due to the partial digestion of blood and therefore indicates blood that has been present in the GI tract for 12–14 hours.
- **LGIB**
  - Patients typically present with bright red blood per rectum (BRBPR), also known as hematochezia.
  - **Caveat:** large (usually >1 L) or brisk UGIB may present with BRBPR or hematochezia as well. Approximately 10–15% of hematochezia is due to UGIB.
- In addition, patients may present with symptoms/signs of associated comorbidities (e.g., encephalopathy due to liver disease, dyspnea due to blood loss, etc.).

Critical presentation

- Higher severity of disease is indicated by:
  - Signs of shock such as hypotension, tachycardia, altered mental status (AMS), decreased urine output (UOP), cool skin, syncope, orthostasis. Change in pulse with posture is more sensitive than hypotension, but may be masked by medications (e.g., beta-blockers).
  - Elderly patient with more than two comorbidities, recurrent hemorrhage, or ischemic chest pain.
  - History of variceal bleed, known liver disease, history of cirrhosis, stigmata of liver disease, excessive alcohol use.
  - Aorto-enteric fistula should be considered if there is a history of aortic graft surgery.
  - The presence of hematemesis, hematochezia in the setting of UGIB is more likely variceal bleed or more significant bleed (both associated with higher mortality).

Diagnosis and evaluation

- **Vital signs**
  - Hypotension, tachycardia, and tachypnea can indicate hemorrhagic shock and requires immediate treatment.

- **History**
  - Ask about history that may be significant for peptic ulcer disease, liver disease, diverticular disease, use of anticoagulation, aortic surgery, etc.
  - Associated risk factors for *peptic ulcer disease:*
    - Nonsteroidal anti-inflammatory drugs (NSAIDs), anticoagulants, glucocorticoid, or aspirin use
    - *Helicobacter pylori* infection
    - Critical illness
    - Gastric acid production.
- **Physical**
  - Vital signs as above.
  - Rectal examination: On examination, evaluate for melena, BRBPR, heme-positive test of stool, hemorrhoids.
  - Abdominal examination: ascites, old surgical scars, pain/tenderness suggesting acute abdomen (e.g., rebound and guarding).
  - Other: check for stigmata of liver disease (e.g., encephalopathy, gynecomastia), bruising suggestive of anticoagulant use or thrombocytopenia.
- **Nasogastric aspiration and lavage** (controversial due to lack of evidence):
  - Procedure causes many false negative results, as well as false positive results.
  - May not be useful for risk stratification.
  - May be helpful in select patients: e.g., patients with hematochezia or melena only without hematemesis to evaluate for potential UGIB.
  - Risk of use among patients with esophageal varices is unknown.
- **Laboratory testing**
  - *Complete blood count:*
    - Hemoglobin/hematocrit (Hgb/Hct) may not reflect the blood loss during the acute bleeding period.
    - Suspected or confirmed significant blood loss OR ongoing bleeding are indications for transfusion.
    - Initial Hct <30% for UGIB portends worse prognosis.
  - *Coagulation profile (PT/PTT/INR):*
    - Initial elevated INR from underlying liver disease portends worse outcomes
    - **Caveat:** Neither coagulation studies nor platelet count reflects the effects of clopidogrel (Plavix) or other new anticoagulants such as dabigatran (Pradaxa) or rivaroxaban (Xarelto).
  - *Type and screen/type and cross:*
    - For critical and potentially critical patients, be sure to have blood preemptively prepared by the blood bank.
  - *Chemistries:*
    - BUN/creatinine ratio >30 is suggestive of GI bleed because digested blood is a source of urea.
    - Use chemistries to evaluate for associated comorbidities such as renal failure or liver disease.

- *Cardiac enzymes:*
  - Use cardiac enzymes to evaluate for signs of cardiac stress and to evaluate for other etiologies (e.g., abdominal pain could be the only symptom of a myocardial infarction).
- **Glasgow-Blatchford score**
  - This score is based on points assigned from the patient's vital signs, blood analysis results, and clinical presentation.
  - It can be used to help assess which patients may be discharged home with outpatient follow-up. Patients **must have all the following criteria** to be considered a score of 0 and potentially safe for outpatient follow-up:
    - Normal Hgb (>12.9 g/dL for men, 11.9 g/dL for women)
    - SBP >109 mmHg
    - Pulse <100 beats/minute
    - No melena, syncope, heart failure, or liver failure.
- **Differentiating UGIB from LGIB**
  - *UGIB is suggested by*
    - History of upper GI bleed or peptic ulcer disease risk factors
    - Melanic stool on examination
    - NG lavage with blood or coffee grounds, and BUN/Cr ratio ≥30 (all of these have specificities over 90%, but low sensitivities).
  - *LGIB is suggested by*
    - History of LGIB, hemorrhoids, diverticular disease
    - Clots in stool
    - Remember, 10–15% of patients presenting with BRBPR have UGIB.

Critical management

- **All patients**
  - Large-bore IV access for volume resuscitation: short, large, peripheral IVs. **Remember, due to smaller size of lumen and length, multilumen central lines are significantly slower and not the best for volume resuscitation!**
  - Secure the airway if indicated.
  - Type and cross for blood products.
  - Transfuse for active bleeding or known low hemoglobin.
  - Correct coagulopathy, thrombocytopenia:
    - Consider indication for the patient's anticoagulation and weigh the risk of further bleeding before reversing anticoagulation.
    - Consider fresh frozen plasma (FFP) or prothrombin complex concentrate (PCC) to reverse warfarin, factor Xa inhibitors, and coagulopathy from liver disease.
    - Consider protamine for patients on heparin.
    - With active bleeding, goal platelet count should be >50 000 cells/microliter.

- Consider platelet transfusion for patients with dysfunctional platelets (e.g., aspirin/clopidogrel).
- Consider desmopressin (DDAVP) in the setting of renal failure to help with uremic platelet dysfunction.
- There are no reversal agents for newer direct thrombin inhibitors.
- There is no evidence to support use of factor VIIa.
- Consider antifibrinolytic agents in the setting of massive bleeding.
- Massive transfusion protocols are helpful for significant bleeding in order to prevent further coagulopathy due to transfusion of high volume of crystalloid or only red cells.
- Consider consulting GI for emergent endoscopy.
- Consider admitting to intensive care unit.
- **Management specifics for UGIB**
  - *Peptic ulcer disease:*
    - Consider proton pump inhibitors (PPIs) if there is suspicion for peptic ulcer disease.
    - H_2-receptor antagonists have not been shown to have the same reduction in rebleeding or transfusion requirements as PPIs.
    - Consider use of erythromycin to promote gastric motility and help improve visualization during endoscopy.
  - *Variceal bleeding:*
    - Decrease splanchnic blood flow (limited evidence supporting use):
      - Octreotide: bolus and infusion.
      - Vasopressin: bolus and infusion.
    - Prophylactic antibiotics (usually fluoroquinolone or third-generation cephalosporin) to prevent spontaneous bacterial peritonitis due to higher risk of bacterial translocation during acute GIB.
    - Insertion of Blakemore/Minnesota tube to tamponade bleeding varices. Can be used for both gastric and esophageal varices and potentially rectal varices as well.
    - Transjugular intrahepatic portosystemic shunt (TIPS):
      - Placement of stent from portal vein to hepatic vein to decrease pressure in the portal system.
      - Usually placed by the interventional radiology team.
      - Can act as a bridge to liver transplantation in the setting of severe or recurrent bleeding.
- **Management specifics for LGIB**
  - There are fewer evidence-based therapies for LGIB than for UGIB.
  - Angiography can identify the site in 40% of LGIB, but must be actively bleeding (usually indicated by unstable vital signs or continued need for transfusion).
  - Consider tagged RBC scan, capsule endoscopy, or push enteroscopy for stable patients.
  - Sigmoidoscopy/colonoscopy is also helpful for stable patients and has the potential benefit of also being therapeutic.
  - Management of LGIB requires surgical intervention more often than UGIB.

Special circumstances

- **Aortoenteric fistula**
  - Suggested by a history of aortic graft (at any time).
  - The fistula usually involves the lower duodenum or jejunum.
  - Emergent surgical consultation is needed as esophagogastroduodenoscopy or colonoscopy will not visualize these areas and will not be therapeutic.
- **Liver disease**
  - Manage as variceal bleeding.
- **Jehovah's Witnesses**
  - It is unlawful to transfuse if the patient expressly forbids it; document the patient's wishes carefully.
  - Manage shock and critical illness according to standard protocols.
  - Experimental use of hemoglobin substitutes is not yet approved by the FDA.
  - Most other treatment options (i.e., erythropoietin, factor VIIa) are not helpful in the short term for acute bleeding.
  - Some patients will accept fractions of whole blood (e.g., albumin) or transfusions.

Vasopressor of choice: give blood products (i.e., massive transfusion) first then consider norepinephrine.

REFERENCES

Alharbi A, Almadi M, Barkun, Martel M. Predictors of a variceal source among patients presenting with upper gastrointestinal bleeding. *Can J Gastroenterol*. 2012; **26**: 187–92.

Barkun AN, Bardou M, Kuipers EJ, *et al.* International consensus recommendations on the management of patients with nonvariceal upper gastrointestinal bleeding. *Ann Intern Med*. 2010; **152**: 101–13.

Berend K, Levi M. Management of adult Jehovah's Witness patients with acute bleeding. *Am J Med*. 2009; **122**: 1071–6.

Chavez-Tapia NC, Barrientos-Gutierrez T, Tellez-Avila FL, *et al.* Antibiotic prophylaxis for cirrhotic patients with upper gastrointestinal bleeding. *Cochrane Database Syst Rev*. 2010; (9): CD 002907.

Hwang JH, Fischer DA, Ben-Menachem T, *et al.* The role of endoscopy in the management of acute non-variceal upper GI bleeding. *Gastrointest Endosc*. 2012; **75**: 1132–8.

Palamidessi N, Sinert R, Falzon L, Zehtabchi S. Nasogastric aspiration and lavage in emergency department patients with hematochezia or melena without hematemesis. *Acad Emerg Med*. 2010; **17**: 126–32.

Sreedharan A, Martin J, Leontiadis GI, *et al.* Proton pump inhibitor treatment initiated prior to endoscopic diagnosis in upper gastrointestinal bleeding. *Cochrane Database Syst Rev*. 2010; (7): CD005415. doi: 10.1002/14651858.CD005415.pub3.

Stabile BE, Stamos MJ. Surgical management of gastrointestinal bleeding. *Gastroenterol Clin North Am*. 2000; **29**: 189–222.

Stanley AJ, Ashley D, Dalton HR, *et al.* Outpatient management of patients with low-risk upper gastrointestinal haemorrhage: multicentre validation and prospective evaluation. *Lancet.* 2009; **373**(9657): 101–13.

Van Ryn J, Stangier J, Haertter S, *et al.* Dabigatran etexilate – a novel, reversible, oral direct thrombin inhibitor: interpretation of coagulation assays and reversal of anticoagulant activity. *J Thromb Haemost.* 2010; **103**: 1116–27.

Vilahur G, Choi BG, Zafar MU, *et al.* Normalization of platelet reactivity in clopidogrel-treated subjects. *J Thromb Haemost.* 2007; **5**: 82–90.

36

Abdominal aortic aneurysms

Marie Carmelle Tabuteau, Payal Modi, and Ted Stettner

Introduction

- Abdominal aortic aneurysm (AAA) refers to aortic dilatations of >3 cm.
- True AAA is a localized dilatation of the aorta caused by weakening of the aorta wall involving all three layers (intima, media, and adventitia).
- AAA most commonly (90% of occurrences) involves descending aorta, especially the infrarenal aorta.
- Pseudoaneurysm is blood flow that communicates with the arterial lumen but is not enclosed by the normal vessel wall. Pseudoaneurysms are contained by adventitia or surrounding soft tissue.
- Aortic dissection is *not* the same as AAA. In aortic dissection, blood enters the media of the aorta and splits the aortic wall.
- AAA causes 15 000 deaths annually in the United States.
  - Screening and early intervention have helped improve death rates and mortality is only 1–2% for electively operated AAAs.
  - On the other hand, mortality is up to 90% for ruptured aneurysms and 50% for those that require emergency surgery. Rupture risk is related to the size of the AAA as detailed in Table 36.1.
- Providers should be aware of the natural history of expansion and rupture of AAA and aggressively advocate repair in any unstable patient with a known AAA. Risk factors for the development of an AAA are listed in Table 36.2.

Practical Emergency Resuscitation and Critical Care, ed. Kaushal Shah, Jarone Lee, Kamal Medlej, and Scott D. Weingart. Published by Cambridge University Press. © Kaushal Shah, Jarone Lee, Kamal Medlej, and Scott D. Weingart 2013.

Table 36.1. AAA size and risk of rupture

AAA diameter (cm)	5-year risk of rupture (%/year)
<4.0 cm	0%
4.0–4.9 cm	0.5–5%
5.0–5.9 cm	3–15%
6.0–6.9 cm	10–20%
7.0–7.9 cm	20–40%
≥8.0 cm	30–50%

Table 36.2. Risk factors for AAA

Male sex (6:1)
Age older than 50 years
History of atherosclerotic disease
Family history of AAA in first-degree relative
Smoking (90% of AAA)
Hypertension
Hyperlipidemia
Previous aortic aneurysm
End-stage syphilis
Mycotic infections (immunosuppression, IV drug use, syphilis)

Presentation

Classic presentation

- The classic triad of ruptured AAA is hypotension, pain, and pulsatile abdominal mass. This occurs in only half of the patients.
- Typical pain is usually described as abdominal or lower back.
- Any patient with these symptoms and a known AAA is at risk for imminent rupture, if rupture has not already occurred.
- Vital sign stability should *not* be reassuring as these patients can deteriorate rapidly.
- Hypotension is the least consistent part of the triad, occurring in as few as one-third of patients.
- Atypical presentations are common. Inflammatory aneurysms may present with fever or weight loss. Patients may complain of pain in the chest, thigh, inguinal area, or scrotum.
- Initial blood loss may be minor and the patient may present with normal vital signs. Vital sign stability should not necessarily be reassuring as these patients can deteriorate rapidly.

Critical presentation

- Rupture is often the first symptom of patients with AAA and is usually experienced as severe abdominal or back pain, especially lumbar pain.
- Pain is often described as severe or abrupt in onset, and characterized as a ripping or tearing sensation radiating to the back.
- Bleeding can lead to hemorrhagic shock with hypotension, altered mental status, syncope, and sudden death.
- Signs of rupture:
  - Hypotension
  - Periumbilical ecchymosis (Cullen's sign)
  - Flank ecchymosis (Grey–Turner's sign)
  - Scrotal or vulvar hematomas.
- Less common but critical presentations of AAA include
  - Extremity ischemia due to peripheral embolization of a thrombus from within the aneurysm
  - Complete aortic occlusion
  - Aortic fistulization:
    - Aortoenteric fistulas within the duodenum can present with unexplained upper or lower GI bleeding.
    - Aortovenous fistulas into the inferior vena cava can present as high-output heart failure with lower-extremity edema, dilated superficial veins, decreased peripheral blood flow, and renal insufficiency with hematuria.
  - Disseminated intravascular coagulation (DIC).

Diagnosis and evaluation

- **Physical examination**
  - As above, vital signs may be normal early in the course of disease but hemodynamic decompensation can occur very rapidly.
  - Physical examination may be unremarkable, and the classic finding of a palpable abdominal mass is not always appreciated.
  - In the lower extremities, a widened pulse pressure may suggest the presence of AAA.
  - A benign clinical examination is not considered reliable enough to rule out AAA. Factors such as size of the AAA and the patient's body habitus may disguise underlying pathology.
- **Diagnostic tests**
  - *Laboratory tests:*
    - No specific laboratory studies exist that can be used to make the diagnosis of abdominal aortic aneurysm.
    - Patients presenting with a ruptured AAA may have anemia, but a normal hemoglobin certainly does not rule out even ruptured AAA.

- In mycotic aneurysms, blood cultures are often positive and reveal the nature of the infecting agent.
- *Abdominal radiography:*
  - Although symptomatic aneurysms are usually large and often calcified, abdominal radiography is not the preferred method as it has low sensitivity and specificity for detecting AAA when compared with ultrasound and CT.
  - If an abdominal aortic aneurysm is appreciated on the radiograph, the most common findings are paravertebral soft tissue mass or calcification of the aortic wall.
- *Ultrasound:*
  - Ultrasound (US) is the preferred method of screening with 100% sensitivity in detecting AAA.
  - Compared with computed tomography, US is low in cost and has no radiation or contrast exposure.
  - In the emergent setting, US can be performed at bedside to evaluate a patient with potential ruptured AAA, averting the need to take an unstable patient to the radiology suite.
  - Bedside US must contain views of the aorta along the entire course for appropriate diagnosis. Patients with a normal diameter throughout the course of the abdominal aorta likely do not have AAA.
  - This technique is limited by obesity, bowel gas, and abdominal tenderness.
  - Operator dependency is a major disadvantage of the US study.
    - Depending on the level of skill and experience the US examination is more prone to interpretive or technical error.
    - Patient habitus may also cause inaccurate results secondary to inconsistent views of the aorta.
  - Although US is sensitive in detecting AAA, it cannot be relied on to determine whether there has been a rupture of the AA. Free intraperitoneal or retroperitoneal blood in the presence of other clinical symptoms may be suggestive of rupture but it is not always appreciated.
- *Computed tomography (CT):*
  - 100% accurate in determining the presence and exact size of AAA.
  - CT is more sensitive than other imaging modalities in detecting retroperitoneal hemorrhage associated with aneurysm.
  - IV contrast is not necessary to identify aneurysm and acute hemorrhage is well visualized on scans done without contrast.
  - During AAA rupture, blood is often seen as retroperitoneal fluid located adjacent to the aneurysm, often tracking into the perinephric space or along the psoas muscle.
  - The crescent sign (layering blood within aorta) indicates an impending rupture.

- *Contrast aortography:*
  - This was the gold standard prior to widespread use of modern CT scanners.
  - Used for evaluation of aneurysms before elective surgery.
  - Carries risk of complications, such as bleeding, allergic reactions, atheroembolism, and nephrotoxicity.
  - Useful in documenting length of the aneurysm, especially upper and lower limits, and the extent of associated atherosclerotic vascular disease.
  - The presence of mural clots may reduce the luminal size; thus, aortography may underestimate the diameter of an aneurysm.
- *Magnetic resonance imaging (MRI):*
  - MRI is minimally invasive and, when combined with magnetic resonance angiography (MRA), can provide excellent details for the preoperative evaluation of AAAs.
  - MRI has 100% sensitivity in detecting aneurysms, and successfully identifies the proximal and distal extent of the aneurysms, the number and origins of renal arteries, and the presence of inflammation.
  - The use of MRI is not realistic for unstable patients due to the length of time required to obtain the images and the difficulty accessing and monitoring the patient.

Critical management

- Ruptured AAA is fatal unless treated surgically. Hemodynamically unstable patients should be taken to the OR as soon as possible and diagnostic testing should be kept to a minimum.
- Unstable patients should have standard resuscitative measures (e.g., large-bore intravenous access, cardiac monitoring, supplemental oxygen, blood type and cross-matching, vasopressors) while preparing for transfer to the operating room.
- Symptomatic patients with known AAA should be evaluated by vascular surgery regardless of the AAA size.
- **Surgical management**
  - Patients may be taken to the OR on the basis of clinical suspicion as testing may delay treatment and increase the risk of death.
  - Patients taken to the OR as soon as possible after arrival in ED have a higher chance of survival than those patients who have had delayed OR times because of stabilization in the ED.
  - There is a 50% operative mortality rate in patients with ruptured AAA.
  - The vascular surgeon may choose to repair via open approach with laparotomy or endovascular technique.
    - Open AAA repair requires direct access to the aorta through an abdominal or retroperitoneal approach.

Table 36.3. Nonemergent treatment and monitoring

Asymptomatic AAA size	Monitoring
3–4 cm	Annual ultrasound
4–4.5 cm	Ultrasound every 6 months
>4.5 cm	Refer to vascular surgeon
5.5	Surgery indicated

- Endovascular repair of an AAA involves gaining access to the lumen of the abdominal aorta, usually via small incisions over the femoral vessels.
- An endograft, typically a cloth graft with a stent exoskeleton, is placed within the lumen of the AAA, extending distally into the iliac arteries.
- **Nonemergent treatment and monitoring**
  - Nonemergent management is summarized in Table 36.3. The patient must be compliant with follow-up in order to be safely managed expectantly.
  - AAAs greater than 5 cm are at greatest risk for rupture and should be referred to a vascular surgeon for prompt evaluation (outpatient evaluation only if asymptomatic).
  - In patients with a small AAA, reduction of the expansion rate and rupture risk can be accomplished with smoking cessation, blood pressure control, and beta blockade.
- **Complications of repair**
  - With more patients living longer after AAA repairs, more and more of these patients will present to the ED with complications from the repair.
  - *Graft infection:*
    - Infection can disrupt the anastomosis between native artery and the graft leading to leakage of blood and pseudoaneurysm formation.
    - Subtle signs of graft infections include low-grade fever, abdominal, or back pain.
    - Patients may also present in florid septic shock due to bacteremia.
    - CT should be performed to evaluate possible infection. Findings consistent with graft infection include fluid or gas collections adjacent to the graft.
  - *Aortoenteric fistula (AEF):*
    - AEF most commonly presents as gastrointestinal bleeding.
    - Severity of bleeding can range from occult to massive.
    - An AEF must be considered in any patient with GI bleeding and history of abdominal aortic surgery.
    - In an unstable patient, diagnostic testing may be averted in lieu of laparotomy or angiography.
    - In a stable patient upper endoscopy and/or CT may be useful diagnostic adjuncts.
    - Patients with AEF may also get secondary graft infection.

- *Pseudoaneurysm:*
  - Occurs at the site of leaking anastomosis.
  - Most commonly it is due to degeneration of the native vessel but can also be seen with both graft infection and AEF.
  - Patients may present with pain or pulsatile mass in the abdomen or groin.
  - Complications of pseudoaneurysm formation include rupture and downstream embolic phenomena.
  - Patients with suspected pseudoaneurysm may be evaluated with CT, US, and/or angiography.
- *Aortocaval fistula:*
  - **Aortocaval fistula is a surgical emergency.**
  - Spontaneous aortocaval fistula is rare and occurs in only 4% of all ruptured AAA.
  - Physical signs may be subtle or vague. The presence of low back pain, machinery-like abdominal murmur, and high-output cardiac failure unresponsive to medical treatment should raise the suspicion.
  - Preoperative diagnosis is crucial, as adequate preparation is needed because of the massive bleeding during surgery.
  - Successful treatment depends on management of perioperative hemodynamics as well as control of bleeding from the fistula.

Sudden deterioration

- In patients with suspected symptomatic AAA, sudden deterioration almost certainly indicates an aneurysm rupture.
- In the absence of immediate intervention, hemorrhagic shock will lead to death in more than 90% of patients.
- Immediate resuscitation should begin with packed red cells infused as quickly as possible.
- Ensure cessation of any prior antihypertensive therapies.
- Concomitant airway management should be initiated.
- **Notably, if patients require ACLS, survival is unlikely.**

Vasopressor of choice: give blood products first then consider norepinephrine.

REFERENCES

Isselbacher EM, *et al*. Diseases of the aorta. In *Braunwald's Heart Disease: A Textbook of Cardiovascular Medicine*. Philadelphia: Saunders; 2005.

Longo D, Fauci A, Kasper D, *et al*., eds. Diseases of the aorta. In *Harrison's Principles of Internal Medicine*. 18th edn. New York: McGraw-Hill; 2012.

Marx JA, Hockberger RS, Walls RM, Adams J, Rosen P, eds. Abdominal aortc aneurysm. In *Rosen's Emergency Medicine: Concepts and Clinical Practice*, 7th edn. Philadelphia, PA: Mosby Elsevier; 2010.

Metcalfe D, Holt PJ, Thompson MM. The management of abdominal aortic aneurysms. *BMJ*. 2011; **342**: 2011.

Schermerhorn ML, *et al*. Endovascular vs. open repair of abdominal aortic aneurysms in the Medicare population. *N Engl J Med*. 2008; **358**: 464.

Tintinalli J, Stapczynski JS, Ma OJ, *et al. Tintinalli's Emergency Medicine Manual*. 7th edn. New York: McGraw-Hill; 2010.

37

Acute pancreatitis

John Woodruff and Abigail Hankin

Introduction

- Pancreatitis has a litany of potential causes (Table 37.1), but within the Western world, alcohol abuse and cholelithiasis account for the overwhelming majority of cases.
- Inappropriate release of the pancreatic enzyme trypsin within the pancreas, causing injury to the pancreas and a widespread inflammatory response.
- The bulk of patients with acute pancreatitis experience a mild and self-limited disease that resolves within a few days, but 15–25% of patients will experience severe pancreatitis (5% mortality).
  - Severe disease may manifest locally within the pancreas as necrosis, hemorrhage, abscess, or pseudocyst.
  - Clinical manifestations remote to the pancreas include renal failure, both bleeding and thromboembolic events, pleural effusion, systemic inflammatory response syndrome (SIRS), shock and hemodynamic collapse, and acute respiratory distress syndrome (ARDS) secondary to loss of surfactant and SIRS.
  - The greatest challenge in emergency department management of acute pancreatitis is separating the rare critically ill patient from the many patients with benign self-limited illness and triaging them to a higher level of care.

Practical Emergency Resuscitation and Critical Care, ed. Kaushal Shah, Jarone Lee, Kamal Medlej, and Scott D. Weingart. Published by Cambridge University Press. © Kaushal Shah, Jarone Lee, Kamal Medlej, and Scott D. Weingart 2013.

Table 37.1. Causes of acute pancreatitis

Toxicological	• Chronic ethanol abuse
	• Toxic alcohols
	• Azathioprine
	• Mercaptopurine
	• Valproic acid
	• Didanosine
	• Corticosteroids
	• Sulfa drugs
	• Scorpion venom
Obstructive	• Gallstones
	• Pancreatic tumors
	• External compression
	• Pancreatic divisum
	• Parasites: clonorchiasis, ascariasis
Trauma	• Classic etiology is blunt trauma of bicycle handlebars to the epigastrium
Metabolic	• Hypertriglyceridemia
	• Hypercalcemia
Infectious	• CMV
	• HIV
	• Mumps
	• Coxsackie
	• Hepatitis A and B
	• Cryptococcus
	• Toxoplasma
	• Mycobacteria

Presentation

Classic and critical presentations

- Historical features of pancreatitis include its characteristic abdominal pain, classically described as epigastric in location and radiating to the back. This is typically associated with nausea and vomiting.
  - Painless disease in awake patients is uncommon but, for reasons that are unclear, painless pancreatitis may be seen more frequently in peritoneal dialysis patients or patients who have undergone renal transplantation.
  - The location of pain may be quite variable depending on which part of the pancreas has the most severe inflammation.
- Findings on physical examination include upper abdominal tenderness, sometimes associated with rebound and guarding.
  - The physical examination in the patient with suspected pancreatitis should involve a thorough search for findings suggestive of severe disease (discussed below): tachycardia, hypotension, acute abdominal findings, including severe

tenderness, guarding, and periumbilical and flank ecchymoses (Cullen's and Grey–Turner's signs, respectively), and an abnormal lung examination, including dyspnea and basilar rales.
- **Predicting severe illness**
  - Severe pancreatitis (which is essentially synonymous with necrotizing pancreatitis) is typically defined using the **Atlanta classification**, which was developed in 1992.

Atlanta classification
Severe pancreatitis is present if any of the following are present:
Local complications
- Necrosis
- Abscess
- Pseudocyst
Organ damage
- Shock: systolic blood pressure <90 mmHg
- Pulmonary insufficiency: PaO_2 ≤60 mmHg
- Renal failure: creatinine >2.0 mg/dL (after rehydration)
- Gastrointestinal bleeding: >500 mL in 24 hours

- **Prognostic scores**
  - Multiple scoring systems have been developed to predict the severity of illness in acute pancreatitis, but none of them should replace regular reassessment of the patient's clinical condition.
  - The most commonly used scoring system is the **Ranson score**, but the utility of this tool for the emergency physician is limited by the fact that its appropriate use requires data that is not available until 48 hours after admission.
    - *Ranson criteria:* One point if any of the following are **present on admission:**
      - Age >55 years
      - Blood glucose levels >200 mg/dL
      - WBC count >16 000/microliter
      - LDH >350 IU/L
      - AST/SGOT >250U.
    - *Ranson criteria:* One point if any of the following are present **within 48 hours of admission:**
      - Calcium <8 mg/dL
      - PaO_2 <60 mmHg
      - Base deficit >4 mEq/L
      - Decrease in hematocrit of more than 10 percentage points
      - Need for >6 L IVF resuscitation.
  - **Scoring:** The presence of three or more of the above Ranson criteria is associated with more severe disease and a higher risk of morbidity and mortality.

- An **APACHE II** score ≥8 at the time of admission has been shown in multiple studies to be predictive of mortality and has been recommended by the American Gastroenterological Association (AGA) to predict severe illness in pancreatitis.
  - Unfortunately, its use in the emergency department is limited by the fact that its appropriate use requires data that is not available until 24 hours after admission. Additionally, because of its complexity, it typically requires imputing the values into a computer for calculation.
- Several **other scoring systems** are available.
  - The **harmless acute pancreatitis score** is the easiest to apply in the emergency department. Patients with a normal serum creatinine, normal hematocrit, and no abdominal rebound or guarding almost universally have a benign course of illness.
  - The **bedside index of severity in acute pancreatitis (BISAP)** is a scoring system that uses data generally available upon admission to predict in-hospital mortality. It has been prospectively validated in multisite study for the prediction of mortality in patients with acute pancreatitis (Table 37.2). Criteria include the following:
    - BUN >25 mg/dL
    - Altered mental status
    - >2 SIRS criteria
    - Age >60
    - Pleural effusion.
- Radiological assessment of severity can be aided by use of the graded **CT Severity Index**; a low severity index score at 4 days has a sensitivity near 100% for ruling out pancreatic necrosis.
  - The CT Severity Index is based on the amount of necrosis found on CT scan. A score of 0–1 is associated with a 0% mortality and morbidity, whereas a score of 7–10 is associated with a 17% mortality and 92% complication rate.
- **Patients whose initial presentation is suggestive of a severe course of disease should be managed in a critical care unit.**

Diagnosis and evaluation

- A frequently cited **definition of pancreatitis is the presence of at least two of the following**
  - Upper abdominal pain
  - Serum lipase at least 3 times greater than the upper limit of normal
  - CT findings suggestive of acute pancreatitis.
- Laboratory findings in acute pancreatitis most importantly include elevated serum levels of **lipase** and **amylase**.

Table 37.2. BISAP criteria

Number of criteria present	Predicted in-hospital mortality
0	0.1%
1	0.5%
2	1.9%
3	5.3%
4	12.7%
5	22.7%

- Elevations of these enzymes are thought to result from local destruction of pancreatic tissue, translocating these exocrine proteins (normally confined to the lumen of the pancreatic ducts and gut) to an ectopic location within the blood.
- An elevated serum lipase is a fairly specific marker for pancreatic injury. Amylase is expressed in a variety of tissues and is notoriously nonspecific; in the appropriate clinical setting, a serum amylase >3 times the upper limit of normal can also be diagnostic of pancreatitis. However, amylase returns to normal within a few days, so a normal amylase does not rule out pancreatitis.
- Of note, **serum amylase and lipase may also be elevated in clinical situations in which there is destruction of pancreatic tissue but where acute pancreatitis is not the primary pathological condition.** Examples of this scenario include perforated peptic ulcers and septic shock.
- **The magnitude of the elevation of serum amylase and lipase does not predict disease severity.**
- If the emergency physician or admitting team are planning to use Ranson criteria, other laboratory values will be needed at the time of admission: CBC, chemistry (including AST), and LDH.
- Radiological studies are generally not needed to diagnose pancreatitis, but may be exploited to rule out other causes of abdominal pain in the setting of diagnostic uncertainty, ascertain the cause of pancreatitis, or further evaluate for the development of severe pancreatitis.
  - **CT of the abdomen** may be indicated at the time of admission if there is concern for other life-threatening causes of abdominal pain. However, a majority of patients with mild pancreatitis will not require a CT at any point during their hospitalization.
    - In patients with severe pancreatitis, abdominal CT can be useful to identify the extent of pancreatic necrosis and identify local complications, but guidelines generally recommend obtaining the CT 2–3 days after initial presentation to maximize probability of identifying necrosis.
    - MRI with gadolinium contrast medium may be an alternative to CT in patients with acute or chronic renal insufficiency, although one must weigh benefits against the risks of nephrogenic systemic fibrosis.

- Patients with a first episode of pancreatitis should receive a **focused abdominal ultrasound** to further evaluate for gallstone disease as a potential etiology of pancreatitis.
  - Ultrasonography is important in this setting because **known gallstone pancreatitis may fundamentally change management**, triggering evaluation for possible cholecystectomy, endoscopic retrograde cholangiopancreatography, and sphincterotomy (discussed below).

Critical management

- **Mild pancreatitis**
  - Generally, patients need supportive care.
  - **Forced anorexia** results in pancreatic rest. Patients are generally able to tolerate oral feeds within three to seven days. Prolonged gut rest should be avoided due to increased risk of superimposed infection that occurs with lack of enteral feeding.
  - **Narcotic analgesia** and **antiemetics** are usually needed.
    - There are hypothetical concerns about morphine paradoxically worsening pain by causing a spasm of the sphincter of Oddi. This is almost never experienced in the clinical setting.
  - **Early, aggressive fluid resuscitation** with close monitoring of volume status is vital but is often neglected in patients with acute pancreatitis. It is needed to address the hypovolemia that is caused by both emesis and a potent systemic inflammatory response. *Sample initial protocol:*
    - Hypovolemic patient: infuse 500–1000 mL/hour fluid
    - Euvolemic patient: infuse 250–350 mL/hour
    - Reassess volume status every 1–4 hours, based on vital signs, urine output, hematocrit, and mental status.
  - Patients should be frequently reevaluated for progression to severe disease or complications of acute pancreatitis.
  - Although infection is a common cause and result of progression to severe disease, **there is no evidence to support prophylactic antibiotics in mild acute pancreatitis.**
  - Although attempt to suppress gland function (decreasing gastric acid production, use of anticholinergics or somatostatin) makes physiological sense, evidence has not shown these therapies to be effective.
- **Gallstone pancreatitis**
  - Surgical and gastroenterological consultations are merited.
  - **Cholecystectomy** is generally indicated in these patients, although the decision for immediate versus delayed cholecystectomy will often depend upon the patient's clinical condition. Patients who are critically ill may benefit from a less invasive procedure (namely, ERCP) until their condition has stabilized.

- **ERCP (endoscopic retrograde cholangiopancreatography)** with sphincterotomy is generally indicated in patients with gallstone pancreatitis in the setting of
  - Severe disease
  - Biliary obstruction
  - Cholangitis
  - Not being a candidate for cholecystectomy
  - Gallstone pancreatitis despite prior cholecystectomy.
- AGA guidelines suggest that ERCP is generally not indicated in patients with mild disease in whom cholecystectomy is anticipated.
- **Pancreatitis with SIRS (systemic inflammatory response syndrome)**
  - Patients presenting with **SIRS** may have
    - Infected pancreatic necrosis
    - Sterile pancreatic necrosis (resulting in systemic inflammation but not infection)
    - An etiology of SIRS not directly related to their pancreatitis (e.g., pneumonia).
  - If SIRS persists beyond the initial fluid resuscitation, consider imaging with CT to search for pancreatic abscess or necrosis.
  - Although antibiotics may be a temporizing measure, **definitive treatment of infected necrotizing pancreatitis involves percutaneous drainage or surgical debridement.**
- **Hemorrhagic pancreatitis**
  - Hypovolemia in the setting of a low or decreasing hemoglobin should be considered concerning for hemorrhagic pancreatitis.
  - Many of these patients will need surgical intervention.
- Other indications for surgical management include exsanguinating hemorrhage (e.g., pseudoaneurysms caused by the pancreatitis), abdominal compartment syndrome, and acute abdomen.

Sudden deterioration

- Sudden *respiratory collapse* is likely secondary to **ARDS** and may require intubation with low-volume ventilation strategies. Other potential etiologies for respiratory collapse include large pleural effusions, but the deterioration associated with pleural effusions is typically subacute.
- Sudden *hemodynamic collapse* usually results from **SIRS or exsanguinating hemorrhage.**
  - Place a central line, initiate volume resuscitation with crystalloid, and begin pressors.
  - Check the patient's hemoglobin immediately, and prepare to transfuse blood products.

- Have a low threshold to begin broad-spectrum antibiotics and seek surgical consultation for operative management.

Vasopressor of choice: norepinephrine.

REFERENCES

Banks PA, Freeman ML. Practice Parameters Committee of the American College of Gastroenterology. Practice guidelines in acute pancreatitis. *Am J Gastroenterol.* 2006; **101**: 2379–400.

Bradley EL 3rd. A clinically based classification system for acute pancreatitis. Summary of the International Symposium on Acute Pancreatitis, Atlanta, GA, September 11–13, 1992. *Arch Surg.* 1993; **128**: 586–90.

Nathens AB, Curtis JR, Beale RJ, *et al.* Management of the critically ill patient with severe acute pancreatitis. *Crit Care Med.* 2004; **32**: 2524–36.

Papachristou GI, Muddana V, Yadav D, *et al.* Comparison of BISAP, Ranson's, APACHE-II, and CTSI scores in predicting organ failure, complications, and mortality in acute pancreatitis. *Am J Gastroenterol.* 2010; **105**: 435–41.

Wu BU, Johannes RS, Sun X, *et al.* The early prediction of mortality in acute pancreatitis: a large population-based study. *Gut* 2008; **57**: 1698–703.

38

Fulminant hepatic failure

Heather Meissen and Matthew Nicholls

Introduction

- Fulminant hepatic failure, synonymous with acute hepatic failure, is defined as a sudden arrest of normal hepatic function.
- The syndrome is identified by the rapid onset, within 8 weeks of injury, of hepatic encephalopathy in an otherwise healthy individual, with no prior liver injury, often in association with coagulopathy, jaundice and multi-system organ failure.
- A number of etiologies can lead to acute hepatic failure (Table 38.1).
- Acetaminophen overdose is the leading cause of fulminant hepatic failure due to both intentional and unintentional overdoses.
- Hepatocyte injury and necrosis can lead to multi-organ failure. The most lethal complication is cerebral edema with subsequent brain herniation.
- The pathogenesis of multi-organ failure associated with acute hepatic failure is complex and not fully understood.

Presentation

Classic presentation

- Typically patients present with nonspecific symptoms:
  - Fatigue
  - Malaise
  - Anorexia
  - Abdominal pain
  - Jaundice.

Practical Emergency Resuscitation and Critical Care, ed. Kaushal Shah, Jarone Lee, Kamal Medlej, and Scott D. Weingart. Published by Cambridge University Press. © Kaushal Shah, Jarone Lee, Kamal Medlej, and Scott D. Weingart 2013.

Table 38.1. Etiologies of acute hepatic failure

Viral	• Hepatitis –A, B, D, E
	• Herpes simplex virus
	• Cytomegalovirus
	• Epstein–Barr virus
	• Herpes varicella zoster
	• Adenovirus
Drugs and toxins	• Acetaminophen
	• Carbon tetrachloride
	• Sulfonamides
	• Tetracycline
	• Isoniazid
	• NSAIDs
	• Rifampicin
	• Valproic acid
	• Disulfiram
	• *Amanita phalloides*
	• *Bacillus cereus* toxin
	• Herbal supplements
Vascular	• Budd–Chiari Syndrome
	• Shock liver
	• Right heart failure
	• Veno-occlusive disorder
Metabolic	• Acute fatty liver of pregnancy
	• HELLP syndrome
	• Wilson disease
	• Reye syndrome
	• Galactosemia
	• Hereditary fructose intolerance
	• Tyrosinemia
	• Alpha-1 antitrypsin deficiency
Miscellaneous	• Primary graft failure/dysfunction of transplanted liver
	• Autoimmune hepatitis

Critical presentation

• Patients can present with:
  • Hypotension due to generalized systemic inflammatory response
  • Coagulopathy
  • Encephalopathy with progression to coma and brain herniation (Table 38.2).

Table 38.2. Grading of hepatic encephalopathy

	Grade 1	Grade 2	Grade 3	Grade 4
Level of consciousness	Awake	Decreased, but opens eyes spontaneously	Asleep, but arousable to verbal stimuli	Comatose, no response
Orientation	Oriented	Disoriented to time events	Complete disorientation	Comatose
Intellectual functions	Mental clouding, slowness to answer questions	Amnesia for past events	Inability to make computations	Comatose
Behavior	Forgetful, restless, irritable	Lethargic	Bizarre behavior, rage	Comatose
Mood	Euphoria, depression	Apathetic, paranoid	Apathy increased	Comatose
Neuromuscular	Tremors, yawning, decreased muscular coordination	Hypoactive reflexes, asterixis, ataxia and slurred speech	Babinski, clonus, decortications, decerebration, rigid, seizures	Seizures
EEG	Mild abnormalities	Moderate abnormalities	Severe abnormalities	Severe abnormalities

Diagnosis and evaluation

- **Diagnosis**
  - Diagnosis is made based on clinical presentation and laboratory findings. Consider the tests listed below (though many will not be reported back within a few hours of the ED stay).
  - *Chemistry:* Acetaminophen level, alpha-1 antitrypsin level, alpha-1 antitrypsin phenotype, ammonia level, amylase, lipase, ceruloplasmin, cholesterol, comprehensive metabolic panel, magnesium, phosphorus, gamma-glutamyl-transferase (GGT), lactate dehydrogenase (LDH), lactic acid, uric acid, pregnancy screen.
  - *Immunology:* Mitochondrial M2 Ab IgG, anti-nuclear Ab screen (ANA, IgG), smooth muscle Ab, IgG, IG heavy chain quantitation, alpha fetoprotein tumor marker.
  - *Hematology/coagulation:* Antithrombin III activity assay, CBC, D-dimer, factor V, VII, and VIII, fibrinogen, MOCHA (markers of coagulation hemostatic activation), PT, PTT, INR.

- *Microbiology/infectious disease:* CMV antibody total (anti-CMV Ab), CMV antibody IGM, IgG, Coxsackie B virus Abs, Epstein–Barr virus Ab profile, hepatitis A Ab total and IgM, hepatitis B DNA quantification, hepatitis B diagnostic profile, hepatitis C Ab, herpes simplex virus DNA by PCR, HIV antigen Ab combo, rapid plasma reagin test.
  - *Urine:* Urine sodium, urine creatinine, 24-hour urine copper level, toxicology drug screen especially acetaminophen, urinalysis.
  - *Imaging:* Abdominal ultrasound (US) with Doppler, noncontrast head CT, abdomen MRI with and without contrast, transthoracic US.
- **Prognosis**
  - *Three possible outcomes:*
    - Spontaneous survival without liver transplantation (>40%)
    - Orthotopic liver transplantation (25%)
    - Death (33%).
  - The shorter the interval between jaundice and the development of hepatic encephalopathy the higher the likelihood of spontaneous survival.
  - *King's College Criteria:*
    - Used to determine prognosis and need for transplant.
    - If the patient satisfies any of the following criteria, they most likely will require a liver transplant to survive.
    - **Acetaminophen-induced disease:**
      - Arterial pH <7.3
      or all of the following:
      - grade III or IV encephalopathy
      - Prothrombin time >100 seconds
      - Serum creatinine >3.4 mg/dL (301 micromol/L).
    - **All other causes of hepatic failure:**
      - Prothrombin time >100 seconds (INR >6.5)
      or any three of the following:
      - Age <10 years or >40 years
      - Etiology: non-A, non-B hepatitis, halothane hepatitis, idiosyncratic drug reactions
      - Duration of jaundice before onset of encephalopathy >7 days
      - Prothrombin time >50 seconds
      - Serum bilirubin >18 mg/dL (308 micromol/L).

Critical management

- **Progression of disease can be quite rapid; patients should be transferred to a transplant center as soon as possible.**
- Critical care management as needed for cardiovascular, pulmonary, and infectious complications and other comorbidities.
- **Acetaminophen toxicity**

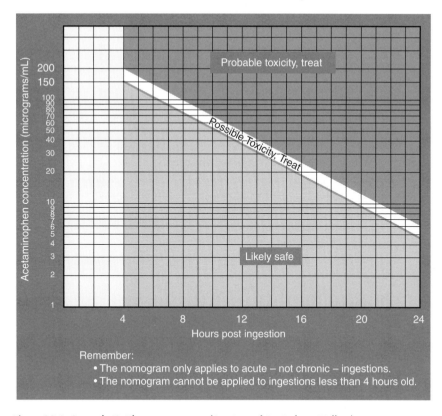

Figure 38.1. Rumack–Matthew nomogram. (Courtesy of Dr. Graham Walker.)

- Prognosis and treatment decisions can be based on Rumack–Matthew nomogram (Figure 38.1).
- It is important to remember that the nomogram is based on a single ingestion and may not apply if the time of ingestion is unknown or in the cases of multiple ingestions.
- *N-Acetylcysteine (NAC):*
  - NAC should always be given in acetaminophen toxicity except for rare occasions.
  - NAC is indicated for all levels where toxicity is possible.
  - Given the limitations of the nomogram, NAC should be administered if there is any doubt of the amount or time of ingestion(s). Furthermore, NAC may be beneficial even late after ingestion.
  - Watch for anaphylactoid reaction with IV NAC. Typically, this reaction will be abated by decreasing the rate of infusion, administering antihistamines, and providing supportive care. If the reaction is severe, stop the infusion,

treat with antihistamines, and consider restarting after the symptoms improve.

- NAC should be continued until the end of the protocol and until evidence of severe liver injury resolves (usually when AST and ALT are <1000).

- **Management of complications related to liver failure**
  - **Neurological**
    - Frequent neurological checks; worsening hepatic encephalopathy may be due to progression to cerebral edema.
    - Minimize sedation to avoid confusing drug effects with clinical deterioration. When needed, choose short-acting agents.
    - *Management of hepatic encephalopathy:*
      - Grade III encephalopathy requires intubation for airway protection.
      - Consider CT scan to evaluate for cerebral edema and rule out other causes of altered mental status; however, *remember that a normal scan does NOT rule out cerebral edema.*
      - Herniation is unlikely with ammonia levels <150 micromol/L.
      - Consider intracranial monitoring in the following patients:
        - Grade III and higher encephalopathy
        - Markedly elevated ammonia levels
      - Unlike with chronic hepatic failure, lactulose has not been proven to have any long-term benefit in acute fulminant hepatic failure
    - *Management of cerebral edema/elevated intracranial pressure (ICP)*
      - Goals ICP <20 mmHg and CPP >60 mmHg (CPP = MAP − ICP). Even if no ICP monitoring available, it is important to manage grade III and higher encephalopathy as if ICP is known to be elevated.
      - **Basic management:**
        - Sedation and muscle relaxation as needed
        - Keep environment calm with little stimulation
        - Position HOB at 30–45 degrees
        - Keep head in midline position to allow the jugular veins to drain
        - Minimize other adjuncts to care such as suctioning or laying supine for turns
        - Consider specific treatments to prevent elevated ICP during intubation (i.e., IV lidocaine and muscle relaxants)
        - Avoid hypoventilation. Hyperventilation is not necessary and may cause cerebral vasoconstriction leading to cerebral ischemia.
        - Correct hyponatremia
        - Control fever and seizures
      - **Osmotic therapy:**
        - Indicated for severe intracranial hypertension defined as sustained ICP>20–25 mmHg for >5–10 min
        - Mannitol
          - Avoid if serum osmolality >320 mOsm/L or with renal failure.
          - Can cause renal toxicity.

- Hypertonic saline
  - May be better osmotic agent than mannitol.
  - No diuretic properties.
  - No renal toxicity.
  - Goal Na = 145–155 mmol/L.
  - Careful when discontinuing hypertonic saline; wean to avoid abrupt drop in sodium and rebound cerebral edema.
- Consider mild hypothermia for refractory cases:
  - Goal 32–33°C
  - Control shivering
  - Burst suppression on EEG/phenobarbital coma.
- Coagulopathy:
  - Typically, clinically important bleeding infrequent despite coagulopathy.
  - FFP for elevated INR with acute bleeding or prior to procedure.
  - Vitamin K may be administered for elevated INR without acute bleeding.
  - Give cryoprecipitate if fibrinogen <100 mg/dL.
  - If actively bleeding, attempt to maintain platelet count >50 000. In the absence of bleeding, maintain platelet count >10 000.
  - Consider activated recombinant factor VII in refractory cases (use *only* if placing an intracranial monitor).
- **Hypoglycemia**
  - Maintain blood glucose >70 mg/dL (3.9 mmol/L).
  - Administer dextrose in the form of bolus and drip as needed.
  - Bolus dextrose 50%, 50 mL via IV push.
  - Start a drip since most of these patients will require a continuous glucose source – D5W, D10W, or D20W and titrate rate to goal blood glucose >70 mg/dL (3.9 mmol/L).
  - Check blood glucose every 30 minutes until the goal is reached.
- **Renal failure**
  - Renal failure occurs in up to 50% of cases, even more frequently in acetaminophen toxicity.
  - Avoid nephrotoxins.
  - Management of hypervolemia is crucial to reducing cerebral edema.
  - In most cases continuous renal replacement therapy is indicated.
  - Avoid intermittent hemodialysis as some evidence suggests rapid fluid shifts lead to brain herniation.

Sudden deterioration

- Transfer to a transplantation facility as soon as possible.

- MARS ("molecular adsorbents recirculation system" or artificial extracorporeal liver support) therapy is being studied in some centers. If a transplantation center is not readily available, consider transfer to a center that utilizes MARS.

Vasopressor of choice: norepinephrine.

REFERENCES

Ford R, Sonali S, Subramanian R. Critical care management of patients before liver transplant. *Transplant Rev.* 2010; **24**: 190–206.

Ostapowicz G, Lee M. Acute hepatic failure: a Western perspective. *J Gastroenterol Hepatol.* 2000; **15**: 480–8.

Polson J, Lee W. AASLD Position Paper: The management of acute liver failure. *Hepatology.* 2005; **41**: 1179–97.

Sass DA, Shakil AO. Fulminant hepatic failure. *Liver Transpl.* 2005; **11**: 594–605.

39

Acute mesenteric ischemia

Carolyn Maher Overman and Jeffrey N. Siegelman

Introduction

- Mesenteric ischemia is a generic term that implies inadequate blood flow to the intestines. It can be both acute and chronic and caused by several different etiologies. The blood supply to the abdominal organs is listed in Table 39.1.
- It is a rare life-threatening vascular emergency, occurring with increasing frequency and with mortality rates between 60% and 80%.
- It affects primarily those older than 50 years with systemic and cardiovascular disease.
- The acute form is more common and results in rapid intestinal ischemia, infarction/necrosis, sepsis, and death. Splanchnic vascular insufficiency in chronic ischemia can also threaten bowel viability.
- Ischemic colitis is much less common than small bowel ischemia.
- Even with advances in diagnostic testing, survival has not significantly improved, largely because of the difficulty of making a timely diagnosis.
- **Pathogenesis**
  - 25% of cardiac output is provided to the splanchnic circulation.
  - Severity of disease is inversely related to mesenteric blood flow and quantity of collaterals.
  - Critical threshold of hypoperfusion leads to intestinal villi ischemia, release of endothelial factors, inflammatory cells, oxygen free radicals, and intraluminal bacteria proliferation.
  - Extent of infarction depends on presence of the collateral circulation and duration of ischemia.
  - Necrosis/infarction may be seen as early as 10–12 hours.

Practical Emergency Resuscitation and Critical Care, ed. Kaushal Shah, Jarone Lee, Kamal Medlej, and Scott D. Weingart. Published by Cambridge University Press. © Kaushal Shah, Jarone Lee, Kamal Medlej, and Scott D. Weingart 2013.

Table 39.1. Arterial supply to abdominal organs

Arterial supply	Target organs
Celiac	Esophagus, stomach, proximal duodenum, liver, gallbladder, pancreas, and spleen
Superior mesenteric artery	Distal duodenum, jejunum, ileum, colon to the splenic flexure
Inferior mesenteric artery	Descending colon, sigmoid, and rectum

- Untreated intestinal ischemia can lead to intestinal gangrene, bowel perforation, diffuse peritonitis, septic shock, cardiac depression, multi-system organ failure, and death.
- **Etiology**
  - *Mesenteric arterial embolism (MAE)*
    - This is the most common and accounts for 40–50% of cases.
    - Median age is 70 years and it is more common in women than men.
    - Most mural thrombi originate from cardiac source and often lodge in a branch of the superior mesenteric artery (SMA).
  - *Mesenteric arterial thrombosis (MAT)*
    - MAT accounts for 25% of cases.
    - Almost all cases are caused by severe atherosclerosis and most often thrombus forms in the SMA.
    - Consequently, patients often have preceding symptoms of chronic mesenteric ischemia:
      - *Intestinal or mesenteric angina:* postprandial abdominal pain that occurs due to inability to augment blood flow that normally is needed after eating
      - Cachexia and malnutrition.
    - Consider MAT in elderly patients with uncontrolled hypertension, atherosclerosis, and vascular disease. It can also be seen in fibromuscular or rheumatological disease.
    - Perioperative mortality ranges from 70% to 100% secondary to delay in timely diagnosis.
    - Differentiation from embolism is important as surgical treatment usually requires bypass with bowel resection, whereas embolic disease requires embolectomy with bowel resection.
  - *Nonocclusive mesenteric ischemia (NOMI)*
    - NOMI accounts for 20% and can occur in all ages of critically ill hospitalized patients.
    - It occurs in diseases that lead to cardiovascular dysfunction (shock, sepsis, burns, trauma, pancreatitis, etc.) with low cardiac output leading to splanchnic vasoconstriction and loss of vascular autoregulation.

- Treatment is usually aimed at correcting the underlying condition, avoiding vasoactive drugs (if possible), systemic anticoagulation if not contraindicated, and broad-spectrum antibiotics.
- *Mesenteric venous thrombosis (MVT)*
  - This is associated with hypercoagulable states, inflammatory conditions, and trauma.
  - The least common form of myocardial infarction, it accounts for only 10% of cases.
  - Often occurs in the younger population with milder symptoms.
  - Mortality rates are lower than with other causes, ranging from 20% to 50%.
  - Venous congestion leads to bowel edema, which can severely limit blood supply.
  - Treatment is systemic anticoagulation.
- **Risk factors**
  - Risk factors for mesenteric ischemia are listed in Table 39.2.

Table 39.2. Risk factors for subtypes of mesenteric ischemia

Etiology	Risk factor
Mesenteric arterial embolism	1. Coronary artery disease: postmyocardial infarction or ischemia 2. Heart disease: congestive heart failure, cardiomyopathies, ventricular aneurysms 3. Valvular disease: rheumatic heart disease, endocarditis 4. Arrhythmias: atrial fibrillation and other atrial tachyarrhythmias 5. Vasculature: aortic aneurysm, aortic dissection 6. Coronary angiography
Mesenteric arterial thrombosis	1. Uncontrolled hypertension 2. Cerebral, coronary, or peripheral vascular disease
Nonocclusive mesenteric ischemia	1. Cardiovascular: congestive heart failure, arrhythmias, cardiogenic shock 2. Hypoperfusion: hypovolemic or septic shock 3. Drugs: vasopressors, α-agonists, vasopressin, digoxin, cocaine
Mesenteric venous thrombosis	1. Hypercoagulable process: pregnancy, oral contraceptives, protein C, S, or antithrombin III deficiencies, polycythemia vera, sickle cell disease, malignancy, systemic lupus erythematosus 2. Abdominal inflammatory conditions: diverticulitis, cholangitis, appendicitis, pancreatitis 3. Trauma: abdominal injuries, venous injuries 4. Other: portal hypertension, congestive heart failure, renal failure

Presentation

Classic and critical presentation

- The diagnosis should be considered in those older than 50 years, presenting with nonspecific abdominal pain and risk factors for the disease.
- The physician must have a high index of suspicion as the history may be difficult to obtain.
- Acute onset of severe poorly localized abdominal pain.
- Often presents with vague complaints and pain out of proportion to the examination.
- Nausea/vomiting and a history of intestinal angina.
- Diarrhea due to cathartic stimulus of ischemia.
- Gross or occult GI bleeding.
- Peritonitis is a late finding and indicates severe bowel ischemia and necrosis.
- Time is bowel: survival is 50% when diagnosed within 24 hours but drops to less than 30% after 24 hours.
- **Subtype presentations**
  - Clinical presentations of the subtypes of mesenteric ischemia are listed in Table 39.3.

Table 39.3. Presentation of the subtypes of mesenteric ischemia

Mesenteric arterial embolism	Mesenteric arterial thrombosis	Nonocclusive mesenteric ischemia	Mesenteric venous thrombosis
• Appears ill • Tachycardia • Acute unrelenting abdominal pain • Nausea/vomiting • Frequent bowel movements	*Acute* • Similar to MAE *Subacute* • Postprandial pain • Weight loss • Nausea	• Critically ill patient with worsening clinical picture or failure to thrive	• Typically late presentation (1–2 weeks) • Nonspecific abdominal pain • Diarrhea • Vomiting

Diagnosis and evaluation

- **Laboratory work**
  - Nonspecific, but may reveal the following:
    - Leukocytosis
    - Hemoconcentration
    - Elevated anion gap metabolic acidosis

- Elevated amylase, CPK, and LDH
- Later findings of elevated lactic acid, hyperphosphatemia, and hyperkalemia.
- Possible future tests that are currently not validated include
  - D-dimer
  - Glutathione *S*-transferase
  - Intestinal fatty-acid binding protein
  - Procalcitonin.
- **Imaging**
  - *Abdominal radiography:*
    - This is the initial test to rule out other possible diagnoses or complications of AMI (i.e., obstruction and perforation).
    - Abnormal findings are noted only 20% of the time.
    - May show adynamic ileus, thumb-printing or thickening of bowel loops, pneumatosis, or late finding of free air or air in the portal venous system.
  - *CT-angiography (CTA):*
    - Contrast-enhanced multidetector CT is now the most commonly used test to diagnose acute mesenteric ischemia.
    - Recent meta-analysis has shown sensitivity of 82.8–97.6% and specificity of 91.2–98.2% comparable with angiography, which remains the gold standard.
    - May show thickened bowel walls, dilated bowel loops, pneumatosis, air in the portal system, infarction, arterial or venous thrombosis.
    - CTA can likely help with diagnosis even if presentation not due to mesenteric ischemia.
    - If CTA is completely normal but there is a high index of suspicion, further angiography or diagnostic laparotomy is recommended.
  - *Ultrasound:*
    - Noninvasive and without radiation.
    - Low sensitivity due to obstruction of the view by gas-filled bowel.
  - *Angiography:*
    - The gold standard, though invasive, not readily available, and rarely employed.
    - Angiography has been largely replaced by CTA.
    - It is used if there is diagnostic uncertainty.
    - Both diagnostic and potentially therapeutic.

Critical management

Establish IV access and begin fluid resuscitation with crystalloid products
Treat the underlying cause if possible
Placement of NG tube
Correct electrolyte abnormalities
Prepare blood and check coagulation factors, preoperative laboratory studies
Discontinue medications with vasoconstrictive properties
Begin broad-spectrum antibiotics
If there are no contraindications, start heparin therapy
Consult general or vascular surgery emergently

- *It is imperative to remember that this diagnosis almost always requires surgical repair.*
- **Surgical management**
  - Emergent laparotomy is indicated, especially if signs of peritonitis are present.
  - Surgery is generally the standard of care for mesenteric arterial embolism and thrombosis.
  - Surgery is done to determine the extent of damage, to find the underlying cause, to revascularize viable bowel, and to resect infarcted bowel.
  - Bowel is often left in discontinuity.
  - Second-look procedures are often performed 24–48 hours after the initial surgery in order to restore continuity, assess for extension of ischemia. This also ensures that at-risk or ischemic bowel is not used for the final anastomosis.
- **Novel treatments**
  - Glucagon drips may decrease vasospasms
  - Papaverine, a phosphodiesterase inhibitor that reduces mesenteric vasoconstriction, can be directly infused into the SMA during angiography.
- **Subtype management**
  - Specific management for each subtype of mesenteric ischemia is listed in Table 39.4.

Vasopressor of choice: norepinephrine.

Table 39.4. Management of the subtypes of mesenteric ischemia

Mesenteric arterial embolism	Mesenteric arterial thrombosis	Nonocclusive mesenteric ischemia	Mesenteric venous thrombosis
• Embolectomy then distal bypass graft • Resect necrotic bowel	• Bypass graft or stenting • Resect necrotic bowel	• Treat the underlying cause • Fewer surgical options • Papaverine or glycerol infusion • Resect necrotic bowel	• Depends on extent of ischemia • Difficult for surgical management if diffuse thrombosis • Mild ischemia: treat with anticoagulation • Severe ischemia: treat with bowel resection of necrotic segments

REFERENCES

Evennett NJ, Petrov MS, Mittal A, Windsor JA. Systematic review and pooled estimates for the diagnostic accuracy of serological markers for intestinal ischemia. *World J. Surg.* 2009; **33**: 1374–83.

Menke J. Diagnostic accuracy of multidetector CT in acute mesenteric ischemia: systematic review and meta-analysis. *Radiology.* 2010; **256**(1): 93–101.

Oldenburg WA, Lau LL, Rodenberg TJ, *et al.* Acute mesenteric ischemia: a clinical review. *Arch Intern Med.* 2004; **164**: 1054–62.

Renner P, Kienle K, Dahlke MH, *et al.* Intestinal ischemia: current treatment concepts. *Langenbecks Arch Surg.* 2011; **396**: 3–11.

Torrey SP, Henneman PL. Disorders of the small intestine. In: Marx JA, Hockberger RS, Walls RM, Adams J, Rosen P, eds. *Rosen's Emergency Medicine: Concepts and Clinical Practice.* 7th edn. Philadelphia, PA: Mosby Elsevier; 2010.

40

The surgical abdomen

Sarah Fisher and Carla Haack

Introduction

- Abdominal pain is the most common reason for emergency department visits and is a leading cause of hospital admissions in the United States.
- Acute abdominal pain is defined as sudden-onset pain lasting less than 7 days. It is a generic term and the pain can be due to many possible causes that range from benign to life threatening.
- Once an etiology that requires surgical intervention is suspected, involvement of appropriate consultants should not be delayed.

Presentation

Classic and critical presentations

- The patient can present with anything from mild to severe abdominal pain. Depending on the etiology and severity of the disease, the pain could be vague and dull, or severe and localized. This is because of the following pathophysiology:
  - Autonomic nerves (sympathetic and parasympathetic) innervate the abdominal viscera; stretching or distension of hollow abdominal viscera generates pain that is described as dull, crampy, or aching and is often poorly localized.
  - Somatic nerves (spinal nerves) innervate the parietal peritoneum, and transmit sharp and severe, localizable signals.
- The **location** and **characterization** of the pain can help distinguish between different etiologies of the abdominal pain (see Figure 40.1).

Practical Emergency Resuscitation and Critical Care, ed. Kaushal Shah, Jarone Lee, Kamal Medlej, and Scott D. Weingart. Published by Cambridge University Press. © Kaushal Shah, Jarone Lee, Kamal Medlej, and Scott D. Weingart 2013.

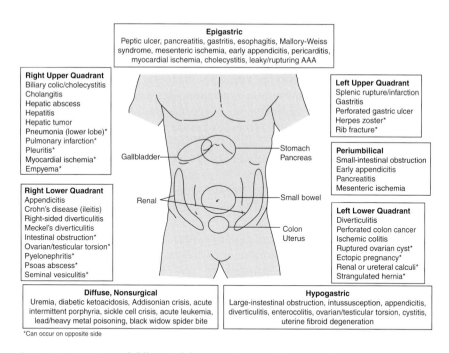

Epigastric
Peptic ulcer, pancreatitis, gastritis, esophagitis, Mallory-Weiss syndrome, mesenteric ischemia, early appendicitis, pericarditis, myocardial ischemia, cholecystitis, leaky/rupturing AAA

Right Upper Quadrant
Biliary colic/cholecystitis
Cholangitis
Hepatic abscess
Hepatitis
Hepatic tumor
Pneumonia (lower lobe)*
Pulmonary infarction*
Pleuritis*
Myocardial ischemia*
Empyema*

Left Upper Quadrant
Splenic rupture/infarction
Gastritis
Perforated gastric ulcer
Herpes zoster*
Rib fracture*

Gallbladder — Stomach
Pancreas

Periumbilical
Small-intestinal obstruction
Early appendicitis
Pancreatitis
Mesenteric ischemia

Right Lower Quadrant
Appendicitis
Crohn's disease (ileitis)
Right-sided diverticulitis
Meckel's diverticulitis
Intestinal obstruction*
Ovarian/testicular torsion*
Pyelonephritis*
Psoas abscess*
Seminal vesiculitis*

Renal — Small bowel

Colon
Uterus

Left Lower Quadrant
Diverticulitis
Perforated colon cancer
Ischemic colitis
Ruptured ovarian cyst*
Ectopic pregnancy*
Renal or ureteral calculi*
Strangulated hernia*

Diffuse, Nonsurgical
Uremia, diabetic ketoacidosis, Addisonian crisis, acute intermittent porphyria, sickle cell crisis, acute leukemia, lead/heavy metal poisoning, black widow spider bite

Hypogastric
Large-intestinal obstruction, intussusception, appendicitis, diverticulitis, enterocolitis, ovarian/testicular torsion, cystitis, uterine fibroid degeneration

*Can occur on opposite side

Figure 40.1. Location and differential diagnosis of acute abdominal pain.

- Additionally patients could present with referred pain, which is pain experienced at a site (or sites) distant from the initiating organ due to a shared neural origin with another body organ, such as right shoulder pain due to biliary colic or back pain due to pancreatitis.
- **Acute-onset pain lasting longer than 6 hours in a previously healthy patient is often due to a surgical condition.**

Diagnosis and evaluation

- **History and physical characteristics**
  - A thorough history will generally narrow the differential diagnosis.
  - **Past medical and surgical histories** and **medication usage** may harbor clues (e.g., prior abdominal surgery may suggest adhesions as an etiology for bowel obstruction) or rule out potential diagnoses (e.g., prior cholecystectomy in the setting of right upper quadrant pain).
  - Always note the **location** and **characterization** of the pain to help with the differential diagnosis (see Figure 40.1).

- **Duration of symptoms**, **mode of onset** (gradual and insidious versus sudden), and **associated symptoms** (nausea, vomiting, anorexia, fatigue, rash) should be noted.
- Change over time should be noted: the temporal transition from poorly described vague abdominal pain to persistent sharp discomfort specific to an area of the abdomen, such as occurs in appendicitis, often signifies the worsening of an intra-abdominal process and might need surgical intervention.
- **Physical examination**
  - Assess the patient overall, including vital signs (derangement of vital signs signifies more serious underlying illness) and demeanor.
  - A focused examination should include not only the gastrointestinal system but also the cardiovascular and respiratory systems.
  - *Abdominal examination:*
    - Begin the abdominal examination away from the area that is most painful.
    - Inspect the abdomen for surgical scars, bulges, pulsations, and other abnormalities (skin discoloration, petechiae).
    - Observe the respiratory movement of the abdomen – in cases of peritonitis the abdominal wall will barely move due to muscle rigidity, which can be localized or generalized.
    - Auscultate for bowel sounds, bruits and abnormal pulsations.
    - Begin the palpation portion of the examination gently, progressing slowly to deeper palpation (remember that the stethoscope can be used to distract and palpate simultaneously). Ask the patient to point with one finger to the area that is most painful, and begin palpating the abdomen far away from that point.
    - Involuntary guarding (physiological contraction of the abdominal wall) denotes an underlying inflammatory process (i.e., peritonitis), which can be localized or generalized.
    - Gentle percussion combined with palpation is more specific than testing for rebound.
    - Muscular rigidity, the extreme of involuntary guarding, can be absent in cases of chronic deconditioning, the severely decompensated patient, or the elderly.
  - Rectal and pelvic examinations should be performed in appropriate patients.
- **Laboratory testing**
  - Results of a selected test should be anticipated to *alter the management plan*; otherwise that test should not be ordered.
  - Initial bloodwork including a **hematocrit** and **electrolytes** can guide initial fluid resuscitation.
  - The white blood cell count (WBC), while useful, is fairly nonspecific as WBCs can be elevated in a variety of nonsurgical conditions, and normal or low in surgical conditions.
  - In the unstable patient, an **arterial blood gas** and/or base deficit may provide more information than blood chemistries and better guide resuscitation.

- **Coagulation studies** and a **type and screen** are generally necessary tests for the patient with acute abdominal pain of suspected surgical etiology. Cross-matched blood should be requested in select patients.
- Females of child-bearing age should have a urine pregnancy test.
- **Radiological testing**
  - Abdominal plain films are rarely diagnostic, although they may identify air–fluid levels (suggestive of a bowel obstruction or ileus), renal or ureteral calculi, and occasionally free intraperitoneal air.
  - The test of choice to identify free intraperitoneal air is the **upright chest radiograph**. For patients who cannot sit upright, consider a lateral decubitus radiograph.
  - **Ultrasound** should be considered for suspected biliary (acute cholecystitis) and gynecological etiologies of acute abdominal pain (tubo-ovarian abscess, ectopic pregnancy).
  - **Computed tomography (CT)** has largely supplanted plain film radiology in many centers, but concerns of cost and the risk of ionizing radiation require judicious use of this modality.
    - When considering abdominal and pelvic CT, the suspected diagnosis should guide the use of IV and oral contrast. Many emergency departments have established protocols to guide the use of contrast.
    - *Water-soluble* oral contrast should be used in cases of suspected obstruction or perforation.
    - The interpretation of findings on CT (or any test) should match the story painted by the history and physical examination. Otherwise, reevaluate the patient.

Critical management

- **The unstable patient**
  - As with the stable patient, a well-formulated differential diagnosis based on careful history and physical examination will guide the plan of care far better than a "shotgun" approach of imaging and laboratory tests.
- **Resuscitation** must begin concurrently with the diagnostic modalities.
  - **Intubation** may be necessary for airway protection.
  - **Large-bore intravenous access** should be secured and electrolyte abnormalities corrected.
  - **Nasogastric decompression** is beneficial in patients with generalized ileus.
  - A **Foley catheter** can be placed to monitor fluid status and guide resuscitation.
  - Hypothermia should be corrected with **warming blankets** and **heated fluids**.
  - **Frequent reassessment** of hemodynamics and acid–base status is necessary.
  - An unstable patient should *never* be transported to the radiology suite without a supervising physician.

- **Pain control**
  - **Early and judicious opioid administration** is recommended.
  - Historically, some clinicians have cautioned against the use of analgesia in the patient with an "acute abdomen" out of concern that opioids would mask presenting symptoms and confound timely diagnosis. Over the past decade, multiple prospective, randomized, controlled trials have failed to show that early analgesia administration impairs diagnostic accuracy.
- **Preparation for the OR**
  - The amount of time allowed for preoperative resuscitation should be balanced with the degree to which the underlying disease process is likely to progress.
  - Patients with an acute abdomen requiring surgical correction should be treated in similar fashion as the unstable patient.
  - Appropriate fluid resuscitation should be given (via large-bore intravenous access), and electrolyte abnormalities should be corrected.
  - In addition to a type and screen, **cross-matched blood** should be available for the operating suite in cases in which the degree of operative intervention is unknown (i.e., the patient with large amounts of free intraperitoneal air, as opposed to the stable patient with early appendicitis).

Special circumstances

- **Special populations**
  - A higher index of suspicion for abdominal catastrophe is necessary in situations in which the history is compromised or in which the physical examination is altered or unreliable.
  - Some patients, including **children, developmentally delayed, or obtunded individuals** (from illness or drugs) cannot give a reliable history.
  - **Patients with spinal cord injuries** and impaired sensation often present in a delayed fashion.
  - **Pregnancy** displaces the abdominal viscera and alters the presentation of common illnesses.
  - **The elderly or immunosuppressed** may not experience symptoms in the same way as most adults.
  - **Morbid obesity** hinders physical examination.

REFERENCES

Ameloot K, Gillebert C, Desie N, Malbrain ML. Hypoperfusion, shock states, and abdominal compartment syndrome (ACS). *Surg Clin North Am.* 2012; **92**(2): 207–20, vii.

Cameron JL. *Current Surgical Therapy.* 9th edn. Philadelphia, PA: Mosby Elsevier; 2008.

McNamara R, Dean AJ. Approach to acute abdominal pain. *Emerg Med Clin North Am.* 2011; **29**: 159–73, vii.

Silen W. *Cope's Early Diagnosis of the Acute Abdomen.* 21st edn. New York: Oxford University Press; 2005.

Townsend CM Jr., Beauchamp RD, Evers BM, Mattox KL. *Sabiston Textbook of Surgery.* 19th edn. Philadelphia, PA: Elsevier Saunders; 2012.

41

Abdominal compartment syndrome

Sarah Fisher and Carla Haack

Introduction

- Increased intra-abdominal pressure (IAP) from fluid or gas accumulation compromises the respiratory and cardiovascular systems and decreases perfusion to abdominal organs.
- Sources of increased IAP include hemorrhage (traumatic or iatrogenic), inflammation (peritonitis, pancreatitis), hollow viscus perforation, ascites, and systemic sources (capillary leak and bowel edema from sepsis, burns, or massive fluid resuscitation).
- The World Society of the Abdominal Compartment Syndrome defines **abdominal compartment syndrome (ACS)** as increased pressure within the abdominal cavity ≥20 mmHg associated with *new* organ dysfunction or failure.
- ACS can be primary (resulting from an intra-abdominal process), or secondary (due to bowel edema from aggressive fluid resuscitation or sepsis) and can occur in patients whose abdomen *has not been surgically altered.*
- IAP measurements >25 mmHg are often associated with significant organ dysfunction requiring surgical decompression, but there is not a universal threshold value applicable to all patients.
- IAP is influenced by respiration, body mass index, position, and severity of illness. In the critically ill hypotensive patient, even slight increases in IAP may compromise abdominal perfusion, leading to worsening acidosis and further clinical decline.

Practical Emergency Resuscitation and Critical Care, ed. Kaushal Shah, Jarone Lee, Kamal Medlej, and Scott D. Weingart. Published by Cambridge University Press. © Kaushal Shah, Jarone Lee, Kamal Medlej, and Scott D. Weingart 2013.

Presentation

Classic and critical presentations

- **Neurological**
  - Increased IAP has been shown to **decrease cerebral perfusion pressure** by decreased cardiac output (CO) and hypotension, as well as via increased thoracic pressure with functional obstruction of cerebral venous outflow.
- **Cardiovascular**
  - Increased IAP directly compresses the vena cava, **decreasing venous return and cardiac output (CO)**, which increases systemic venous congestion and edema. The diaphragm bulges upward, displacing the heart and compromising diastolic filling, which further decreases CO.
- **Respiratory**
  - The cephalad displacement of the diaphragm also **decreases pulmonary compliance**, leading to segmental alveolar collapse and subsequent ventilation/perfusion mismatches. In patients on ventilators (majority of patients), an **increase in peak airway pressures and peak inspiratory pressures** will be observed in addition to increased difficulty in ventilating overall. The increase in thoracic pressure artificially increases central venous pressure (CVP) and pulmonary capillary wedge pressure (PCWP), compromising the value of these markers for guiding resuscitation.
- **Renal**
  - Direct compression of the kidneys combined with decreased vascular inflow and outflow can create **oliguria** and compromise renal function even in the setting of maintained hemodynamics.
- **Gastrointestinal**
  - Direct compression within the abdominal cavity **decreases splanchnic blood flow** leading to bowel ischemia and necrosis. This also contributes to the formation of bowel edema, which in turn increases IAP.
- **Musculoskeletal**
  - **Musculoskeletal dysfunction**, both within the abdominal wall and in the extremities, is also observed as a result of decreased CO, global ischemia, and reperfusion injury.

Diagnosis and evaluation

- The most efficient way to recognize and treat ACS is by recognizing and correcting predisposing factors before ACS occurs.
- In the closed abdomen, the gold standard approach to measuring IAP uses a urinary bladder catheter ("**bladder pressures**") with the patient in **full supine position**.

- Normal IAP ranges from 0 to 5 mmHg, with IAP after uncomplicated surgical procedures ranging between 3 and 15 mmHg.
- A maximum of 20–25 mL of sterile saline is injected into the catheter, which is then clamped and connected to a transducing device.
- The pubic symphysis is used as the zeroing point on a supine patient.
- Time should be allowed for the detrusor muscle of the bladder to accommodate the volume before the pressure is measured.
- IAP should be measured at end expiration.

- IAP may be artificially elevated by abdominal wall contraction (such as in an awake patient or in situations of inadequate analgesia), body habitus (obesity), or patient positioning (raising the head of the bed). In intubated patients, pharmacological paralysis may enhance the accuracy of IAP measurements as well as provide therapeutic benefit.

Critical management

- **Early recognition** of risk factors and delaying definitive abdominal wall closure remains the best therapy for ACS. In cases in which the abdominal wall is already closed or the decompression is inadequate, timely intervention can be life-saving.
- Any patient suspected of having ACS should have frequent measurements of IAP.
- The definitive treatment for a patient with ACS is **decompressive laparotomy**.
- There is some evidence to support the use of percutaneous decompression using a diagnostic peritoneal lavage catheter as an alternative treatment prior to decompressive laparotomy.
- There is **no standard consensus** on when to intervene. The decision is made based on clinical judgment, presence of end-organ failure, and serial measurements of IAP.
- Aggressive **fluid resuscitation** to maintain hemodynamics may overcome some of the deleterious effects of increased IAP; however, others have recommended conservative resuscitation to avoid excess third-spacing, bowel edema, and subsequent worsening of IAP. In trauma patients and other select groups, consider the use of blood products and colloids over crystalloids.
- **CVP and PCWP are unreliable** in the setting of increased IAP. Determination of right ventricular end-diastolic volume with pulmonary artery catheters has been suggested as a surrogate endpoint, as has maintenance of abdominal perfusion pressure (mean arterial pressure – IAP) above 50 mmHg, but neither has been tested in prospective, randomized clinical trials.
- If the underlying insult causing ACS is expected to resolve within a relatively short time period, temporizing measures other than surgical decompression can be adopted. **Liberal analgesia** and **sedation** as well as **pharmacological paralysis** are adjunct measures that may decrease abdominal wall tension. Paracentesis

and renal replacement therapy can be used in appropriately selected patients to normalize fluid balance.

- When the decision to surgically decompress is made, **resuscitation to a euvolemic status** is imperative, as surgical decompression results in the following:
  - Decreased systemic vascular resistance
  - Increased respiratory tidal volumes
  - Washout of byproducts of anaerobic metabolism, releasing acid, potassium, and other potentially arrhythmogenic byproducts into the circulation.
- Remember that ACS can occur even in the already decompressed abdomen – either due to an incision that is too small or due to an abdominal closure system that is too tight.

REFERENCES

Ameloot K, Gillebert C, Desie N, Malbrain ML. Hypoperfusion, shock states, and abdominal compartment syndrome (ACS). *Surg Clin North Am.* 2012; **92**(2): 207–20, vii.

Cameron JL. *Current Surgical Therapy.* 9th edn. Philadelphia, PA: Mosby Elsevier; 2008.

Silen W. *Cope's Early Diagnosis of the Acute Abdomen.* 21st edn. New York: Oxford University Press; 2005.

Townsend CM Jr., Beauchamp RD, Evers BM, Mattox KL. *Sabiston Textbook of Surgery.* 19th edn. Philadelphia: Elsevier Saunders; 2012.

42

Esophageal perforation and mediastinitis

Kathryn A. Seal and Sarvotham Kini

Introduction

- Esophageal rupture (perforation) is a potentially life-threatening condition. It carries a mortality rate of nearly 20%, which can be even higher with delays in recognition and treatment.
- The incidence of esophageal perforation is approximately 3 in 100 000. Most of these are secondary to diagnostic or therapeutic esophagoscopy or esophageal dilation. Although esophageal perforation is less common with flexible endoscopy, the number of perforations has increased due to an increased total number of procedures. Other less frequent causes are listed in Table 42.1.
- Unlike the rest of the gastrointestinal tract, the esophagus lacks a serosal layer. As a result, any tear will cause direct communication with the mediastinum.
- Small esophageal tears rarely cause mediastinitis but large tears can lead to intense mediastinitis with a massive inflammatory response, pleural contamination from leaking gastric and bacterial contents, and ultimately death from sepsis.
- The common sites of perforation depend on the etiology (Table 42.2).

Presentation

Classic presentation

- Pain or fever after recent esophageal instrumentation is esophageal perforation until proven otherwise.
- **Pain is almost always present** and can be in the chest, abdomen, back, or neck.

Practical Emergency Resuscitation and Critical Care, ed. Kaushal Shah, Jarone Lee, Kamal Medlej, and Scott D. Weingart. Published by Cambridge University Press. © Kaushal Shah, Jarone Lee, Kamal Medlej, and Scott D. Weingart 2013.

Table 42.1. Less frequent causes of esophageal perforation

Foreign bodies (button batteries)
Caustic ingestions
Trauma (blunt or penetrating)
Violent emesis (Boerhaave syndrome)
Valsalva (cough, heavy lifting, childbirth)
Severe esophagitis
Peptic esophageal ulcer
Spontaneous
Other iatrogenic causes (nasogastric tube placement, postoperative
    anastomosis breakdown)

Table 42.2. Common sites of perforation

Etiology	Perforation site
Spontaneous/forceful emesis	Distal posterolateral wall of the esophagus just above the diaphragm
Foreign bodies	Cervical esophagus or site of stricture
Blunt trauma to neck/thorax	Proximal and middle thirds of the esophagus
Caustic ingestions	Diffuse injury: Alkali burns tend to cause more severe disease than acidic burns because of the liquefactive necrosis
Iatrogenic injuries	Any of the following sites: 1. Pharyngoesophageal junction (thinnest wall with no serosal layer) 2. Esophagogastric junction (acute curve as esophagus enters abdomen) 3. Sites of known strictures

- **Meckler's classic triad** includes sharp chest or epigastric pain, violent vomiting, and subcutaneous emphysema; however, it is only present in a minority of cases.
- **Subcutaneous emphysema** can be found on careful examination of the neck and chest wall in approximately 60% of cases.
- **Hamman's sign** can be present and is the "crunching" sound heard during auscultation of the chest with pneumomediastinum.

Critical presentation

- About a third of patients present with atypical symptoms or signs including sepsis, peritonitis, respiratory distress, fever, pneumo/hydrothorax, fulminant shock, and multi-system organ failure.
- Approximately 17% of esophageal perforations are diagnosed only at autopsy.

Diagnosis and evaluation

- A high index of suspicion is of paramount importance.
- The differential diagnosis is listed in Table 42.3.
- **Chest radiography**
  - 90% of patients will have findings suggestive of perforation on simple chest radiography; signs to look for (see Figure 42.1) are
    - Left pleural effusion
    - Mediastinal air
    - Subcutaneous emphysema
    - Widened mediastinum
    - Pneumothorax
    - Pulmonary infiltrate.
- **Additional imaging studies**
  - A contrast study such as esophagography with Gastrograffin should be performed if perforation is suspected. Although barium has superior sensitivity, it will cause a worsened mediastinal/peritoneal inflammatory response if a leak is present. In addition, Gastrograffin is recommended because it will not obscure visualization during endoscopy. A second study with dilute barium may be considered if an initial study with Gastrograffin is negative (see Figure 42.2).
  - Computed tomography (CT) of the chest and abdomen with oral contrast may better define the leak, assess complications, and exclude other diagnoses. With increased availability and improved resolution, CT is often used as first-line imaging modality. CT findings of perforation include
    - Mediastinal air
    - Subcutaneous emphysema
    - Pleural effusion
    - Pneumopericardium
    - Pneumoperitoneum.
- **Laboratory studies**
  - Laboratory studies are nonspecific and unreliable, especially initially on presentation.
- **Pleurocentesis**
  - Examination of pleural fluid will reveal gastric contents, an elevated amylase, and a low pH (generally <7.4).
- **Adjunctive upper endoscopy**
  - Flexible upper endoscopy to confirm negative esophagram findings is controversial.
  - While it can be helpful if initial contrast study is negative, it carries the risk of worsening small tears or causing new perforation.

Table 42.3. Differential diagnosis

Acute myocardial infarction
Aortic dissection
Pulmonary embolism
Perforated peptic ulcer
Acute pancreatitis
Cholecystitis
Mesenteric ischemia
Pneumothorax
Pneumonia/lung abscess
Pericarditis

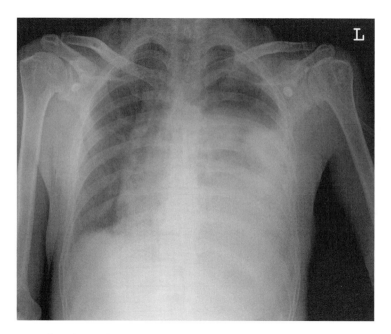

Figure 42.1. Plain chest radiograph showing left pleural effusion, left pneumothorax with tracheal deviation, subcutaneous emphysema in the neck and probable pneumomediastinum. (Courtesy of Dr. Steven Schabel.)

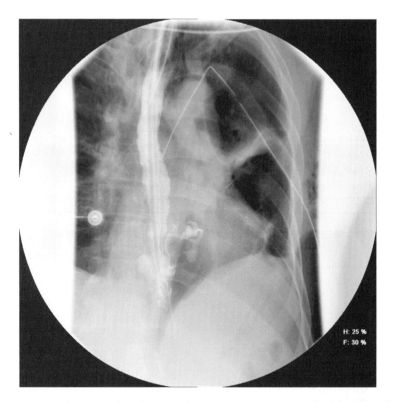

Figure 42.2. Esophagram with oral contrast demonstrates active contrast leak from site of esophageal perforation into the left chest. (Courtesy of Dr. Steven Schabel.)

Critical management

Establish IV access and begin fluid resuscitation with crystalloid products
Make the patient NPO
Administer a proton pump inhibitor
Give IV pain control
Begin broad-spectrum antibiotics
Check preoperative laboratory work
Consult general or thoracic surgery urgently

- Initial management of this potentially fatal condition must be aggressive.
- Give broad-spectrum antibiotics to cover Gram-positive, Gram-negative, and anaerobic organisms.
- **Surgical treatment**
  - **Early surgical consultation**, as primary repair within 24 hours is generally indicated.

- Indications for surgical repair include sepsis, shock, respiratory failure, pneumothorax, pneumoperitoneum, mediastinal emphysema.
- Surgical treatment may include tube thoracostomy, exploration, and drainage as well as primary repair of the esophageal perforation. Surgeons may choose repair or resection, diversion or stent placement at their discretion.
- **Medical treatment**
  - Nonoperative medical treatment may be feasible in clinically stable patients in the following circumstances:
    - Small iatrogenic tear
    - Minimal to no symptoms
    - Absence of infection
    - Delay (>24 hours) in diagnosis without adverse effect
    - High surgical risk.
- Many of these patients will require an **admission to the intensive care unit**
- **Poor prognostic factors** include
  - Delayed treatment
  - Underlying severe esophageal disease
  - Need for major surgical repair
  - Thoracic location of perforation.

Vasopressor of choice: norepinephrine.

REFERENCES

Bhatia P, Fortin D, Inculet RI, Malthaner RA. Current concepts in the management of esophageal perforations: a twenty-seven year Canadian experience. *Ann Thorac Surg.* 2011; **92**(1): 209–15.

Brewer LA, Carter R, Mulder GA, Stiles QR. Options in the management of perforations of the esophagus. *Am J Surg.* 1986; **152**: 62–9.

Jaworski A, Fischer R, Lippmann M. Boerhaave's syndrome. Computed tomographic findings and diagnostic considerations. *Arch Intern Med.* 1988; **148**: 223–4.

Sreide J. Esophageal perforation: diagnostic work-up and clinical decision-making in the first 24 hours. *Scand J Trauma Resusc Emerg Med.* 2001; **19**: 66–72.

Wu J, Mattox K, Wall M. Esophageal perforations: new perspectives and treatment paradigms. *J Trauma.* 2007; **63**: 1173.

Young C, Menias CO, *et al.* CT features of esophageal emergencies. *MD Radiographics.* 2008; **28**: 1541–53.

43

Small bowel obstruction

Byron Pitts, John Lemos, and Kevin McConnell

Introduction

- Small bowel obstruction (SBO) results from the interruption of normal intestinal flow. Severely ill patients may present with SIRS criteria, peritonitis, bowel ischemia, and frank bowel necrosis.
- Table 43.1 details the specific types of small bowel obstruction.
- Common causes of small bowel obstruction include hernias, neoplasms, intussusception, and others (see Table 43.2).

Presentation

Classic presentation

- Crampy, paroxysmal abdominal pain with abdominal distension, vomiting, and inability to pass flatus in a patient with prior abdominal surgery, abdominal neoplasm, or hernia.
- Vomiting may only occur if the obstruction is proximal.
- Bowel dilatation causes increased secretory activity that causes accumulation of fluid in the proximal bowel and increased peristalsis. As a result, frequent loose stools and flatus may be seen in early bowel obstructions.
- Loss of flatus is a late finding.

Critical presentation

- Increased bowel distension causes increased bowel wall edema that results in significant fluid shifts. This may lead to:

Practical Emergency Resuscitation and Critical Care, ed. Kaushal Shah, Jarone Lee, Kamal Medlej, and Scott D. Weingart. Published by Cambridge University Press. © Kaushal Shah, Jarone Lee, Kamal Medlej, and Scott D. Weingart 2013.

Table 43.1. Etiology of small bowel obstruction

Type	Etiology
Mechanical	A physical barrier exists that blocks normal intestinal flow
Closed-loop	Two sequential sites of obstruction block a portion of bowel, usually through a hernia or adhesive band
Functional obstruction/ adynamic ileus	Disturbance in gut motility, failure of peristalsis, most often caused by laparotomy, critical illness, or prolonged opiate use
Pseudo-obstruction	Disturbance of gut motility associated with an underlying condition, but without an underlying lesion. Examples: amyloidosis, hyperthyroidism, hypokalemia, etc.

Table 43.2. Common causes of SBO (percent of all cases)

Postoperative adhesions	50%
Hernias	15%
Neoplasms	15%
Intussusception	5%
Other	15%

- Hypovolemic shock
- Electrolyte abnormalities
- Severe acidosis.
- Bowel perforation and peritonitis:
  - Bowel perforation may be due to increased intraluminal pressure. In addition, if the arterial supply to the bowel is compromised (severe edema, physical obstruction of mesenteric pedicle), bowel wall ischemia and necrosis will follow.
- Severe septic shock due to bacterial translocation.
- Multi-organ system failure due to primary SIRS response or subsequent shock states.
- Age, treatment delay, and preexisting comorbidities are all associated with a worse prognosis.

Diagnosis and evaluation

- **History**
  - A thorough history should be taken, with particular attention paid to prior SBOs, abdominal surgeries, hernias, cancer, and opiate use.
- **Physical examination**
  - *Vital signs:* Fever, tachycardia, hypotension, tachypnea (compensate for metabolic acidosis or in response to pain).

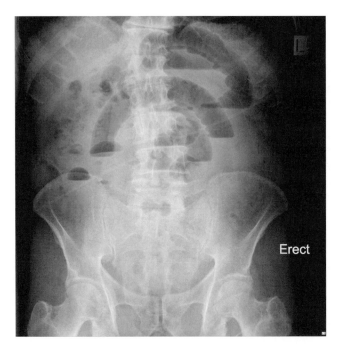

Erect

Figure 43.1. Small bowel obstruction on plain film demonstrates multiple air–fluid levels in dilated loops of bowel with no air in the rectum. (Image by Mike Cadogan from the Global Medical Education Project [GMEP.org]. This image is protected under a Creative Commons CC BY-NC-SA 3.0 license.)

- *Abdominal examination:*
  - Visually inspect the abdomen for scars and distension.
  - Auscultate for high-pitched bowel sounds.
  - Assess for peritoneal findings and distension.
  - Palpate and visually inspect for hernias.
- *Rectal examination:* Consider a rectal examination with evaluation for occult blood, although diagnostic yield may be low and classically the rectal vault will be empty.
- **Laboratory evaluation**
  - Findings will not be specific to bowel obstruction. Results may show evidence of dehydration, acidosis, renal failure, leukocytosis, etc.
- **Imaging**
  - *Plain films* (Figure 43.1)
    - Plain radiography has poor sensitivity and specificity (46% sensitivity, 66% specificity).
    - Indicated in almost all patients with clinically suspected SBO.

- Findings include multiple air–fluid levels, dilated loops of bowel, and absent colonic gas. (Figure 43.1)
- As good as CT scan for "high-grade" obstruction.
- Poor sensitivity for "low-grade" obstruction.
- Cannot differentiate between strangulation and simple obstruction.
- *CT scan:*
  - CT has 80–90% sensitivity, 70–90% specificity.
  - Can often diagnose obstruction when plain radiography is inconclusive.
  - May be helpful to further characterize previously diagnosed obstruction.
  - May show cause of obstruction, such as a mass or occult hernia.
  - Findings not present on simple radiography may include bowel wall thickening, pneumatosis, portal venous gas.
  - Allows determination of "transition point" which aids in surgical planning.
  - May show alternative diagnoses.
  - Does not necessarily need oral contrast as intraluminal fluid will serve this purpose.
  - One must weigh the benefit of CT against potential risks of traveling for a sick patient and possible delay in surgical intervention.
- *Ultrasonography:*
  - US has 93% sensitivity, 100% specificity.
  - With proper training, bedside ultrasound compares favorably with traditional plain radiography.
  - Advantages include that it can be done rapidly at the bedside, it is less costly and less invasive, and there is no need for risky patient travel.
  - Findings include
    - Fluid-filled bowel loops >2.5 cm (90% sensitivity, 83% specificity)
    - Decreased peristalsis (27% sensitivity, 97% specificity).
- SBO that is confirmed with radiography or ultrasound in the setting of a good clinical presentation or with distinct clinical signs of obstruction or peritonitis will likely need operative management. *Further imaging should not be necessary.*

Critical management

Establish IV access and begin fluid resuscitation with crystalloid products
Monitoring equipment (cardiac, blood pressure, pulse oximetry, etc.)
Placement of NG tube
Analgesia
Anti-emetics
NPO
Surgical consult

- **Antibiotics** are indicated with evidence of ischemia, perforation, or severe disease, although there is no good evidence supporting or refuting the use of empiric broad-spectrum antibiotics.
- **Nonoperative management**
  - Includes bowel decompression with NGT, NPO status, IVF, and serial examinations watching for resolution of obstruction and return of normal bowel function.
  - A trial of 3 days is usually appropriate before proceeding to surgical intervention.
  - Indicated only for patients who are hemodynamically stable without any evidence of severe decompensation or strangulation.
- **Operative management**
  - Urgently indicated for any evidence of strangulation.
  - May be indicated with signs of severe disease or decompensation (acidosis, fever, tachycardia, etc.).
  - Also indicated after failure of conservative measures.

Vasopressor of choice: norepinephrine.

REFERENCES

Jang BT, Schindler D, Kaji AH. Bedside ultransonography for the detection of bowel obstruction in the emergency department. *Emerg Med J.* 2011; **28**: 676–8.

Marx JA, Hockberger RS, Walls RM, Adams J, Rosen P, eds. *Rosen's Emergency Medicine: Concepts and Clinical Practice.* 7th edn. Philadelphia, PA: Mosby Elsevier; 2010.

Suri S, Gupta S, Sudhakar PJ, *et al.* Comparative evaluation of plain films, ultrasound and CT in the diagnosis of intestinal obstruction. *Acta Radiol.* 1999; **40**: 422–8.

44

Acid–base interpretation

Chanu Rhee

Introduction

- Acid–base disturbances are common in critically ill patients, and correct interpretation is crucial to proper management. The arterial blood gas (ABG) is the gold standard for determining acid–base status.
- Acidemia refers to a pH ≤7.35, alkalemia refers to a pH ≥7.45. Acidosis refers to a *process* that increases hydrogen ion concentration, while alkalosis refers to a *process* that decreases hydrogen ion concentration. Patients are either acidemic or alkalemic, but can have multiple simultaneous acid–base processes.
- Normal values from an ABG are pH of 7.36–7.44, HCO_3^- of 21–27, $PaCO_2$ of 35–45 mmHg, and pO_2 of 80–100 mmHg. The pH, $PaCO_2$, and pO_2 are measured directly, while the HCO_3^- is calculated from the Henderson-Hasselbach equation.
- Venous blood gases (VBG) are increasingly being used for convenience. Compared to an ABG, the VBG pH is lower by approximately 0.02–0.04, the $PaCO_2$ is higher by 3–8 mmHg, the HCO_3^- concentration is 1–2 mEq/L higher, and the pO_2 is not useful. In general, VBG values correlate well with ABGs, but periodic correlation with ABGs should be performed if serial VBGs are used.

The following is a **basic approach for ABG interpretation**.

Step 1: Look at pH and $PaCO_2$ to determine the primary disorder. The calculated HCO_3^- should be examined to ensure proper interpretation:
- Low pH with low HCO_3^- → Metabolic acidosis
- Low pH with high $PaCO_2$ → Respiratory acidosis

Practical Emergency Resuscitation and Critical Care, ed. Kaushal Shah, Jarone Lee, Kamal Medlej, and Scott D. Weingart. Published by Cambridge University Press. © Kaushal Shah, Jarone Lee, Kamal Medlej, and Scott D. Weingart 2013.

Table 44.1. Compensation formulas for primary acid–base disorders

Primary disorder	Expected compensation
Metabolic acidosis	1. Expected $PaCO_2 = 1.5 \times [HCO_3^-] + 8 \pm 2$ (Winter's formula) 2. Alternatively, the last two digits of pH should approximate $PaCO_2$
Metabolic alkalosis	$PaCO_2 = 0.7 \times [HCO_3^-] + 20 \pm 5$
Respiratory acidosis	1. Acute: ↓pH by 0.08 for every ↑10 $PaCO_2$ 2. Chronic: ↓pH by 0.03 for every ↑10 $PaCO_2$
Respiratory alkalosis	1. Acute: ↑pH by 0.08 for every ↓10 $PaCO_2$ 2. Chronic: ↑pH by 0.03 for every ↓10 $PaCO_2$

- High pH with low $PaCO_2$ → Respiratory alkalosis
- High pH with high HCO_3^- → Metabolic alkalosis

Step 2: Determine if appropriate compensation is present (based on formulas specific to each disorder). Remember that compensation never fully corrects the pH (see Table 44.1).

Step 3: If degree of compensation is not appropriate, determine whether multiple disorders are present.

- Metabolic acidosis or alkalosis:
  - $PaCO_2$ lower than expected = concomitant respiratory alkalosis.
  - $PaCO_2$ higher than expected = concomitant respiratory acidosis.
- Respiratory acidosis or alkalosis:
  - pH lower than expected = concomitant metabolic acidosis.
  - pH higher than expected = concomitant metabolic alkalosis.

Step 4: If a metabolic acidosis is present, determine whether it is an anion-gap metabolic acidosis. If an anion-gap metabolic acidosis is present, calculate the delta-delta gap (see below).

Step 5: If normal pH, consider other possibilities:

- High $PaCO_2$ and high HCO_3^- : respiratory acidosis + metabolic alkalosis.
- Low $PaCO_2$ and low HCO_3^-: respiratory alkalosis + metabolic acidosis.
- Normal $PaCO_2$ and HCO_3^-, but elevated anion gap: anion gap metabolic acidosis + metabolic alkalosis.
- Normal $PaCO_2$, HCO_3^-, and anion gap: no acid–base disturbance, or non–anion-gap acidosis + metabolic alkalosis.

Metabolic acidosis

Presentation

Classic presentation
- Symptoms depend on the severity and etiology of the underlying acidosis, and are often nonspecific. Altered mental status, weakness, nausea, and abdominal pain are common.

- Hyperkalemia is often present due to transcellular shift of K^+ out of cells and H^+ into cells.
- Kussmaul respirations are classically associated with diabetic ketoacidosis (DKA), and refer to rapid, deep breathing.

Critical presentation
- Extreme acidemia leads to neurological dysfunction (severe obtundation, coma, and seizures) as well as cardiovascular complications (arrhythmias, decreased cardiac contractility, arteriolar vasodilation, and decreased responsiveness to catecholamines). Profound hypotension and shock can result, which can complicate management since hypotension and shock are often the cause of the acidosis.

Diagnosis and evaluation

History and physical examination
- History and physical are generally revealing (e.g., a patient with a history of DKA who presents with nausea, weakness, and signs of dehydration).

Diagnostic tests
- Calculate the anion gap ($Na^+ - [Cl^- + HCO_3^-]$). The expected anion gap is 2.5 × [Albumin].
- If an elevated anion gap (AG) is present, check *delta-delta gap* ($\Delta\Delta$) to evaluate for secondary metabolic derangement. The basic concept behind the $\Delta\Delta$ is to examine whether the observed change in anion gap is matched by an equivalent change in serum bicarbonate level.
- $\Delta\Delta$ = (Calculated AG – Expected AG)/(24 – Measured HCO_3^-).
  - $\Delta\Delta$ <1 = simultaneous non-AG acidosis.
  - $\Delta\Delta$ >2 = simultaneous metabolic alkalosis.
  - $\Delta\Delta$ 1–2 = pure AG metabolic acidosis.
- Alternate method of measuring $\Delta\Delta$:
  (Measured AG – Expected AG) + measured HCO_3^- = "New HCO_3^-"
  "New HCO_3^-" >28 = simultaneous metabolic alkalosis, <20 = a simultaneous non–anion-gap acidosis.
- If an anion-gap acidosis is present, check urine and/or serum for possible etiologies: ketones, lactate, and metabolic panel to assess renal function for evidence of uremia (Table 44.2). If unrevealing, consider toxin screen and serum osmolality to check osmolal gap.
- Osmolal gap (OG) = measured osmoles – calculated osmoles (2 × Na^+ + Glucose/18 + BUN/2.8 + EtOH/4.6).
  - OG >10 suggests ingestion leading to unmeasured osmoles. The major ingestions that cause an elevated OG include various alcohols (ethanol, methanol, ethylene glycol, acetone, isopropyl alcohol), formaldehyde, paraldehyde, and diethyl ether. However, smaller ingestions can be missed and serum volatiles screen should also be checked.

Table 44.2. Etiologies of anion-gap acidosis

Lactic acidosis – common and feared cause of metabolic acidosis in critically ill patients. Degree of elevation correlates with mortality
- **Type A lactic acidosis** (impaired systemic perfusion/oxygenation) – shock (any type), severe hypoxemia, severe anemia
- **Type B lactic acidosis** (no impaired system perfusion/oxygenation)
  Type B1 (systemic processes): liver and/or renal dysfunction (decreased clearance of lactate), seizures, hypothermic shivering, severe exercise, severe asthma exacerbation, ischemic bowel (increased production of lactate), malignancy, diabetic ketoacidosis
  Type B2 (drugs): metformin, isoniazid, linezolid, HIV meds, cyanide, carbon monoxide
  Type B3 (congenital/inborn errors of metabolism)
Ketoacidosis – diabetic ketoacidosis, alcoholism, starvation
Renal failure – decreased excretion of organic anions (phosphates, sulfates, urate)
Ingestions – methanol, ethylene glycol, salicylates, toluene

- If a non–anion-gap acidosis is present and history is unrevealing, check urine anion gap = Urine Na^+ + Urine K^+ – Urine Cl^-. Causes of non–anion gap acidosis are listed in Table 44.3.
- Urine anion gap is an indirect measurement of renal ammonium (NH_4^+) excretion, which is excreted with Cl^-. The normal renal response to acidemia is to increase NH_4^+ excretion.
  - A negative urine anion gap suggests increased renal NH_4^+ excretion consistent with diarrhea, type II renal tubular acidosis (RTA), or dilutional acidosis.
  - A positive urine anion gap suggests impaired renal excretion of NH_4^+ consistent with type I or IV RTA or chronic kidney disease.

Critical management

- The most important step is to identify and treat the underlying etiology. For example, if acidosis is due to DKA, treatment requires insulin and IV fluid resuscitation. For toxic ingestions, antidotes if appropriate (e.g., fomepizole for methanol and ethylene glycol) and hemodialysis can be helpful. If type A lactic acidosis from sepsis is the problem, management includes antibiotics and reversal of shock with fluids and vasopressors.
- Potassium levels should be followed carefully, as initial hyperkalemia will normalize or shift to hypokalemia once acidosis is corrected.
- Critically ill patients with metabolic acidosis often require intubation and mechanical ventilation for airway protection, hemodynamic instability, etc. Once intubated, hyperventilation to compensate for acidosis can be accomplished with the ventilator.
- Alkaline therapy with intravenous sodium bicarbonate is controversial; if used, it should only be done as a temporizing measure in those with severe

Table 44.3. Etiologies of non–anion-gap acidosis

Diarrhea – due to loss of sodium bicarbonate. Most common cause of non-AG acidosis

Dilutional – from rapid infusion of saline that lacks bicarbonate and contains an excess of chloride. Normally causes no more than a mild metabolic acidosis

Renal tubular acidosis

- Type I (distal): impaired distal H^+ secretion. Severe acidosis, positive urine anion gap, associated hypokalemia. *Etiologies:* idiopathic, familial, medications (amphotericin B, lithium), Sjögren syndrome, renal transplantation, obstructive uropathy, sickle cell anemia, rheumatoid arthritis
- Type II (proximal): impaired proximal HCO_3^- reabsorption. Moderate acidosis, negative urine anion gap, associated hypokalemia. *Etiologies:* idiopathic, familial, multiple myeloma, medications (ifosfamide, tenofovir, acetazolamide), amyloidosis, heavy metals, renal transplantation, vitamin D deficiency, paroxysmal nocturnal hemoglobinuria
- Type III: rare autosomal recessive syndrome with features of both distal and proximal RTA.
- Type IV (hypoaldosteronism): decreased ammonium excretion. Mild acidosis, positive urine anion gap, associated hyperkalemia. *Etiologies:* chronic kidney disease (most often diabetic nephropathy), NSAIDs, calcineurin inhibitors, ACE inhibitors/ARBs, potassium-sparing diuretics (spironolactone, eplerenone, amiloride), TMP-SMX, primary adrenal insufficiency, heparin

Acetazolamide – carbonic anhydrase inhibitor causes impaired HCO_3^- reabsorption

Hyperalimentation (TPN) – NH_4Cl and amino acids metabolized to HCl

Ureteral diversion – i.e., ureterocolonic fistula. Urinary Cl^- absorbed by colonic mucosa in exchange for HCO_3^-, leading to increased GI loss of HCO_3^-

Pancreatic fistula – HCO_3^--rich fluid excreted into and lost in the intestines

Posthypocapnia – patients with preexisting, prolonged respiratory alkalosis have compensatory decrease in HCO_3^-. If respiratory alkalosis resolves rapidly (i.e., with sedation and mechanical ventilation), underlying non–anion-gap acidosis will be "unmasked"

---

acidemia and pH <7.10–7.15. The theoretical benefits of raising cardiac output and blood pressure and increasing responsiveness to catecholamine vasopressors are unproven in lactic acidosis. Potential risks include volume overload, paradoxical worsening of intracellular acidosis, and conversion of HCO_3^- to CO_2 which can cause respiratory acidosis in those with inadequate ventilation.

- An alternative to sodium bicarbonate is THAM (tromethamine), a direct proton chelator. Compared to sodium bicarbonate, THAM does not increase $PaCO_2$, making it useful in patients with respiratory acidosis. However, THAM is cleared by the kidneys and must be used cautiously in patients with renal failure.
- Severe acidosis that is refractory to medical management is an indication for hemodialysis.

Table 44.4. Etiologies of metabolic alkalosis

Saline-responsive (urine Cl⁻ <20)
- GI losses of H⁺: vomiting, nasogastric tube suctioning
- Contraction alkalosis from diuresis (extracellular fluid contracts around a fixed amount of HCO_3^-)
- Posthypercapnia: patient with preexisting, chronic respiratory acidosis develops compensatory increase in HCO_3^- over time; rapid correction of respiratory acidosis to a "normal" $PaCO_2$ (usually with mechanical ventilation) "unmasks" compensatory metabolic alkalosis

Saline-resistant (urine Cl⁻ >20)
- Hyperaldosteronism: *primary* (Conn syndrome) = aldosterone secreting adenoma; *secondary* = exogenous mineralocorticoids, Cushing syndrome, renovascular disease
- Hypokalemia: induces a shift of K⁺ out of cells and H⁺ into cells, and intracellular acidosis in renal tubular cells promotes H⁺ secretion and HCO_3^- reabsorption
- Exogenous alkali load (i.e., intravenous sodium bicarbonate)
- Bartter syndrome (defective NaCl reabsorption in ascending loop of Henle)
- Gitelman syndrome (defective NaCl cotransporter in distal tubule)

Metabolic alkalosis

Presentation

Classic presentation
- As for metabolic acidosis, symptoms are nonspecific and usually related to the underlying etiology. Signs of volume depletion are present in many patients with contraction alkalosis or protracted vomiting.

Critical presentation
- Although not as common as severe metabolic acidosis, severe alkalemia can be equally devastating. Neurological symptoms include altered mental status, coma, and seizures. Cardiovascular symptoms include increased risk of arrhythmias and arteriolar vasoconstriction, which can cause decreased coronary blood flow. Alkalemia can also induce hypokalemia, hypocalcemia, and hypophosphatemia.

Diagnosis and evaluation

History and physical examination
- History and physical are generally revealing (i.e., multiple episodes of emesis with signs of dehydration).

Diagnostic tests
- Urine chloride: a urine Cl⁻ <20 suggests saline-responsive etiology (conditions in which chloride is lost). A urine Cl⁻ >20 suggests saline-resistant etiology (see Table 44.4).

- Blood pressure: hypertension with a saline-resistant metabolic alkalosis suggests hyperaldosteronism.

Critical management

- The cornerstone for most patients with saline-responsive metabolic alkalosis is correction of volume depletion with isotonic sodium chloride.
- In patients with concurrent hypokalemia, potassium repletion will improve alkalosis due to transcellular H^+/K^+ exchange. For patients with metabolic alkalosis in whom saline administration is contraindicated (i.e., CHF patients who require diuresis), potassium repletion is still useful. Acetazolamide can help correct both alkalosis and fluid overload.

Respiratory acidosis

Presentation

Classic presentation
- Mild to moderate compensatory hypercapnia, especially when chronic, usually has minimal symptoms, but patients may be anxious or complain of dyspnea.

Critical presentation
- As hypercarbia worsens, patients become progressively confused, somnolent, and obtunded ("CO_2 narcosis"). Elevated $PaCO_2$ leads to cerebral vasodilation and can cause papilledema.
- Cardiovascular complications of acute hypercarbia include tachycardia/arrhythmias and hypertension (mediated by sympathetic nervous system hyperactivity), pulmonary vasoconstriction, and exacerbation of right heart dysfunction.
- Other manifestations are those of severe acidemia, regardless of etiology, and include neurological and cardiovascular complications (seizures, vasodilation, hypotension).

Diagnosis and evaluation

History, physical examination, and diagnostic tests
- History and physical examination may be revealing (e.g., COPD with chronic CO_2 retention), but most patients will warrant a drug and toxicology screen, chest radiograph, and sometimes neuroimaging if routine studies are nondiagnostic. Table 44.5 lists causes of respiratory acidosis.

Critical management

- If medications are a suspected culprit, or the etiology is unclear, reversal (e.g., with naloxone for opiate overdose or flumazenil for benzodiazepines) is warranted.

Table 44.5. Etiologies of respiratory acidosis

CNS depression: sedating medications (opiates, benzodiazepines), CNS pathology or trauma

Lower airway obstruction: COPD, asthma

Upper airway obstruction: laryngospasm, laryngeal edema, tracheal stenosis, obstructive sleep apnea, foreign body

Chest wall disorders: severe kyphoscoliosis, flail chest, ankylosing spondylitis, pectus excavatum

Neuromuscular disorders: Guillain–Barré, myasthenia gravis, poliomyelitis, amyotrophic lateral sclerosis, muscular dystrophy, diaphragmatic dysfunction, botulism

Obesity-hypoventilation syndrome

Lung parenchymal disease (i.e., pneumonia, pulmonary edema, interstitial lung disease): usually causes hypoxia, tachypnea, and respiratory alkalosis, but may progress to muscle fatigue and respiratory acidosis

---

- Noninvasive positive-pressure ventilation with Bi-PAP can be useful in those with mild to moderate respiratory acidosis with a quickly reversible condition. The evidence of benefit for Bi-PAP is strongest for moderate to severe COPD exacerbations, in which mortality is clearly decreased; benefit is also seen with pulmonary edema, although effect on mortality is less clear. Bi-PAP also appears to be useful for asthma exacerbations, and some cases of pneumonia.
- If severe acidemia is present, or the patient is obtunded, intubation may be indicated.

Respiratory alkalosis

Presentation

Classic presentation
- As respiratory alkalosis is most commonly due to hypoxia leading to hyperventilation, dyspnea and anxiety will often be apparent.

Critical presentation
- Acute hypocapnia can cause cerebral vasoconstriction, leading to confusion, dizziness, syncope, and seizure.
- Respiratory alkalosis causes an increase in binding of calcium to albumin, and many of the symptoms of severe respiratory alkalosis are due to hypocalcemia (paresthesias, perioral numbness, and tetany). Hypokalemia and hypophosphatemia also occur due to intracellular shifts.
- Other critical symptoms are those of severe alkalemia, including systemic and coronary vasoconstriction, and arrhythmias.

Table 44.6. Etiologies of respiratory alkalosis

Hypoxia (leading to hyperventilation; most common cause)
Psychiatric conditions: anxiety, pain
Fever
Medications: salicylates (mixed metabolic acidosis and respiratory alkalosis),
   methylxanthines, progesterone, nicotine
Pregnancy (due to progesterone excess)
Hyperthyroidism
Liver failure
Sepsis

Diagnosis and evaluation

History, physical examination, and diagnostic tests

- Assess for causes of tachypnea (i.e., fever, anxiety). Table 44.6 lists causes of respiratory alkalosis.
- In patients with hypoxemia, chest radiography is warranted to evaluate for pulmonary pathology.
- Serum chemistries should be checked (importantly potassium, calcium, and phosphorus).

Critical management

- Treatment is primarily directed at correcting the underlying disorder and managing hypoxemia (if present) as respiratory alkalosis itself is rarely life threatening. Careful attention should be paid to calcium, potassium, and phosphate levels.

Sudden deterioration

- Acute changes in any patient with an acid–base disorder require a rapid reevaluation of the patient's mental status and vital signs, as well as repeat ABG determination.
- If the patient is mechanically ventilated, note any recent ventilator settings changes that might explain a change in CO_2 levels.

Critical care considerations

Review the relevant chapters on the evaluation and management of Mechanical ventilation, The boarding ICU patient in the emergency department, and Common electrolyte disorders.

REFERENCES

Cooper DJ, Walley KR, Wiggs BR, Russell JA. Bicarbonate does not improve hemodynamics in critically ill patients who have lactic acidosis: a prospective, controlled clinical study. *Ann Intern Med*. 1990; **112**: 492.

Gray A, Goodacre S, Newby D, *et al*. Noninvasive ventilation in acute cardiogenic pulmonary edema. *N Engl J Med*. 2008; **359**: 142–151.

Hoste EA, Colpaert K, Vanholder RC, *et al*. Sodium bicarbonate versus THAM in ICU patients with mild metabolic acidosis. *J Nephrol*. 2005; **18**: 303.

Maletesha G, Singh NK, Bharija A, Rehani B, Goel A. Comparison of arterial and venous pH, bicarbonate, PCO_2 and O_2 in initial emergency department assessment. *Emerg Med J*. 2007; **24**(8): 569.

Ram FS, Picot J, Lightowler J, Wedzicha JA. Noninvasive positive pressure ventilation for treatment of respiratory failure due to exacerbations of chronic obstructive pulmonary disease. *Cochrane Database Syst Rev*. 2004; (1): CD004104.

45

Common electrolyte disorders (sodium, potassium, calcium, magnesium)

John E. Arbo

DISORDERS OF SODIUM METABOLISM

Introduction

- Serum sodium (Na) concentration is mediated by free water intake, circulating levels of antidiuretic hormone (ADH), and renal filtration of sodium.
- **Hyponatremia** is defined as serum sodium level of <135 mEq/L, and is due to a deficit of sodium relative to free water. It occurs most commonly in the setting of intravascular volume depletion, where increased secretion of ADH and volume replacement with free water will create a hypotonic state in the process of restoring volume.
- **Hypernatremia** is defined as a serum sodium level of >150 mEq/L, and is due to a deficit of free water relative to sodium. It occurs most commonly from loss of free water due to impaired access. Since most people are able to respond to their thirst stimulus with free water intake, hypernatremia is a rare condition, and is typically only seen in patients with limited mobility or impaired thirst mechanisms. Hypernatremia also occurs in the setting of diabetes insipidus, defined as a loss of free water due to either a deficiency of or insensitivity to ADH.

Practical Emergency Resuscitation and Critical Care, ed. Kaushal Shah, Jarone Lee, Kamal Medlej, and Scott D. Weingart. Published by Cambridge University Press. © Kaushal Shah, Jarone Lee, Kamal Medlej, and Scott D. Weingart 2013.

Hyponatremia

Presentation

Classic presentation
- Signs and symptoms of moderate hyponatremia are nonspecific: generalized weakness, lethargy, nausea, vomiting, and muscle cramps are common.

Critical presentation
- Severe hyponatremia (<120 mEq/L), or rapid drops in serum sodium level, may present with confusion and seizure.

Diagnosis and evaluation

- Hyponatremia is most commonly caused by an excess of ADH released in response to intravascular volume depletion, exacerbated by volume replacement with hypotonic fluids (the body will sacrifice tonicity in order to restore volume). This results in a *hypotonic hyponatremia* (serum osmolarity <280 mOsm/L).
- Hyponatremia in the setting of normal serum osmolarity, or *isotonic hyponatremia* (serum osmolarity = 280 mOsm/L), is referred to as pseudohyponatremia, and represents artifact due to hyperlipidemia or hyperproteinemia. Hyponatremia in the setting of elevated serum osmolarity, or *hypertonic hyponatremia* (serum osmolarity >280 mOsm/L), is due to the presence of another effective osmole such as glucose or mannitol drawing water into the intravascular space. Serum osmolality can be approximated with the following expression: $2 \times$ serum Na^+ + BUN/2.8 + glucose/18.
- The evaluation of **hypotonic hyponatremia** (the majority of cases) begins with an assessment of total body volume status.
- **History**
  - Inquire about total body volume loss (diarrhea, emesis, fever, polyuria) or gain (edema, ascites, oliguria), changes in medications (i.e., diuretics), and symptoms of hypothyroidism or adrenal insufficiency such as weakness and fatigue (increased ADH secretion occurs in both glucocorticoid deficiency and hypothyroidism).
- **Physical examination**
  - Check blood pressure, pulse, mucous membranes, skin turgor, and capillary refill.
  - Perform a bedside cardiac ultrasound looking for inferior vena cava diameter and degree of inspiratory collapse to estimate intravascular volume status.
- **Diagnostic tests**
  - Chemistry panel, TSH, A.M. cortisol, urine sodium, serum and urine osmolality. Urine sodium is a useful diagnostic test in the workup of hypotonic hyponatremia because it serves as an indicator of the body's efforts to restore intravascular volume. If a patient is volume depleted, the kidneys should

retain sodium, and with sodium, water. If the urine sodium >20 mEq/L in this setting, it signals a problem with the kidneys. Total body volume status assessment coupled with urine sodium (mEq/L) helps narrow the diagnosis.

- **Hypovolemic** hypotonic hyponatremia (most common):
  - Urine sodium <20 = extrarenal losses = vomiting, diarrhea, hemorrhage, pancreatitis.
  - Urine sodium >20 = renal losses = diuretics, salt-wasting nephropathy.
- **Euvolemic** hypotonic hyponatremia:
  - Urine sodium <20 = primary polydipsia, beer potomania, "tea and toast"
  - Urine sodium >20 = SIADH, adrenal insufficiency, hypothyroidism.
- **Hypervolemic** hypotonic hyponatremia:
  - Urine sodium <20 = congestive heart failure, cirrhosis, nephritic syndrome
  - Urine sodium >20 = renal insufficiency (inability to excrete free water).
- Euvolemic hypotonic hyponatremia describes a state in which the clinical assessment of volume status is indeterminate. The majority of these cases are caused by SIADH (syndrome of inappropriate antidiuretic hormone secretion). SIADH has multiple etiologies, including disorders of the pulmonary system (COPD, asthma, pneumonia, pneumothorax) and central nervous system (stroke, hemorrhage, mass effect, trauma), drugs (antidepressants, antipsychotics, vasopressin), stress, and pain.
- SIADH is a *diagnosis of exclusion*. The following conditions must be met to make a diagnosis:
  - Hypotonic hyponatremia
  - Clinical euvolemia
  - Urine sodium >20 mEq/L
  - No diuretic use, or evidence of hypothyroidism or adrenal insufficiency
  - Urine osmolality >100 mOsm/kg.
- **A word about urine osmolality (Uosm):** Uosm will almost always be >200 mOsm/kg, and so is rarely useful in the diagnostic process. A Uosm of <100 mOsm/kg is seen in two instances (1) primary polydipsia: a disorder in which free water intake overwhelms the kidneys' excreting capacity, seen in patients in whom medications (neuroleptics) stimulate thirst, and (2) beer potomania or "tea and toast": diets that are mostly water, with limited dietary osmoles.

Critical management

- **Hypovolemic hypotonic hyponatremia:** Management is focused on the use of sodium-containing fluids to replace intravascular volume, replenish serum sodium, and eliminate the stimulus for ADH. If the patient is hypotensive, normal saline boluses should be given as with any patient. Otherwise, unless the patient has altered mental status or is seizing, care should be taken to not raise the serum sodium level by more than 0.5 mEq/hour or a total of 8 mEq/day.

- To ensure an appropriate rate of replacement, calculate the following:
  - Total body water (TBW) in liters = 0.6 (male) or 0.5 (female) × weight in kg.
  - Target serum sodium level (based on 0.5 mEq/hour or 8 mEq/day).
  - Sodium deficit (mEq of sodium needed to reach target) = TBW × (Na target – Na serum).
  - Total replacement fluid needed to provide sodium deficit = Na deficit (mEq)/Na replacement fluid (mEq/L).
  - Hourly infusion rate: Amount of fluid/total replacement time.
- Replacement fluid options include normal saline (154 mEq/L), 2% saline (342 mEq/L), or 3% saline (513 mEq/). 3% saline requires central venous access.
- **Note**: These examples assume a constant urine osmolality. In reality, Uosm will typically decrease as intravascular volume is replaced, the stimulus for ADH is removed, and free water is once again excreted. As this occurs, there can be an unintended increase in the rate of sodium correction.
- To ensure a safe and accurate rate, recheck serum sodium levels frequently, especially if using normal saline. If sodium levels are accidentally overcorrected, consider using DDVAVP (desmopressin) + D5W to re-lower serum level.
- **Euvolemic hypotonic hyponatremia**: Restrict free water and treat underlying cause. In cases where Uosm is high, be careful not to give isotonic fluids (e.g., normal saline) unless the patient is hypotensive, as this can result in a net gain of free water and an unintended worsening of the hyponatremia. Recheck serum sodium levels frequently.
- **Hypervolemic hypotonic hyponatremia**: Restrict free water and treat underlying cause. Recheck serum sodium levels frequently.

Sudden deterioration

- For most cases of hyponatremia, raising the serum sodium by 0.5 mEq/L/hour is appropriate. In severe cases, or when the patient presents with altered mental status or seizure, the initial sodium correction should be 2 mEq/hour until symptoms resolve.
  - Overly rapid correction (>10–12 mEq/L/day of low sodium may cause *central pontine myelinosis* and should be avoided at all costs.

Hypernatremia

Presentation

Classic presentation
- As with hyponatremia, signs and symptoms of moderate hypernatremia are nonspecific. Generalized weakness and nausea are common.

Critical presentation
- Severe hypernatremia, or rapid increases in serum sodium level, may present with confusion and seizure.

Diagnosis and evaluation

- **History**
  - Inquire about sources of insensible losses (fever, tachypnea), diuretic use, osmotic diuresis (glycosuria), osmotic diarrhea (malabsorption, lactulose), and emesis.
- **Physical examination**
  - As with hyponatremia, perform a physical examination assessing volume status, with an additional focus on mental status and mobility.
- **Diagnostic tests**
  - Chemistry panel, urine osmolality, and urine sodium. Hypernatremia is due to a loss of free water relative to sodium. Urine osmolality is a useful diagnostic test in the work-up of hypernatremia because an appropriate response to a relative increase in serum sodium is to concentrate the urine and retain free water. Urine sodium (mEq/L) is useful in *hypovolemic hypernatremia* as an indicator of the body's efforts to restore intravascular volume. Total body volume status assessment coupled with urine sodium and urine osmolality will help narrow the diagnosis.
    - Hypovolemic hypernatremia (most common):
      - Urine will be concentrated, Uosm >600 mOsm/kg.
      - Urine sodium <20 = extrarenal loss = diarrhea, emesis, insensible losses.
      - Urine sodium >20 = renal loss = diuretics use or osmotic diuresis.
    - Euvolemic hypernatremia:
      - Euvolemic hypernatremia results from increased insensible losses (tachypnea or sweating), or loss of free water due to diabetes insipidus (DI).
      - In patients with hypernatremia, the urine should be concentrated. In DI, a condition caused by either a deficiency of or insensitivity to ADH, the urine osmolality (Uosm) will be inappropriately low, often <300 mOsm/kg.
      - The diagnosis of DI is confirmed by testing the response to fluid restriction (urine osmolality should increase by >30 mOsm/kg with this challenge). Once the diagnosis of DI is confirmed, distinguishing between central and nephrogenic DI requires administration of desmopressin (synthetic ADH) and rechecking urine osmolality. In central DI, desmopressin will make the urine more concentrated.
    - Hypervolemic hypernatremia (rare):
      - Hypertonic saline administration.
      - Mineralocorticoid excess which causes suppression of ADH secretion.

Critical management

- Management centers on replacement of the free water deficit. As with hyponatremia, the rate of correction must be carefully monitored. Care should be taken to not lower the serum sodium level by more than 0.5 mEq/hour, or by 8 mEq/day.
- To ensure an appropriate rate of replacement, calculate the following:
  - Total body water (TBW) in liters = 0.6 (male) or 0.5 (female) × weight in kg.
  - Target serum sodium level (based on 0.5 mEq/hour or 8 mEq/day).
  - Liters of water required to reach target (water deficit) = TBW × [(Na serum/Na target) − 1].
  - Hourly infusion rate: Amount of fluid/total replacement time.
- Emergency treatment of diabetes insipidus centers on replacement of free water deficit. Definitive treatment of DI requires treatment of underlying cause and use of desmopressin.

Sudden deterioration

- Overly rapid correction of hypernatremia may lead to **cerebral edema** and seizure. As with hyponatremia, to ensure a safe and accurate replacement rate, recheck serum sodium levels frequently.

DISORDERS OF POTASSIUM METABOLISM

Introduction

- Disorders of potassium, especially hyperkalemia, are the most feared electrolyte disorders due to their ability to cause life-threatening cardiac arrhythmia.
- Hypokalemia is defined as a serum potassium level of <3.5 mEq/L.
- Hyperkalemia is defined as a serum potassium level of >5.5 mEq/L.

Hypokalemia

Presentation

Classic presentation
- Mild hypokalemia is usually asymptomatic.
- Table 45.1 lists causes of hypokalemia.

Critical presentation
- Severe hypokalemia (<2.5 mEq/L) can present with cardiac, gastrointestinal, and neuromuscular abnormalities.

Table 45.1. Etiologies of hypokalemia

Renal losses: diuretics, RTA, DKA, Bartter's and Gittleman's syndromes
Gastrointestinal losses: diarrhea, emesis, gastric suction, laxative abuse, malabsorption
Transcellular shift: alkalemia, insulin, beta-agonists/bronchodilators, catecholamines,
Hyperaldosteronism

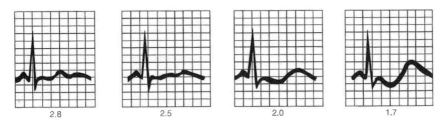

Figure 45.1 ECG changes associated with hypokalemia.

- **Cardiovascular**: classic ECG changes follow a distinct pattern: flattened T waves > ST depression > U waves > QT interval prolongation > ventricular arrhythmia (Figure 45.1).
- **Gastrointestinal**: ileus.
- **Neuromuscular**: nausea, weakness, muscle cramps.

Diagnosis and evaluation

- Chemistry panel including magnesium, urine potassium, 24-hour urine potassium, urine and serum osmolality, and arterial pH.
  - Identify possible causes of transcellular shifts.
  - Measure urine potassium (Up) and calculate transtubular potassium gradient (TTKG) = (Up/Pike)/(Uosm/Poem) where Pike and Poem are plasma potassium and plasma osmolality:
    - Up >30 mEq/day or Up >15 mEq/L or TTKG >7 = renal losses
    - Up <25 mEq/day or Up <15 mEq/L or TTKG <3 = extrarenal loses
- Normally functioning kidneys will respond to hypokalemia with a low TTKG (i.e., decreased excretion of potassium).
- If there are renal loses, check blood pressure and acid–base status. If hypertensive, consider hyperaldosteronism. If normotensive and acidemic, consider DKA or RTA (total body potassium depletion, *not transcellular shift*). If alkalemic, consider diuretics, Bartter syndrome and Gittleman syndrome.

Critical management

- Correct the causes of transcellular shift. If it is a true deficit (*i.e., not transcellular shift*), provide potassium supplementation with potassium chloride (KCl) or potassium phosphate.
- Oral dose of 10 mEq of KCl should raise serum potassium by 0.1 mEq. Use KCl 20 mEq/hour until normalized.
- Correct serum magnesium: hypokalemia is difficult to correct in the setting of hypomagnesemia.

Sudden deterioration

- Cardiac instability: 10 mEq/hour of KCl IV, preferably through a central venous catheter.

Hyperkalemia

Presentation

Classic presentation
- Mild hyperkalemia is usually asymptomatic.
- Table 45.2 lists causes of hyperkalemia.

Critical presentation
- Severe hyperkalemia can present with cardiac and neuromuscular abnormalities.
  - **Cardiovascular**: Classic ECG changes follow a distinct pattern: peaked T waves > widening of the QRS > AV conduction blocks > sine waves > ventricular fibrillation (Figure 45.2).
  - **Neuromuscular**: Paresthesias and weakness of the extremities, flaccid paralysis.

Diagnosis and evaluation

- **Diagnostic tests**
  - Chemistry panel, urine potassium, urine and serum osmolality.
  - Identify and correct causes of pseudohyperkalemia.
  - Identify possible causes of transcellular shifts.
  - Assess for renal dysfunction (GFR and creatinine).
  - If there is renal dysfunction, calculate the transtubular potassium gradient (TTKG) as described above.
  - Normally functioning kidneys will respond to hyperkalemia with an elevated TTKG (i.e., increased excretion of potassium). A low (<7) TTKG in the setting of hyperkalemia and normal functioning kidneys suggests hypoaldosteronism.

Table 45.2. Etiologies of hyperkalemia

Impaired excretion: renal insufficiency, potassium sparing diuretics, ACE-inhibitors
Transcellular shift: acidemia, lack of insulin, burns, tumor lysis, digoxin toxicity, beta-blockers, trauma, rhabdomyolysis, succinylcholine
Hypoaldosteronism
Excess intake
Pseudohyperkalemia: hemolysis of blood sample, elevated WBC or platelet count

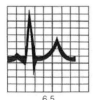 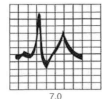 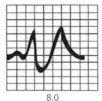 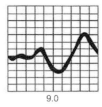

| 6.5 | 7.0 | 8.0 | 9.0 |

Figure 45.2. ECG changes associated with hyperkalemia.

Critical management

- **Stabilize cardiac cell membrane:** for hyperkalemia with ECG changes, or any K >7.0 mEq/L, give calcium chloride 1 g through a central venous catheter, otherwise use calcium gluconate (remember that the chloride:gluconate ratio is 1:3).
- **Drive potassium into cells:**
  - Regular insulin 10 units IV with 1 ampule D50 to prevent hypoglycemia.
  - Sodium bicarbonate 50 mEq (1 ampule).
  - Albuterol 10–20 mg inhaled (note this is 2–4 times the regular adult dose).
- **Decrease total body potassium:**
  - Sodium polystyrene sulfonate (Kayexalate) 30–90 g PO.
  - Loop diuretics (furosemide) 40 mg IV.
  - Hemodialysis for refractory hyperkalemia or unstable patients.

Sudden deterioration

- Cardiac instability: IV calcium chloride via a central venous catheter.
- Emergent hemodialysis.

DISORDERS OF CALCIUM METABOLISM

Introduction

- Release of calcium stores into the circulation is regulated by extracellular calcium concentration, parathyroid hormone (PTH), vitamin D metabolites, and calcitonin.

- 40% of serum calcium is bound to protein, primarily albumin. 45% is physiologically free (not bound to albumin) and is measured as ionized calcium (iCa). 15% is bound to other anions.
- Normal serum calcium measures 8.5–10.5 mg/dL and reflects total calcium (bound and unbound). Normal ionized calcium measures 2.1–2.6 mEq/L (1.05 to 1.3 mmol/L).
- Decreases in albumin lower total serum calcium without affecting ionized calcium. Corrected calcium (mg/dL) = measured calcium + [0.8 × (4 − albumin)].
- Since ionized calcium is the biologically active fraction, it is always best to measure it directly in patients with low serum albumin.

Hypocalcemia

Presentation

Classic presentation
- Mild hypocalcemia is usually asymptomatic.
- Table 45.3 lists causes of hypocalcemia.

Critical presentation
- Severe hypocalcemia (ionized calcium <1.6 mEq/L or <0.8 mmol/L) can affect the cardiovascular and neuromuscular systems.
  - **Cardiovascular symptoms**: may impair cardiac contractility resulting in hypotension and cardiac dysrhythmias. Hypocalcemia-related hypotension does not respond to vasopressors or plasma volume expansion. Hypocalcemia prolongs the QTc interval, which can result in ventricular dysrhythmia.

Table 45.3. Etiologies of hypocalcemia

Hypoparathyroidism
- Primary: due to radiation therapy, surgery, infiltrative diseases, or genetic disorders
- Secondary (pseudohypoparathyroidism): end-organ resistance to parathyroid hormone (PTH)

Vitamin D deficiency
- Renal disease
- Hepatic disease
- Decreased intake/malabsorption
- Hypomagnesemia (decreased sensitivity to PTH)

Calcium sequestration/precipitation
- Massive blood transfusion (calcium binds to citrate anticoagulant)
- Hyperphosphatemia
- Alkalosis
- Pancreatitis
- Sepsis

- **Neuromuscular symptoms**: may include paresthesias (classically fingertips and perioral), seizures, muscle spasms, and tetany. Classic findings include **Chvostek's** sign (twitching of the facial muscles after tapping of the facial nerve, seen in 10–30% of cases) and **Trousseau's** sign (carpopedal spasm when blood flow to the hand is decreased by inflating a blood pressure cuff above systolic pressure for 3 minutes).

Diagnosis and evaluation

- **Diagnostic tests**
  - Serum and ionized calcium, serum albumin, parathyroid hormone (PTH), phosphate (PO_4), magnesium, and renal function studies.
  - Low calcium/elevated PTH/elevated PO_4: chronic renal failure, pseudohypo-parathyroidism.
  - Low calcium/elevated PTH/low PO_4: vitamin D deficiency.
  - Low calcium/low PTH/elevated PO_4: hypoparathyroidism.

Critical management

- Treat severe ionized hypocalcemia, and any symptomatic hypocalcemia with IV calcium gluconate or calcium chloride.
- One 10-mL ampule of 10% calcium gluconate contains 90 mg (4.6 mEq) of calcium, and will raise total serum calcium levels by 0.5 mg/dL. For symptomatic patients, follow the bolus with an infusion. Check iCa at regular intervals.
- Replete magnesium if low.

Sudden deterioration

- Hypotension, ventricular tachycardia, or seizures: cardiac monitor and rapid correction with IV calcium chloride (requires central venous access).

Hypercalcemia

Presentation

Classic presentation
- Mild cases are usually asymptomatic.
- Table 45.4 lists causes of hypercalcemia.

Critical presentation
- Severe hypercalcemia (serum calcium level greater than 14 mg/dL) can produce acute neuropsychiatric, gastrointestinal, cardiovascular, renal, and skeletal symptoms.

Table 45.4. Etiologies of hypercalcemia

Hyperparathyroidism (excessive release of PTH)
• Typically due to a single adenoma, occasionally hyperplasia
Malignancy
• Osteolysis: multiple myeloma, breast and bone cancer
• Malignancy-associated PTH-related peptide
Familial hypocalciuric hypercalcemia (FHH)
• Genetic mutation in Ca-detecting receptor in parathyroid and kidney
Vitamin D excess
• Granulomatous disorders (tuberculosis, sarcoidosis, Wegener's syndrome)
• Vitamin D intoxication
Other
• Immobilization, thiazide diuretics, calcium antacids, milk-alkali syndrome

---

- Remember: *"stones, bones, abdominal groans, and psychic overtones."*
  - **Neuropsychiatric symptoms**: confusion, delirium, psychosis, weakness, and coma.
  - **Gastrointestinal symptoms**: abdominal pain, nausea, emesis, constipation, or ileus.
  - **Cardiovascular symptoms**: hypertension, bradycardia, shortened QT interval.
  - **Renal symptoms**: polyuria (with associated hypovolemia) and nephro-lithiasis
  - **Skeletal**: osteopenia and associated fractures.

Diagnosis and evaluation

- **Diagnostic tests**
  - Serum and ionized calcium, parathyroid hormone (PTH), and albumin.
  - Elevated calcium/elevated PTH: hyperparathyroidism, familial hypocalciuric hypercalcemia.
  - Elevated calcium/low PTH: malignancy, all other causes.

Critical management

- Treat symptomatic patients, and any serum level greater than 14 mg/dL. Mainstays of treatment include hydration and diuresis with loop diuretics.
- Since hypercalcemia produces an osmotic diuresis, be careful to correct hypo-volemia before giving diuretics. Goal urine output is 100–200 mL/hour.
- Long-term management (e.g., malignancy) includes use of calcitonin and other inhibitors of bone resorption such as bisphosphonates.

DISORDERS OF MAGNESIUM METABOLISM

Introduction

- Normal serum concentration is 1.5–2.5 mg/dL.

Hypomagnesemia

Presentation

Classic presentation
- Mild hypomagnesemia is usually asymptomatic, but failure to correct low serum magnesium may contribute to refractory hypokalemia and hypocalcemia.
- Table 45.5 lists causes of hypomagnesemia.

Table 45.5. Etiologies of hypomagnesemia

Chronic alcoholism, malnutrition, malabsorption (decreased intake)
Pancreatitis
Diarrhea, sepsis, burns
Diuretics
Large-volume fluid resuscitation

Critical presentation
- Severe hypomagnesemia (serum levels less than 1 mg/dL) may affect the cardiovascular and neurological systems.
  - **Cardiovascular**: prolonged QT, ventricular tachycardia, torsades de pointes.
  - **Neurological**: muscle weakness, tetany, and seizure.

Diagnosis and evaluation

- ECG, serum electrolytes with magnesium and calcium.

Critical management

- Dose and route of magnesium repletion varies with the severity of symptoms.
- For mild hypomagnesemia, begin repletion with magnesium sulfate ($MgSO_4$) 2 g IV over 2 hours.

Sudden deterioration

- Seizure: 4 g IV $MgSO_4$ as needed (q4h prn).
- Ventricular arrhythmias: 2–6 g $MgSO_4$ IV over several minutes.

Hypermagnesemia

Presentation

Classic presentation
- Most cases are asymptomatic.
- Table 45.6 lists causes of hypermagnesemia.

Table 45.6. Etiologies of hypermagnesemia

Renal insufficiency
Excessive intake

Critical presentation
- Severe hypermagnesemia (serum levels >4.0 mg/dL) may affect the cardiovascular and neurological systems.
  - **Cardiovascular**: bradycardia, hypotension, heart block.
  - **Neurological**: hyporeflexia, somnolence.

Diagnosis and evaluation

- ECG, serum electrolytes with magnesium and calcium.

Critical management

- Intravenous fluids and loop diuretics.

Sudden deterioration

- If the patient becomes hemodynamically unstable, calcium gluconate 1 g IV over 2–3 minutes should be given in addition to IV fluids and loop diuretics.
- If the patient is in renal failure, hemodialysis may be required.

Vasopressor of choice: none.

REFERENCES

Freda BJ, Davidson MB, Hall PM. Evaluation of hyponatremia: a little physiology goes a long way. *Cleveland Clin J Med.* 2004; **71**: 639–50.

Hatton KW, Fuhrman T. Electrolyte disorders: derangements of sodium, potassium, calcium, and magnesium. In: Rehm G., ed. *Adult Multi-professional Critical Care Review.* Mount Prospect, IL: Society of Critical Care Medicine, 2009.

Londner M, Hammer D, Kelen GD. Fluid and electrolyte problems. In: Tintinalli J, Kelen GD, Stapczynski JS, eds. *Emergency Medicine: A Comprehensive Study Guide*. New York: McGraw-Hill Companies, Inc., 2004.

Marino PL. Renal and electrolyte disorders. In: *The ICU Book*. 3rd edn. Philadelphia, PA: Lippincott Williams & Wilkins, 2007.

Perianayagam A, Sterns RH, Silver SM, *et al.* DDAVP is effective in preventing and reversing inadvertent overcorrection of hyponatremia. *Clin J Am Soc Nephrol.* 2008; **3**:331–6.

46

Acute kidney injury and emergent dialysis

Feras H. Khan

Introduction

- Acute kidney injury (AKI) is defined as a fall in glomerular filtration rate (GFR) and the accumulation of nitrogenous wastes.
- The Kidney Disease Improving Global Outcomes (KDIGO) group defines AKI as
  - Increase in serum creatinine by ≥ 0.3 mg/dL within 48 hours, or
  - Increase in serum creatinine to ≥ 1.5 times baseline within the prior 7 days, or
  - Urine volume <0.5 mL/kg/hour for 6 hours.
- There are three classes of AKI:
  - Prerenal: inadequate perfusion of the kidney (most common) (see Table 46.1)
  - Renal: diseases intrinsic to the kidney (see Table 46.2)
  - Postrenal: obstruction distal to the kidney (see Table 46.3).

Presentation

Classic presentation

- Since the etiology of AKI varies greatly, findings on initial examination may be vague.
- Common signs and symptoms include:
  - Decreased urine output
  - Signs and symptoms of reduced kidney function: lethargy, fatigability, anorexia, nausea, and vomiting
  - Dark or turbid urine
  - Pulmonary and peripheral edema.

Practical Emergency Resuscitation and Critical Care, ed. Kaushal Shah, Jarone Lee, Kamal Medlej, and Scott D. Weingart. Published by Cambridge University Press. © Kaushal Shah, Jarone Lee, Kamal Medlej, and Scott D. Weingart 2013.

Table 46.1. Etiologies of prerenal AKI: the most common cause of renal failure

Dehydration
Hemorrhage
Gastrointestinal losses
Diuretics
Hyperglycemia
Burns
Heart failure
Cirrhosis
Drugs (angiotensin-converting enzyme inhibitors, NSAIDs)

Table 46.2. Etiologies of renal AKI: most commonly caused by acute tubular necrosis, or acute interstitial nephritis

Acute interstitial nephritis: beta-lactams, sulfa-based drugs, NSAIDs
Renal ischemia
Antimicrobials: aminoglycosides, amphotericin B
Intravascular hemolysis: hemolytic uremic syndrome and thrombotic thrombocytopenic purpura
Rhabdomyolysis
Other toxic agents: cisplatin, cyclosporine A, contrast dye

Table 46.3. Etiologies of postrenal AKI: the least common cause of AKI, due to obstruction distal to the renal parenchyma

Papillary necrosis
Retroperitoneal mass
Prostatic hypertrophy
Urethral stricture

Critical presentation

- Altered mental status and seizure.
- Hyperkalemia with associated arrhythmias.
- Pulmonary edema causing respiratory failure.

Diagnosis and evaluation

- **History and physical examination**
  - A careful patient history will frequently reveal etiology of renal failure (e.g., medications or recent administration of contrast dye).

Table 46.4. Urine microscopy/urinary sediment findings: probable etiology

Hyaline casts: prerenal (hypovolemia)
Muddy brown casts: ATN
White blood cell casts and eosinophils: AIN
Pigmented casts: myoglobinuria

- **Diagnostic tests**
  - Urine studies: urinalysis, microscopy, creatinine, osmolality, and electrolytes (Table 46.4).
  - Bladder catheter: enables hourly monitoring of urine output, and treats post-renal obstruction.
  - Renal ultrasound: demonstrates signs of urinary obstruction including hydronephrosis and evaluates kidney size to determine acuity of injury.
  - Calculate the following:
    - Fractional excretion of sodium (FENA):
      - FENA = (U Na/P Na)/(U Cr/P Cr).
      - <1% indicates prerenal causes of AKI.
      - >2% indicates intrinsic causes including acute tubular necrosis (ATN).
    - A sodium level <20 mEq/L suggests a prerenal condition in a patient with oliguria.
    - Creatinine clearance (CrCl) may be calculated to assess general kidney function:
      - CrCl = (140 − age [years]) × weight (kg)/72 × Cr (mg/dL) × 0.85 (in women)
- **KDIGO AKI Severity Score** is used to define the degree of kidney injury.
  - **Stage 1:** 1.5–1.9 times baseline, *or* ≥0.3 mg/dL increase in the serum creatinine, *or* urine output <0.5 mL/kg/hour for 6–12 hours.
  - **Stage 2:** 2.0–2.9 times baseline increase in the serum creatinine, *or* urine output <0.5 mL/kg/hour for 6–12 hours.
  - **Stage 3:** >3 times baseline increase in the serum creatinine, *or* increase in serum creatinine to ≥4.0 mg/dL, *or* urine output of <0.3 mL/kg/hour for >24 hours, *or* anuria for ≥12 hours, *or* the initiation of renal replacement therapy, *or*, in patients <18 years old, decrease in estimated GFR to <35 mL/minute per 1.73 m^2.
- The clinical utility of AKI scoring systems is uncertain, but they help predict mortality. As the stage of AKI worsens, the risk of death and need for renal replacement therapy increases.

Critical management

- A careful patient history and appropriate laboratory testing should reveal the cause of AKI.

- Once AKI is diagnosed, all drugs that cause renal injury should be discontinued.
- Airway management:
  - Volume overload due to AKI can lead to pulmonary edema, which may require respiratory support including noninvasive positive-pressure ventilation or intubation.
- Hemodynamic management:
  - Correcting hemodynamic instability is paramount to preserve renal function.
  - Patients with prerenal failure and hypotension require IV fluids to normalize blood pressure.
  - Vasopressors such as norepinephrine, dopamine, and vasopressin may be used in patients with persistent shock following appropriate volume resuscitation.
  - Low-dose dopamine is not helpful in patients with oliguric AKI.
  - Bolus doses of furosemide or other diuretics to promote urinary output have not been shown to be useful. Diuretics may provide symptomatic improvement in patients who are volume overloaded.
- Renal replacement therapy (RRT):
  - If AKI is present, consider consulting nephrology to help decide whether the patient requires dialysis, and if so, what type of RRT.
  - Indications for emergent dialysis include
    - Volume overload
    - Metabolic acidosis
    - Uremia (encephalopathy, pericarditis)
    - Hyperkalemia.
  - Vascular access must be placed for dialysis. Traditionally, a large-bore venous catheter is placed in either the internal jugular vein or femoral vein.
- Types of renal replacement therapy (RRT): the type of dialysis that a patient will receive varies based on institution and familiarity with each technique.
  - *Hemodialysis (HD):* Blood flows alongside dialysate across a semipermeable membrane in opposite directions (countercurrent mechanism). Solutes are removed by diffusion.
    - Disadvantages: critically ill patients with hypotension may not tolerate HD due to the high flow rates required to achieve diffusive clearance.
    - Advantages: solutes are cleared rapidly, so it requires less time to complete.
  - *Hemofiltration/continuous veno-venous hemofiltration (CVVH)*
    - Uses convection to remove solutes.
    - Fluid balance is controlled closely through continuous changing of the amount of fluid given back to the patient.
    - Causes less hypotension as lower flow rates result in less hypotension.
    - Advantages: hemodynamic stability, slower fluid shifts, volume control.
    - Disadvantages: requires continuous monitoring; patient must remain immobile during therapy; hypothermia.
  - *Sustained low-efficiency dialysis (SLED)*

- Similar to HD except that this modality uses slower blood-pump speeds and low dialysate flow rates for 6–12 hours daily.
- Advantages: high solute clearance, requires less time than CVVH, uses the same machines as HD.
- Disadvantages: longer time requirement than HD.

Sudden deterioration

- Patients with AKI who suddenly decompensate should be rapidly evaluated for electrolyte imbalances. Hyperkalemia, which can cause cardiac arrhythmias, is the most concerning.
- AKI resulting in metabolic acidosis can cause hypotension. Temporary treatment includes volume resuscitation and vasopressors. A sodium bicarbonate infusion can be considered while preparing for dialysis.
- Any patient with uremia and hypotension should be evaluated with echocardiography for pericardial tamponade from uremic pericarditis.

Special circumstances

- **Acute interstitial nephritis:** an inflammatory reaction that impairs kidney function, typically caused by a medication hypersensitivity reaction.
  - Common causes include antibiotics (aminoglycosides, cephalosporins, penicillins), NSAIDs, and diuretics.
  - Fever, rash, and eosinophilia may be seen but are not always present.
  - WBC casts and eosinophils may be seen on urinalysis.
  - Renal biopsy can be used to make a definitive diagnosis.
  - Treated by stopping offending agent and consider steroids.
- **Contrast-induced nephropathy:** an acute injury to the renal tubular epithelial cells caused by iodinated radiocontrast agents used in radiological procedures.
  - Risk factors include advanced age, diabetes, dehydration, congestive heart failure, and underlying renal disease.
  - A rise in creatinine is typically seen 48–72 hours following contrast administration.
  - Pretreatment is the best strategy for patients who require contrast study:
    - Isotonic saline 6 hours prior to the procedure and continued for 6 hours after the procedure.
    - N-acetylcysteine: 600 mg PO twice daily before and after the procedure.
    - Reduced osmolality dyes and decreased dye loads for at-risk patients.
    - Some centers also consider bicarbonate infusions.
- **Rhabdomyolysis** occurs when myoglobin released by injured muscle damages the renal tubular epithelial cells.
  - Diagnosis is confirmed by testing for CK and urine myoglobin.

- Aggressive volume administration with isotonic fluids is the standard of care.
- Severe cases may require hemodialysis.

REFERENCES

Bellomo R, Chapman M, Finfer S, *et al.* Low-dose dopamine in patients with early renal dysfunction: a placebo-controlled randomized trial. Australian and New Zealand Intensive Care Society (ANZICS) Clinical Trials Group. *Lancet.* 2000; **356**: 2139–43.

Gauthier PM, Szerlip HM. Metabolic acidosis in the intensive care unit. *Crit Care Clin.* 2002; **18**: 289–308.

Ho KM, Sheridan DJ. Meta-analysis of furosemide to prevent or treat acute renal failure. *BMJ.* 2006; **333**: 420.

Kidney Disease: Improving Global Outcomes (KDIGO) Acute Kidney Injury Work Group. KDIGO Clinical Practice Guideline for Acute Kidney Injury. *Kidney Int Suppl.* 2012; **2**: 1–138.

McCullough PA. Contrast-induced acute kidney injury. *J Am Coll Cardiol.* 2008; **51**: 1419–28.

Mehran R, Nikolsky E. Contrast-induced nephropathy: definition, epidemiology, and patients at risk. *Kidney Int Suppl.* 2006: S11–15.

Stevens MA, McCullough PA, Tobin KJ, *et al.* A prospective randomized trial of prevention measures in patients at high risk for contrast nephropathy: results of the P.R.I.N.C.E. Study. Prevention of Radiocontrast Induced Nephropathy Clinical Evaluation. *J Am Coll Cardiol.* 1999; **33**: 403–11.

47

Rhabdomyolysis

Jeremy Gonda

Introduction

- Rhabdomyolysis is a condition of acute skeletal muscle injury and breakdown that results in the release of toxic intracellular contents into the bloodstream.
- There are multiple etiologies of rhabdomyolysis (Table 47.1). The common end-point of muscle injury is disruption of the sodium–potassium–ATPase pump, resulting in elevated intracellular calcium that is harmful to muscle.
- Presentation ranges from asymptomatic elevation in muscle enzymes to a life-threatening condition characterized by acute kidney injury (AKI), dehydration, metabolic acidosis, and electrolyte disarray.
- AKI is the most serious complication of rhabdomyolysis. The combination of volume depletion, acidemia, and the release of nephrotoxins from damaged muscle leads to:
  - Renal vasoconstriction and ischemia
  - Tubular obstruction
  - Direct injury of the proximal tubules.
- Alcohol and drugs are contributing factors in up to 80% of adult cases of rhabdomyolysis.

Presentation

Classic presentation

- Triad of myalgias, weakness, and dark urine (classically reddish brown, or "tea-colored").
- Myalgias occur most commonly in the proximal muscle groups.

Practical Emergency Resuscitation and Critical Care, ed. Kaushal Shah, Jarone Lee, Kamal Medlej, and Scott D. Weingart. Published by Cambridge University Press. © Kaushal Shah, Jarone Lee, Kamal Medlej, and Scott D. Weingart 2013.

Table 47.1. Etiologies of rhabdomyolysis

Traumatic	Nontraumatic
Multitrauma/crush injury	Environmental heat illness/dehydration
Burns	Seizures
Vascular or orthopedic surgery	Hereditary myopathies
Coma	Malignant hyperthermia
Immobilization	Neuroleptic malignant syndrome
Envenomation (snake, black widow)	Drugs
Extreme exertion	Infections (typically viral)
Electrical injury	Electrolyte abnormalities: hypokalemia, hypophosphatemia
Drugs: statins, colchicine, salicylates, neuroleptics, antipsychotics	Endocrine abnormalities: diabetic ketoacidosis (DKA), hyperosmolar hyperglycemic state (HHS), hypothyroidism

- Physical examination may reveal muscle swelling and tenderness, with occasional skin changes including discoloration, induration, and blistering.
- It is possible for rhabdomyolysis to present without any of these signs or symptoms, making serum markers essential to the diagnosis.

Critical presentation

- Severe cases may present with hypovolemic shock, AKI, metabolic acidosis, disseminated intravascular coagulation (DIC), compartment syndrome, hyperkalemia, and cardiac arrhythmias.
- Compartment syndrome occurs due to swelling and edema of the injured muscle: classic physical examination findings include pain, paresthesias, paralysis, pallor, and pulselessness.

Diagnosis and evaluation

- **History and physical examination**
  - Take a history to elicit traumatic and nontraumatic causes of rhabdomyolysis. Always inquire about drug and alcohol use.
  - Physical examination may reveal muscle swelling and tenderness with overlying skin changes including discoloration, induration, or blistering.
  - Affected muscle should be evaluated for signs of compartment syndrome.
- **Diagnostic tests**
  - Serum creatine kinase (CK):
    - CK elevated >5 times normal value is the hallmark of rhabdomyolysis.
    - CK rises in 2–12 hours and peaks in 24–72 hours.

- The CK-MM fraction (found in skeletal and cardiac muscle) predominates.
- If serum CK levels fail to stabilize with appropriate therapy, or continue to rise for longer than 72 hours, consider ongoing muscle injury or compartment syndrome.
- Urine myoglobin:
  - Myoglobin released from damaged muscle produces the classic reddish-brown urine color.
  - Results as (+) "blood" on urine dipstick without RBCs on the microscopic urine analysis.
- Urine studies:
  - Urine electrolytes are typically consistent with a prerenal picture as a result of volume depletion.
  - Granular casts may also be seen and suggest acute tubular necrosis.
- Serum AST, ALT, LDH, and aldolase:
  - Elevated levels of these intramyocyte enzymes may appear following release from damaged muscle cells.
- Serum electrolytes with calcium, phosphate, and uric acid:
  - Hyperkalemia, hyperphosphatemia, and hyperuricemia: serum levels will be elevated due to release from damaged muscle cells.
  - Hypocalcemia: serum levels will be low due to calcium influx into damaged muscle cells, precipitation with excess serum phosphate, and decreased bone responsiveness to parathyroid hormone in the setting of AKI.
  - Creatinine, blood urea nitrogen (BUN), and glomerular filtration rate (GFR) may demonstrate renal dysfunction.
- DIC panel: platelets, fibrinogen, PTT, D-dimer, blood smear:
  - DIC is a pathological activation of clotting seen during severe illness, inflammation, or infection, and is a known complication of rhabdomyolysis.
- ECG:
  - If electrolyte disturbances are present, an ECG is needed to screen for arrhythmias and conduction abnormalities.
- The following **specialized tests** may be utilized when the diagnosis is unclear:
  - Electromyography (EMG), muscle biopsy, and magnetic resonance imaging (MRI).

Critical management

- The cornerstone of management includes discontinuation of inciting factors and aggressive management of fluid and electrolyte abnormalities.
- **Volume repletion**
  - Intravenous fluids enhance renal perfusion and increase urinary flow in order to prevent AKI and increase potassium excretion.

- Early and aggressive resuscitation (studies have not determined the ideal rate or total amount) using isotonic fluids (normal saline or lactate ringer) with the following clinical markers as guides of adequate resuscitation:
  - Serum CK nadirs or decreases to <5000 U/L *and*
  - Urine output 200–300 mL/hour *and*
  - Initial (+) urine dipstick for "blood" (myoglobin) becomes (−), *or*
  - The patient is unable to tolerate volume of fluid given.
- **Electrolyte management**
  - Hyperkalemia: anticipate and treat aggressively as indicated.
  - Hypocalcemia: supplement calcium if symptomatic (weakness, tetany, seizures, prolonged QTc interval, cardiac arrhythmias), but otherwise use with caution as rebound hypercalcemia may occur as rhabdomyolysis resolves.
  - Hyperuricemia: treat with allopurinol 300 mg every 8–12 hours if uric acid >8 mg/dL.
- **Sodium bicarbonate**
  - No definitive evidence of benefit over isotonic volume repletion.
  - Potential benefit: urine alkalinization (maintaining a urine pH >6.5) may help prevent AKI.
  - Risk: may induce calcium-phosphate precipitation resulting in hypocalcemia.
  - Recommendation: use in severe cases, if calcium levels are normal, arterial pH <7.50, and serum bicarbonate is <30 mEq/L.
  - A bicarbonate infusion consists of 3 ampules of sodium bicarbonate (150 mEq) in 1 liter of D5W. Infuse at 200 mL/hour to maintain urinary pH >6.5.
- **Loop diuretics**
  - No definitive evidence of benefit.
  - Potential benefit: may be helpful in patients with volume overload and evidence of ongoing rhabdomyolysis.
  - Risk: may worsen hypocalcemia.
- **Mannitol**
  - No definitive evidence of benefit. A trend toward improved success has been observed in patients with CK levels >30 000 U/L.
  - Potential benefit: may be protective in encouraging diuresis, and in its role as a free radical scavenger.
  - Risk: volume depletion, hypernatremia, and acute kidney injury if >200 g/day is given.
  - Contraindicated in patients with low urine output (<0.5 mL/kg/hour for more than 24 hours).
- **Dialysis**
  - Indicated in cases of severe rhabdomyolysis complicated by
    - Persistent metabolic acidosis
    - Volume overload
    - Uremia
    - Severe electrolyte disorders.

- Dose or type of dialysis is dependent on the hemodynamic stability of the patient and the desired speed of solute (potassium, urea, myoglobin) clearance. If the patient is hemodynamically stable and rapid solute clearance is preferred (i.e., critical hyperkalemia), then intermittent hemodialysis (iHD) is the method of choice. If the patient is hemodynamically unstable or there is concern for too rapid solute clearance, then continuous veno-venous hemodiafiltration (CVVHD) is chosen.

Sudden deterioration

- Sudden deterioration suggests worsening metabolic acidosis secondary to renal failure, compartment syndrome, or arrhythmias due to severe electrolyte disturbance.
- **Metabolic acidosis**: consider bicarbonate infusion while waiting to initiate renal replacement therapy in consultation with nephrology. Intubation may be needed if significant pulmonary edema has occurred in the setting of aggressive fluid repletion and worsening kidney function.
- **Compartment syndrome**: elevate the affected limb and request surgical consultation for fasciotomy.
- **Arrhythmias**: recheck serum electrolytes, ECG, and treat accordingly using ACLS protocols.

Vasopressor of choice: none.

REFERENCES

Bosch X, Poch E, Grau JM. Rhabdomyolysis and acute kidney injury. *N Engl J Med*. 2009; **361**: 62.

Brown CV, Rhee P, Chan L, *et al.* Preventing renal failure in patients with rhabdomyolysis: do bicarbonate and mannitol make a difference? *J Trauma*. 2004; **56**: 1191.

Counselman FL. Rhabdomyolysis. In: Tintinalli J, Kelen GD, Stapczynski JS, eds. *Emergency Medicine: A Comprehensive Study Guide*. New York: McGraw-Hill Companies; 2004.

Huerta-Alardin AL, Varon J, Marik PE. Bench-to-bedside review: rhabdomyolysis – an overview for clinicians. *Crit Care*. 2005; **9**: 158.

Lameire N, Van Biesen W, Vaholder R. Acute renal failure. *Lancet*. 2005; **365**: 417–30.

Hematology–oncology emergencies

48

Reversal of anticoagulation

Calvin E. Hwang

Introduction

- Nearly 60 million people in the United States are on some form of anticoagulation or antiplatelet therapy, including 4 million on warfarin, 50 million on aspirin, and 1.4 million on clopidogrel.
- These patients often present to the emergency department (ED) with various bleeding diatheses including intracranial hemorrhages, gastrointestinal bleeding, and trauma-associated bleeding.
- Patients on therapeutic warfarin have twice the risk of developing an intracerebral hemorrhage compared with those not on anticoagulation. This risk is even higher in those with supratherapeutic INR values.
- Common anticoagulants and their mechanism of action are presented in Table 48.1.

Presentation

Classic presentation

- Patients on anticoagulation who fall may have no immediate sequelae of an intracranial hemorrhage (ICH). Symptoms can develop over days or even weeks.
  - The most common presentation of intracranial hemorrhage is an insidious onset of headache, light-headedness, nausea, and vomiting.

Practical Emergency Resuscitation and Critical Care, ed. Kaushal Shah, Jarone Lee, Kamal Medlej, and Scott D. Weingart. Published by Cambridge University Press. © Kaushal Shah, Jarone Lee, Kamal Medlej, and Scott D. Weingart 2013.

Table 48.1. Mechanism of action of common anticoagulants

Warfarin	Inhibits the synthesis of vitamin K-dependent coagulation factors (II, VII, IX, X) and proteins C and S
Heparin	Activates antithrombin III, leading to inactivation of thrombin and other coagulation factors
Enoxaparin	Similar to heparin, activates antithrombin III, but preferentially inhibits factor Xa
Dabigatran	Direct thrombin inhibitor
Aspirin	Inhibits cyclooxygenase-1 and -2 enzymes, leading to inhibition of platelet aggregation
Clopidogrel	Inhibits platelet ADP receptors, preventing platelet aggregation

- Emergency physicians must maintain a high level of suspicion for intracranial bleeding in patients on anticoagulation, even in the absence of trauma, and particularly in those patients with a supratherapeutic INR.
- Patients on anticoagulation (and antiplatelet therapy in particular) also commonly present with gastrointestinal bleeding.
- Other patients may have less critical sources of bleeding but may present with insufficient hemostasis, as with epistaxis or superficial lacerations.

Critical presentation

- Patients with more significant head trauma can present acutely with altered mental status and obtundation, or with abnormal neurological findings such as hemiplegia, cranial nerve deficits, or seizures.
- Patients may also present in shock from life-threatening bleeds such as gastrointestinal bleeds, massive hemoptysis, epistaxis, or internal bleeding from trauma.

Diagnosis and evaluation

- **Imaging**
    - In anticoagulated patients with altered mental status or possible head trauma, a non-contrast computed tomography (CT) is key in identifying intracranial hemorrhage.
    - Acute intracranial hemorrhages will appear bright on CT while chronic hemorrhages will appear dark.
    - Anticoagulated patients with head trauma, no loss of consciousness, and a negative initial head imaging should be observed for at least 6 hours (the exact number of hours is controversial) from the onset of the trauma. A repeat CT scan after this observation period is also controversial.

- Those with large intracranial hemorrhages (greater than 30 mL), midline shift, or extension into the ventricles have particularly poor prognoses.
  - The Intracerebral Hemorrhage Score is a clinical tool that can help predict prognosis. It uses GCS, age, ICH volume, location, and intraventricular extension to help determine prognosis and estimate mortality.
- **Laboratory tests**
  - All patients with serious bleeding should receive a complete blood count, electrolyte levels, renal function testing, coagulation tests (PT/INR/aPTT), and type and cross-match.
  - For ED patients on warfarin, PT/INR is crucial to assess the degree of hypercoagulability.
  - There is no readily available laboratory test that can identify ED patients on dabigatran. The aPTT test is the most sensitive in determining the presence of the anticoagulant effect of dabigatran, but can often be normal depending on the timing of the test.
  - ED patients treated with heparin can be monitored using the aPTT or heparin activity level.
  - The aPTT test is not reliable for ED patients on enoxaparin and an anti-Xa activity level should be obtained instead. This test is not readily available everywhere, however, and may be difficult to interpret depending on the timing of the patient's last dose of enoxaparin.

Critical management

- Initial management should start with the ABCs. Undertake airway management for patients with suspected intracranial hemorrhage who are not protecting their airway.
- Obtain adequate intravascular access with two large-bore intravenous lines for possible massive transfusion of blood products.
- **Patients on warfarin**
  - All patients with serious or life-threatening bleeding should receive vitamin K 10 mg IV for sustained reversal of warfarin-induced anticoagulation.
    - While there are concerns about IV vitamin K-induced anaphylaxis, more recent literature suggests the incidence to be similar to that of anaphylaxis with penicillin, and slow administration (over 1 hour) may further decrease this risk.
  - If available, prothrombin complex concentrates (PCCs) have been shown to result in faster correction of INR and require less total volume of infusion than fresh frozen plasma.
  - In institutions where PCC is not available, these patients should receive fresh frozen plasma, initially dosed at 10–15 mL/kg. This may be difficult in patients with medical comorbidities such as heart failure.
- **Patients on dabigatran**
  - No research study to date has been able to show reversibility of dabigatran.

- If available and clinically feasible, dialysis can remove approximately 60% of dabigatran at 2 hours.
- Additional studies are still pending on the efficacy of PCC and recombinant factor VIIa in reversing dabigatran.
- **Patients on heparin**
  - Heparin can be reversed emergently in patients with serious bleeding through the use of protamine sulfate at a ratio of 1 mg protamine sulfate/100 units heparin.
  - This may need to be titrated further in patients on subcutaneous heparin as its absorption will be slower.
- **Patients on enoxaparin**
  - Although protamine sulfate does not reverse the anti-Xa activity of enoxaparin, its administration at a ratio of 1 mg/mg of enoxaparin may reduce clinical bleeding.
- **Patients on antiplatelet medications**
  - For critical bleeding, platelet transfusion may be beneficial, as antiplatelet medicines frequently irreversibly inactivate platelets.
  - Desmopressin (DDAVP) can be also administered to these patients as it enhances platelet adhesion to the vessel walls, and increases factor VIII and von Willebrand factor (vWF).

Sudden deterioration

- Deterioration in these patients usually occurs because of worsening intracranial bleed or from hemorrhage and anemia.
  - For patients with suspected or confirmed ICH, a neurosurgical consult should be obtained immediately for drainage and/or craniotomy in the operating room.
  - Patients that are continuing to hemorrhage should be aggressively reversed and transfused with packed red blood cells. A surgical consultation may also be needed to help control the source of bleeding.

Pressor of choice: Patients on anticoagulants presenting in shock will need to be aggressively resuscitated with blood products. Infusion of crystalloids and use of pressors such as phenylephrine and norepinephrine can be initiated as a temporizing measure.

REFERENCES

Bershad EM, Suarez JI. Prothrombin complex concentrates for oral anticoagulant therapy-related intracranial hemorrhage: a review of the literature. *Neurocrit Care*. 2010; **12**: 403–13.

Itshayek E, Rosenthal G, Fraifeld S, *et al.* Delayed posttraumatic acute subdural hematoma in elderly patients on anticoagulation. *Neurosurgery*. 2006; **58**: E851–6.

Massonnet-Castel S, Pelissier E, Bara L, *et al.* Partial reversal of low molecular weight heparin (PK 10169) anti-Xa activity by protamine sulfate: in vitro and in vivo study during cardiac surgery with extracorporeal circulation. *Haemostasis.* 1986; **16**: 139–46.

Van Ryn J, Stangier J, Haertter S, *et al.* Dabigatran etexilate – a novel, reversible, oral direct thrombin inhibitor: interpretation of coagulation assays and reversal of anticoagulant activity. *Thromb Haemost.* 2010; **103**: 1116–27.

Vigué B. Bench-to-bedside review: Optimising emergency reversal of vitamin K antagonists in severe haemorrhage – from theory to practice. *Crit Care.* 2009 ;**13**: 209.

49

Disseminated intravascular coagulation and thrombotic thrombocytopenic purpura/ hemolytic uremic syndrome

Joseph E. Tonna

Introduction

- Thrombotic thrombocytopenic purpura/hemolytic uremic syndrome (TTP/ HUS) and disseminated intravascular coagulation (DIC) share many characteristics making it difficult to differentiate them, especially early on.
- The differential diagnoses of TTP/HUS and DIC include other imminently life-threatening diseases. It is essential for the emergency physician to consider and recognize these conditions, as the treatment for one may be harmful in another (Table 49.1).
- TTP and HUS are now considered spectrum manifestations of one disease. They are caused by direct platelet thrombosis and fibrin deposition with resultant microvascular red blood cells (RBCs) thrombosis, hemolysis, and anemia. They do not directly involve the coagulation cascade, and therefore do not prolong clotting times. The characteristics of the disease are a result of the manifestations of the formation and effects of microthrombi:
  - Thrombocytopenia
  - Anemia
  - Intracerebral thrombosis resulting in fluctuating mental status, seizures, cerebral vascular infarcts (CVA), and coma
  - Renal thrombosis resulting in renal dysfunction.
- DIC is a consumptive coagulopathy initiated by blood exposure to foreign antigens (Table 49.2), resulting in ongoing simultaneous activation of the coagulation and fibrinolytic cascades on a disseminated level.
  - The consumption of coagulation factors leads to increased clotting times.
  - Simultaneous fibrin deposition and fibrinolysis leads to fibrinogenemia, and increased D-dimer and fibrin split products (FSP).

Practical Emergency Resuscitation and Critical Care, ed. Kaushal Shah, Jarone Lee, Kamal Medlej, and Scott D. Weingart. Published by Cambridge University Press. © Kaushal Shah, Jarone Lee, Kamal Medlej, and Scott D. Weingart 2013.

Table 49.1. Differential diagnosis of systemic atraumatic purpura

Disseminated intravascular coagulation
Thrombotic thrombocytopenic purpura/hemolytic uremic syndrome
Meningococcemia, pneumococcemia, staphylococcemia, gonococcemia
Rocky Mountain spotted fever
Immune thrombocytopenic purpura
Henoch–Schönlein purpura
Hemorrhagic drug reaction
Stevens–Johnson syndrome/toxic epidermal necrolysis
Viral hemorrhagic fever (Hanta, Lassa, dengue)

Table 49.2. Conditions associated with DIC

Severe infection/sepsis
Trauma (including neurotrauma)
Solid and myeloproliferative malignancies
Transfusion reactions
Rheumatological conditions (adult-onset Still's disease, systemic lupus erythematosus)
Obstetric complications (amniotic fluid embolism, abruptio placentae, HELLP, eclampsia)
Vascular abnormalities (Kasabach–Merritt syndrome, large vascular aneurysms)
Liver failure
Envenomations
Hyperthermia/heatstroke
Hemorrhagic skin necrosis (purpura fulminans)
Transplant rejection

HELLP, hemolysis, elevated liver enzymes, and low platelet count.

- Platelet activation leads to thrombocytopenia.
- Microvascular thrombosis leads to a consumptive and destructive anemia.
- Decreased procoagulant reserves lead to impaired hemostasis, seen as systemic microhemorrhages (petechiae, purpura, mucous membrane bleeding, oozing at intravenous sites).
- DIC is not a disease in itself, but rather a reaction to another physiological insult. As such, the effects of DIC can be mitigated, but treatment is predicated upon identification and treatment of the initiating condition (Table 49.2).
- Both TTP/HUS and DIC are conditions in which there is microvascular thrombosis and fibrin deposition. The resultant microvascular meshwork inflicts damage on passing red blood cells (RBCs), resulting in the formation of schistocytes and a microangiopathic hemolytic anemia (MAHA).

Presentation

Classic presentation of DIC

- DIC develops 6–48 hours after a physiological insult. Many of the patients developing this condition are already hospitalized.
- Patients will have diffuse petechiae, purpura, bleeding from their mucous membranes, and oozing from intravenous or surgical sites.
- Laboratory investigations will show:
  - Thrombocytopenia
  - Anemia
  - Increased international normalized ratio (INR), prothrombin time (PT), and activated partial thromboplastin time (aPTT)
  - Increased D-dimer
  - Increased fibrin split products (FSP)
  - Decreased fibrinogen (may be normal since fibrinogen is an acute-phase reactant).

Critical presentation of DIC

- Patients with DIC may present with life-threatening conditions associated with a **coagulopathy**:
  - Pericardial tamponade
  - Massive gastrointestinal bleeding
  - Pulmonary hemorrhage
  - Intracranial hemorrhage.
- They may also present with life-threatening conditions attributed to a **hypercoagulable** state:
  - Cerebrovascular accident (CVA)
  - Mesenteric ischemia and thrombosis
  - Venous thromboembolic events (VTEs) such as pulmonary embolus (PE) or deep vein thrombosis (DVT).

Classic presentation of TTP/HUS

- The classic presentation of TTP involves a pentad of symptoms that include fever, neurological signs, anemia, thrombocytopenia, and renal dysfunction. This collection of symptoms is only seen in 20–30% of cases and it is strongly recommended to suspect the condition and manage it as such if a patient exhibits three or more of those features (Table 49.3).
- The disease is termed HUS when renal failure predominates over neurological symptoms.
- HUS is most commonly seen in children and often follows an infectious illness, usually diarrhea. It is classically associated with E. coli O157:H7.

Table 49.3. Symptoms associated with TTP

Finding	Mechanism
Fever	Acute-phase reaction
Altered mental status	From cerebral microvascular thrombosis
Anemia	From MAHA *and* thrombosis
Thrombocytopenia	From direct platelet activation
Renal dysfunction	From renal microvascular thrombosis

Critical presentation of TTP/HUS

- Morbidity and mortality in patients with TTP/HUS is usually attributed to thrombosis rather than anemia and bleeding.
- Patients with TTP can present with neurological symptoms that can be life-threatening themselves or complicated by a life-threatening event:
  - Seizures
  - CVA resulting in falls or aspiration
  - Myocardial infarction
  - Arrhythmias.
- Patients (usually children) presenting with HUS may have significant renal dysfunction requiring dialysis.

Diagnosis and evaluation

- DIC is suspected in the individual who has suffered a physiological insult and is showing signs of bleeding:
  - Petechiae, purpura, or ecchymoses
  - Bleeding from mucous membranes including the gastrointestinal tract
  - Oozing or bleeding from intravascular access sites, surgical sites, or drains.
- No single laboratory test is sensitive or specific enough to diagnose DIC. Together with a strong clinical suspicion, however, certain findings on serial laboratory examinations can help make the diagnosis.
  - A complete blood count should be sent to rule out significant anemia.
  - Thrombocytopenia should be present as it is seen in up to 98% of DIC patients.
  - A peripheral blood smear can show evidence of schistocytes.
  - Coagulation studies will usually show elevated PT/INR and aPTT.
  - D-dimer and FSP will be elevated but are very nonspecific.
  - Fibrinogen levels can be low or normal as it is an acute-phase reactant.
  - A basic metabolic profile should be sent to assess renal function and electrolytes.

- The diagnosis of TTP/HUS should be suspected in patients presenting with three or more of the classic pentad of symptoms (Table 49.3).
- Laboratory investigations can help strengthen the diagnosis of TTP/HUS and assess for possible complications of the condition.
  - A complete blood count will reveal mild to moderate anemia and thrombocytopenia.
  - A peripheral blood smear will show schistocytes. The latter are considered by some to be essential to make the diagnosis of TTP/HUS.
  - Coagulation studies (PT/INR, aPTT) should be within the normal range.
  - D-dimer and FSP are usually normal or mildly elevated.
  - Fibrinogen will be normal or elevated.
  - BUN and creatinine should be measured to assess renal function. This will also help differentiate TTP from HUS.
  - Lactate dehydrogenase (LDH) and direct/indirect bilirubin can help determine the presence and degree of hemolysis.
  - Given the strong association between TTP/HUS and the human immunodeficiency (HIV), HIV testing should be offered to patients in which the diagnosis is entertained.
- Imaging:
  - Imaging does not help diagnose TTP/HUS or DIC.
  - Computed tomography (CT), radiography and ultrasonography may be used if clinically indicated to help identify complications arising from:
    - Pulmonary hemorrhage
    - Intracranial hemorrhage
    - Cerebrovascular accident
    - Mesenteric ischemia
    - Pulmonary embolism
    - Cardiac tamponade.

Critical management

DIC

- The initial management of DIC should be directed at treating the underlying disorder.
- Administration of blood products should be guided by clinical necessity such as active bleeding or the need to perform an invasive procedure.
  - Platelet administration should be considered in the bleeding patient if the platelet count falls below 50×10^6/mL. A prophylactic transfusion should also be considered in the nonbleeding patient with a platelet level less than 10×10^6/mL.
  - Routine administration of platelets and coagulation factors is not indicated despite low platelet counts and increased coagulation times.

- Bleeding patients with an elevated INR (>2), a 2-fold prolongation of aPTT, or a fibrinogen level below 100 mg/dL should receive FFP at a starting dose of 10–15 mL/kg.
- Cryoprecipitate lacks several clotting factors and should only be administered as an adjunct to FFP in bleeding patients with low fibrinogen (<100 mg/dL).
- Prothrombin concentrates (PCCs) allow for administration of selected factors for DIC but do not contain all the factors lost in the consumptive coagulopathy. They also do not contain the ADAMTS-13 protein, a large protein involved in blood clotting that is necessary in TTP/HUS.
- Low-dose heparin (5–10 units/kg/hour) without a bolus may be considered for DIC if there is purpura fulminans, ongoing ischemia, skin infarction, a clinically significant limb thrombus (arterial or venous), or other thromboembolic events. The decision to initiate anticoagulation in these patients should be done after consultation with a hematologist and an intensivist.

TTP/HUS

- Since the mortality from TTP/HUS can decrease from 90% to 10% with appropriate management, treatment should be initiated after consultation with a hematologist on all patients exhibiting three or more criteria for the condition (Table 49.3).
- The therapy of choice for TTP/HUS is plasmapheresis and plasma exchange with fresh frozen plasma. Patients can be effectively temporized by FFP transfusions until these modalities are available.
- Platelet transfusion should be avoided in patients suspected of having TTP/HUS as they can provide further substrate for intravascular thrombosis. They may be considered for life-threatening bleeds such as intracranial hemorrhage, but the decision to transfuse should be made after consultation with a hematologist and a surgeon or neurosurgeon.
- In children, HUS can often be managed without blood product transfusion, plasmapheresis, or plasma exchange. This is not usually the case with adult patients presenting with HUS.
- Patients with HUS may require dialysis if the renal dysfunction is severe.
- Corticosteroids are commonly administered to patients with TTP/HUS.

Sudden deterioration

- **Acute change in mental status**
  - Consider obtaining a CT head to rule out an intracranial hemorrhage.
  - A hematologist and neurosurgeon should be consulted to help guide reversal of anticoagulation in these patients.

- **Hemorrhage in DIC**
  - Patients with life-threatening hemorrhage should be managed by massive transfusion while ensuring appropriate replacement of clotting factors, fibrinogen, and platelets.
- **Life- or limb-threatening thromboembolism**
  - Consider heparin infusion without bolus at 5–10 units/kg/hour in consultation with a hematologist and an intensivist.
  - For large vessel thrombi, consider consulting an interventional radiologist or a vascular surgeon for directed thrombolysis or thrombectomy.
- **Worsening hypoxia**
  - Obtain a chest radiograph to rule out pulmonary hemorrhage.
  - If the patient requires intubation, lung-protective ventilation should be initiated.
  - Pulmonary embolism should remain high on the differential for these patients.
- **Hypotension**
  - An ECG should be performed quickly to rule out ischemia/infarction.
  - Perform a bedside echocardiography to rule out cardiac tamponade.
  - The heart should also be assessed for focal hypocontractility.
  - A digital rectal examination should be performed to rule out gastrointestinal bleeding.

Pressor of choice: the hypotensive patient in DIC will need to be resuscitated with blood products.

Phenylephrine or norepinephrine can be initiated along with crystalloids to temporize these patients until blood products are available.

REFERENCES

Levi M. Disseminated intravascular coagulation. *Crit Care Med.* 2007; **35**: 2191–5.

Levi M, Ten Cate H. Disseminated intravascular coagulation. *N Engl J Med.* 1999; **341**: 586–92.

Levi M, Toh CH, Thachil J, *et al.* Guidelines for the diagnosis and management of disseminated intravascular coagulation. *Br J Haematol.* 2009; **145**: 24–33.

Scott SB. Emergency department management of hematologic and oncologic complications in the patient infected with HIV. *Emerg Med Clin North Am.* 2010; **28**: 325–33.

50

Neutropenic fever

Nolan Caldwell

Introduction

- Neutropenia is characterized by an abnormally low number of polymorpho-nuclear leukocytes (neutrophils). They are the most abundant component of total circulating white blood cells, and an essential phagocytic component of the innate immune system.
- Neutropenia can occur as an isolated cell line abnormality or as a larger cytopenia.
- Febrile neutropenia only yields a microbiological etiology in 10–30% of cases. However, it must be assumed to be infectious in nature, with other potential causes left as diagnoses of exclusion (Table 50.1).

Presentation

Classic presentation

- Without adequate neutrophils, patients can have a blunted inflammatory response to infections. Examples of this are:
  - Urinary tract infection without pyuria
  - CNS infection without nuchal rigidity or focal neurological signs
  - Pneumonia without chest radiograph abnormalities
  - Skin and soft tissue infections without erythema.
- Patients can present with relatively mild symptoms, sometimes with little more than a fever.
- The majority do not present with a clear etiology on history or physical examination.

Practical Emergency Resuscitation and Critical Care, ed. Kaushal Shah, Jarone Lee, Kamal Medlej, and Scott D. Weingart. Published by Cambridge University Press. © Kaushal Shah, Jarone Lee, Kamal Medlej, and Scott D. Weingart 2013.

Table 50.1. Etiologies of neutropenia

Chemotherapy
Radiation therapy to the bone marrow
Genetic mutations
Transient infections
Autoimmune
Drug induced
Nutritional deficiency
Marrow infiltration and destruction
Reticuloendothelial sequestration

- The most common sources of infection are
  - The urinary tract
  - The gastrointestinal tract
  - The lungs
  - Indwelling vascular access sites.
- Febrile neutropenia is most common 7–14 days after chemotherapy, as this is typically the nadir of a patient's white cell count in response to the chemotherapy.
- The most commonly cultured bacteria in febrile neutropenia are Gram-negative aerobes (e.g., *Escherichia coli*, *Klebsiella* species, and *Pseudomonas aeruginosa*), frequently from GI translocation. Antibiotic coverage appropriate for *Pseudomonas* is always necessary.

Critical presentation

- The initial presentation of the critically ill with neutropenic fever may be overt with a clinical presentation similar to that of septic shock and including hypotension, respiratory failure, or any other major organ dysfunction.
- It may also be cryptogenic with isolated confusion, coagulopathy, or cardiac arrhythmias.
- Elderly patients and those taking steroids may present as hypothermic or euthermic. Any unexplained acute clinical deterioration should be considered a fever equivalent.
- Critically ill patients with neutropenic fever will most frequently present with common infections. However, their immunocompromised state places them at risk for more complex disease processes of almost any organ system.
- Although less commonly, these patients are at increased risk of infection from disseminated tuberculosis, candidiasis, *Nocardia*, Aspergillosis, *Fusarium* species, and *Pneumocystis jiroveci*.

Diagnosis and evaluation

- Fever is defined by one temperature reading higher than 38.5°C (101.3°F) or two temperatures >38°C (100.4°F) 1 hour apart. Fevers documented at home by a patient should be accepted as true temperatures.
- Neutropenia is stratified by varying degrees of absolute neutrophil count (ANC):
  - ANC = WBC count × percentage of neutrophils and bands
  - Mild neutropenia: ANC = 1000–1500
  - Moderate neutropenia: ANC = 500–1000
  - Severe neutropenia: ANC <500
- Most inpatient treatment guidelines quantify clinical neutropenia as an ANC <500 or 500–1000 with an anticipated fall to <500.
- The risk of invasive infection increases with the degree of neutropenia, with 20–50% of patients with an ANC <100 developing bacteremia.
- Physical examination should be complete to localize possible sources of infection, and include the mouth and pharynx, back, anogenital region, eyes, and any indwelling catheters.
- Avoid rectal thermometer and digital rectal examination given the risk of bacterial translocation.
- Laboratory investigations should include:
  - Complete blood count with differential.
  - Sputum cultures.
  - Two sets of blood cultures (for patients with indwelling catheters take one blood culture from a peripheral site and one from the central catheter. A differential time to positivity analysis should be performed).
  - Urinalysis and urine culture.
  - Complete metabolic panel.
    - Cerebrospinal fluid (CSF) studies depending on clinical suspicion (CSF may be acellular despite active CNS infection and often shows a lymphocytic pleocytosis with normal protein and glucose levels).
    - Lactic acid if there is a concern for early sepsis.
- Radiographic investigation should include:
  - Chest radiograph (a good initial screening for active pulmonary process; however, high-resolution computed tomography (CT) may reveal evidence of pneumonia in half of febrile neutropenic patients with an unremarkable chest radiograph).
- Ultrasound/CT/magnetic resonance imaging (MRI) can be ordered as needed.

Critical management

- Immediate assessment of systemic compromise should guide initial management and resuscitation. Rapid collection of blood cultures followed by administration

of antibiotics should be achieved within 30 minutes of presentation in the unstable patient, and within 1 hour in the stable patient.
- Options for initial antibiotic selection are presented in Table 50.2.
- In the stable patient, routinely adding vancomycin in the first 72 hours does not reduce mortality and increases nephrotoxicity. Indications for adding vancomycin to the antibiotic regimen are:
  - Catheter-related infection

Table 50.2. Initial antibiotic regimen for patients with febrile neutropenia.

Absence of systemic compromise[a]	Use cefepime 2 g IV every 8–12 hours (monotherapy) *or* ceftazidime 2 g IV every 8–12 hours (monotherapy) *or* piperacillin–tazobactam 4.5 g IV every 6–8 hours (monotherapy) *or* imipenem–cilastatin 500–750 mg IV every 6 hours (monotherapy)
Absence of systemic compromise in a penicillin-allergic patient	Use aztreonam 1–2 g IV every 12 hours *and* vancomycin 1 g IV every 12 hours *or* ciprofloxacin 500 mg IV every 12 hours *and* vancomycin 1 g IV every 12 hours
Presence of systemic compromise[a]	Start monotherapy regimen as in the absence of systemic compromise (above) Add gentamicin 2 mg/kg IV every 8 hours *or* 5 mg/kg IV every 24 hours *or* amikacin 15 mg/kg IV every 24 hours *or* tobramycin 2 mg/kg IV every 8 hours
Add vancomycin in selected patients[b]	Add vancomycin 25–30 mg/kg IV (loading dose), max 2 g/dose
Suspected abdominal or perineal infection *and* receiving monotherapy with cefepime or ceftazidime	Add flagyl 500 mg IV every 12 hours *or* switch to monotherapy with piperacillin–tazobactam 4.5 g IV every 6–8 hours *or* switch to monotherapy with imipenem–cilastatin 500–750 mg IV every 6 hours
Suspected or proven *C. difficile* infection	Add flagyl 500 mg IV every 12 hours and consider oral vancomycin 125 mg PO every 6 hours

[a] Features of systemic compromise include: (1) systolic BP <90 mmHg or >30 mmHg below patient's usual BP, or requirement for pressor support; (2) room air arterial PaO_2 <60 mmHg, saturation <90%, or requirement for mechanical ventilation; (3) confusion or altered mental state; (4) disseminated intravascular coagulation or abnormal PT/aPTT; (5) cardiac failure or arrhythmias, renal failure, liver failure, or any major organ dysfunction.
[b] Indications for adding vancomycin: (1) catheter-related infection; (2) known colonization with MRSA or multidrug-resistant streptococci; (3) blood cultures positive for Gram-positive bacteria and susceptibilities unknown; (4) hypotension.

- Known colonization with methicillin-resistant *Staphylococcus aureus* (MRSA) or multidrug-resistant streptococci
  - Blood cultures positive for Gram-positive bacteria and susceptibilities unknown
  - Hypotension.
- Initially starting antifungal or antiviral therapy is not recommended. However, a lower threshold for broadened initial therapy should be maintained in the critically ill, and based on medical history (prior use of antibiotics, steroids, etc.).
- Current management guidelines of severe sepsis/septic shock (central line with early goal-directed therapy, ARDS network lung protective ventilation, and glycemic control) should be instituted in septic neutropenic patients.
- Many neutropenic patients are concomitantly anemic. No clear optimal transfusion level is known and packed red blood cell administration should be guided by evidence of tissue perfusion.
- There is currently insufficient evidence to support or refute the use of colony-stimulating factor. Most studies agree its use does not change immediate mortality.
- Platelet transfusion guidelines are similar to other disease processes, frequently when less than 10×10^9/L, or less than 50×10^9/L if the patient is actively bleeding.
- Patients with neutropenic fever at low risk for serious complications can potentially be managed as outpatients. Validated tools such as the Multinational Association for Supportive Care in Cancer Risk Index (MASCC risk score) can be used to help select appropriate candidates for discharge. These decisions are institution dependent, however, and should never be made without close discussion with a hematologist/oncologist consultant.

Sudden deterioration

- Many neutropenic patients have impaired physiological responses (lung dysfunction, deficient stress hormones, cardiac impairment) to illness from iatrogenic cancer treatment and are prone to rapid critical deterioration.
- The pathophysiology of the decompensating patient with neutropenic fever is similar to that of a patient in septic shock. Those patients should be resuscitated similarly by the rapid and aggressive administration of crystalloids.
- After appropriate fluid resuscitation, pressor support can be initiated for the persistently hypotensive patient.
- Patients receiving steroids as part of chemotherapy are at higher risk of relative adrenal insufficiency when septic. If the patient is hypotensive and unresponsive to pressor support, consider early stress dose steroids (hydrocortisone 100 mg given intravenously).

Pressor of choice: norepinephrine.

REFERENCES

Freifeld AG, Bow EJ, Sepkowitz KA, *et al.* Clinical Practice Guideline for the Use of Antimicrobial Agents in Neutropenic Patients with Cancer: 2010 Update by the Infectious Diseases Society of America. *Clin Infect Dis.* 2011; **52**: 427–31.

Meckler G, Lindemulder S. Fever and neutropenia in pediatric patients with cancer. *Emerg Med Clin North Am.* 2009; **27**: 525–44.

Paul M, Borok S, Fraser A, Vidal L, Leibovici L. Empirical antibiotics against Gram-positive infections for febrile neutropenia: systematic review and meta-analysis of randomized controlled trials. *J Antimicrob Chemother.* 2005; **55**: 436–44.

Tam CS, O'Reilly M, Andresen D, *et al.* Use of empiric antimicrobial therapy in neutropenic fever. *Intern Med J.* 2011; **41**: 90–101.

Thirumala R, Ramaswamy M, Chawla S. Diagnosis and management of infectious complications in critically ill patients with cancer. *Crit Care Clin.* 2010; **26**: 59–91.

51

Tumor lysis syndrome

Casey Grover

Introduction

- Tumor lysis syndrome (TLS) is a clinical syndrome characterized by the lysis of tumor cells. It may occur spontaneously or in response to chemotherapy.
- It is most commonly seen in patients with hematological malignancies, especially acute leukemia and non-Hodgkin lymphoma, or in any patient with rapidly proliferating tumors.
- In pediatric patients, tumor lysis syndrome is most likely to occur 6 to 72 hours after initiation of chemotherapy.
- Risk factors for the development of TLS include:
  - Intravascular volume depletion
  - Rapidly progressive malignances
  - Renal insufficiency
  - Large tumor burden
  - Hyperuricemia.
- Risk for tumor lysis syndrome can be stratified into high, intermediate, and low (Table 51.1).
- Hyperuricemia may cause precipitation of uric acid crystals in multiple tissues within the body, particularly the kidneys, which may lead to renal failure.

Presentation

Classic presentation

- Cancer cells lyse, releasing their intracellular contents. This leads to the following hematological and electrolyte derangements:

Practical Emergency Resuscitation and Critical Care, ed. Kaushal Shah, Jarone Lee, Kamal Medlej, and Scott D. Weingart. Published by Cambridge University Press. © Kaushal Shah, Jarone Lee, Kamal Medlej, and Scott D. Weingart 2013.

Table 51.1. Risk for tumor lysis syndrome

High risk	Non-Hodgkin lymphoma
	Burkitt lymphoma
	Lymphoblastic lymphoma
	B-cell acute lymphoblastic leukemia (ALL)
	ALL with white blood cell count (WBC) >100 000/microliter
	Acute myelogenous leukemia (AML) with white blood cell count >50 000/microliter, monoblastic cell type
Intermediate risk	Diffuse large B-cell lymphoma
	ALL with WBC 50 000–100 000/microliter
	AML with WBC 10 000–50 000/microliter
	Chronic lymphocytic lymphoma (CLL) with WBC 10 000–100 000 after treatment with fludarabine
	Hematological malignancy with rapid proliferation after initiation of therapy
Low risk	Indolent non-Hodgkin lymphoma
	ALL with WBC <50 000/microliter
	AML with WBC <10 000/microliter
	CLL with WBC <10 000/microliter

- Release of intracellular potassium leads to hyperkalemia.
- Release of intracellular phosphorus leads to hyperphosphatemia.
- Elevated phosphorus causes secondary hypocalcemia.
- Release of intracellular uric acid leads to hyperuricemia.
- Primary hyperkalemia may result in:
  - Cardiac arrhythmias
  - Muscle cramps or weakness
  - Paresthesias
  - Fatigue
  - Nausea, vomiting, and diarrhea.
- Primary hyperphosphatemia may result in:
  - Lethargy
  - Nausea, vomiting, and diarrhea
  - Seizures.
- Secondary hypocalcemia can result in:
  - Neuromuscular irritability or tetany
  - Prolonged QT interval
  - Cardiac dysrhythmias
  - Seizures.
- Primary hyperuricemia may result in:
  - Acute kidney injury, including oliguria and anuria
  - Lethargy.

Critical presentation

- Life-threatening cardiac arrhythmias.
- Renal failure.
- Lethargy requiring intervention for airway protection.
- Seizures.
- Multi-system organ failure.

Diagnosis and evaluation

- The physical symptoms of TLS are usually related to an underlying electrolyte abnormality.
- **Laboratory studies**
  - The laboratory diagnosis of tumor lysis syndrome is made by two or more of the following derangements between 3 and 7 days after the onset of therapy for a hematological malignancy:
    - Hyperuricemia (uric acid >8.0 mg/dL in adults)
    - Hyperkalemia (potassium >6.0 mmol/L)
    - Hyperphosphatemia (phosphorus >4.5 mg/dL in adults, >6.5 mg/dL in children)
    - Hypocalcemia (corrected serum calcium <7.0 mg/dL, or ionized calcium <1.12 mmol/L)
      - Corrected calcium = Serum calcium + [0.8 × (Normal albumin – Serum albumin)].
- **Clinical diagnosis:** Laboratory diagnosis + renal failure, seizure, cardiac arrhythmia, or death.
  - Acute kidney injury is defined as an increase in the serum creatinine (increase by 0.3 mg/dL or more), or oliguria (urine output <0.5 mL/kg/hour).

Critical management

- Prevent acute kidney injury:
  - Acute kidney injury is usually related to hyperuricemia. Therapy is therefore aimed at reducing serum uric acid.
    - Intravenous hydration will improve glomerular filtration and minimize acidosis:
      - Bolus 1–2 liters of crystalloids.
      - Follow with a crystalloid infusion at two times the maintenance rate, with a goal urine output of 1.5–2 mL/kg/hour.
      - Consider loop diuretics in patients with a low urine output despite aggressive hydration.
    - Therapies that decrease serum uric acid level:
      - **Allopurinol** inhibits xanthine oxidase, preventing production of uric acid.

- Give 600–800 mg/day PO in 2–3 divided doses *or* 200–400 mg/m^2/day intravenously (IV) in 1–4 divided doses.
- **Rasburicase** prevents breakdown of uric acid into allantoin, which facilitates renal excretion. It is more efficacious at reducing the serum uric acid level than allopurinol.
  - Administer 0.2 mg/kg IV once, infused over 30 minutes.
- **Urinary alkalinization** may or may not be beneficial and is currently not recommended as a routine intervention. Its use should be discussed in consultation with a hematologist/oncologist. It should be avoided if allopurinol is used as the alkaline environment may cause the precipitation of xanthine and calcium phosphate in the renal tubules.
  - Add 3 ampules (amps) of 8.4% sodium bicarbonate (150 mEq total) to 1 liter of D5W. Start an infusion at twice the maintenance rate and titrate to a urine pH of 7.1–7.5.
- Note: for pediatric dosages for hyperuricemia treatments, we recommend consultation with the on-call pediatric oncologist or pharmacist.
- Prevent cardiac dysrhythmia and neuromuscular irritability.
  - Patients with no evidence of cardiac arrhythmias on ECG can be managed conservatively by limiting potassium and phosphorus intake.
  - Maintain continuous cardiac monitoring for arrhythmias.
- Treat hyperphosphatemia ≥4.5 mg/dL or 25% increase from baseline.
  - **Furosemide** 20–40 mg IV.
  - **Aluminum hydroxide** 50–150 mg/kg/day in 4 divided doses.
  - Severe or symptomatic hyperphosphatemia may require renal replacement therapy.

Sudden deterioration

Patients with TLS usually decompensate because of worsening electrolyte abnormalities. Interventions should target both the developing condition (cardiac arrhythmia, seizure, etc.) and the underlying electrolyte disorder.
- **Obtain a 12-lead ECG immediately to rule out a life-threatening arrhythmia.**
- **Cardiac arrhythmias**:
  - May be due to either hypocalcemia or hyperkalemia.
  - Administer IV calcium:
    - **Calcium gluconate** 1–3 ampules (1 g [4.5 mEq] per 10-mL ampule)
      - 100–200 mg/kg for pediatric patients.
    - **Calcium chloride** 1 ampule (1 g [13.5 mEq] per 10-mL amp) through central line.
    - *Note:* The use of calcium supplementation in TLS may cause precipitation of calcium phosphate.
  - If potassium is elevated:
    - **Albuterol** 10–20 mg nebulized.
    - **Insulin** 10 units IV bolus with 1–2 ampules of **D50W** IV.

- **Insulin** 0.1 units/kg IV with 2 mL/kg of **D25W** IV in pediatric patients.
- **Sodium polystyrene sulfonate (Kayexelate)** 30 g PO or PR.
- Note that the use of Kayexalate is controversial.
  - 0.5–1 g/kg per dose in pediatric patients.
- **Acute kidney injury**:
  - **Renal replacement therapy (dialysis)** is indicated in the case of:
    - Volume overload with pulmonary edema that is refractory to medical therapy
    - Persistent hyperkalemia despite medical therapy
    - Metabolic acidosis despite medical therapy
    - BUN >100 mg/dL
    - Rapidly rising BUN
    - Symptomatic uremia or electrolyte imbalances.
- **Seizures**:
  - Can be caused by severe hypocalcemia or hyperphosphatemia:
    - **Lorazepam** 2–4 mg IV
    - **Diazepam** 5–10 mg IV

Vassoressor of choice: none.

REFERENCES

Behl D, Hendrickson AW, Moynihan TJ. Oncologic emergencies. *Crit Care Clin.* 2010; **26**: 181–205.

Givens ML, Wethern J. Renal complications in oncologic patients. *Emerg Med Clin North Am.* 2009; **27**: 283–91.

Howard SC, Jones DP, Pui CH. The tumor lysis syndrome. *N Engl J Med.* 2011; **364**: 1844–54.

Zonfrillo MR. Management of pediatric tumor lysis syndrome in the Emergency Department. *Emerg Med Clin North Am.* 2009; **27**: 497–504.

52

Sickle cell emergencies

Charles Lei

Introduction

- Sickle cell disease (SCD) is caused by a genetic mutation in the β-globin chain of hemoglobin A (HbA). The mutated hemoglobin is referred to as HbS.
- The mutation causes red blood cells (RBCs) to distort under deoxygenated conditions and produce the characteristic sickled shape.
- Sickled RBCs increase the viscosity of blood and cause sludging and obstruction within the microvasculature. The resulting hypoperfusion worsens hypoxia and acidosis, which contributes to further sickling.
- The distorted sickle cell is less deformable and more susceptible to premature destruction within the microcirculation, shortening its life span from 120 days to about 20 days.
- The overall effect of SCD is chronic hemolysis with periodic episodes of vascular occlusion, resulting in tissue ischemia that can affect almost every organ system.
- Patients with SCD typically do not become symptomatic until around 4 months of age, when fetal hemoglobin (HbF) is replaced by the abnormal HbS.
- Patients with sickle cell trait have a normal life span and are usually asymptomatic.

Presentation

Classic presentations

Vaso-occlusive crisis
- Vaso-occlusive crisis (VOC) is the most common acute manifestation of SCD.

Practical Emergency Resuscitation and Critical Care, ed. Kaushal Shah, Jarone Lee, Kamal Medlej, and Scott D. Weingart. Published by Cambridge University Press. © Kaushal Shah, Jarone Lee, Kamal Medlej, and Scott D. Weingart 2013.

- Sickled RBCs can restrict blood flow and cause ischemic pain to any part of the body. The lower back and the extremities are most commonly affected.
- Triggers include infection, dehydration, change in weather or altitude, and stress, but often there is no identifiable precipitant.
- The pain in VOC is usually diffuse, with variable tenderness. Patients may have slight temperature elevations without true fever.
- Warmth, swelling, redness, or high fever are more typical of an infection such as cellulitis or osteomyelitis. Limited range of motion of a joint should raise suspicion for septic arthritis.
- Young children may present with dactylitis or "sausage digit," which consists of painful swelling of the hands and feet as a result of obstruction of the nutrient arteries of the metacarpals and metatarsals.
- The abdomen is the second most common site of ischemic pain from VOC. Patients typically present with sudden onset of poorly localized abdominal pain. On physical examination, they may have tenderness or guarding, but should not have evidence of peritonitis.

Transient red cell aplasia
- Aplastic crisis is characterized by a rapid decline in RBC production, which results in acute anemia.
- It is most commonly caused by an acute infection with parvovirus B19.
- Patients generally present with fatigue, dyspnea on exertion, and pallor. They may have symptoms of a recent viral infection.

Priapism
- Priapism is a sustained penile erection in the absence of sexual desire.
- It occurs in up to 30% of males with SCD.
- Recurrent episodes can lead to fibrosis and impotence.
- Patients present with a painful, swollen penis. They may have difficulty urinating.

Infection
- Patients with SCD are functionally asplenic after early childhood and are in a persistent immunocompromised state, placing them at increased risk for serious infections from encapsulated organisms.
- Common infections associated with SCD include pneumonia (from *Streptococcus pneumoniae*, *Haemophilus influenzae*, and *Mycoplasma pneumoniae*), meningitis, and osteomyelitis (from *Salmonella typhimurium*, *Staphylococcus aureus*, and *Escherichia coli*).
- A fever of 38.5°C or higher suggests an underlying bacterial infection.

Table 52.1. Causes of acute chest syndrome

Common causes	Possible causes
Pulmonary infection	Thromboembolism
Fat embolism	In situ thrombosis
Rib infarction	Lung sequestration
	Iatrogenic (excessive hydration, excessive narcotic use)

Critical presentations

Acute chest syndrome
- Acute chest syndrome (ACS) is the leading cause of death in patients with SCD.
- ACS is defined as a new infiltrate on chest radiography plus one other new symptom or sign: pleuritic chest pain, cough, shortness of breath, hemoptysis, fever >38.5°C, tachycardia, tachypnea, hypoxia, rales, or wheezing.
- Up to 50% of patients are initially admitted to the hospital for another reason (most often VOC) and subsequently develop ACS.
- The potential etiologies of ACS are listed in Table 52.1.

Splenic sequestration
- Splenic sequestration, or intrasplenic trapping of RBCs, is a major cause of morbidity and mortality in SCD. It is more common in children who have not yet undergone splenic auto-infarction.
- It results in a sudden enlargement of the spleen accompanied by an acute fall in the hemoglobin level.
- Symptoms include fatigue, abdominal fullness, and left upper quadrant abdominal pain.
- Physical examination may reveal tachycardia, pallor, and splenomegaly.
- Patients can rapidly deteriorate and develop altered mental status, hypotension, and cardiovascular collapse secondary to anemia and hypovolemic shock. The condition can be fatal within hours.

Stroke
- Stroke is one of the most devastating complications of SCD.
- Children with SCD have a 200-fold higher risk of stroke than those without SCD. Approximately 10% of patients experience a stroke before the age of 20 years.
- Patients with ischemic stroke typically present with hemiparesis or focal deficits. Vague symptoms consistent with a transient ischemic attack may be warning signs of an impending stroke.
- Patients with hemorrhagic stroke may exhibit headache, vomiting, or altered mental status.

Eye trauma

- Even minor trauma to the eye can cause hemorrhage (hyphema) into the anterior chamber in patients with sickle cell disease. Patients with sickle cell trait are also at increased risk for hyphema and its complications.
- When hyphema develops, sickled RBCs may clog the trabecular meshwork resulting in acute angle-closure glaucoma.
- Patients with SCD are also more susceptible to rebleeding and delayed complications such as optic nerve atrophy and central retinal artery occlusion.
- Symptoms include pain and decreased visual acuity in the affected eye.
- Physical examination may reveal hyphema and elevated intraocular pressure.

Diagnosis and evaluation

- Obtain a complete blood count to assess the degree of anemia.
- A reticulocyte count can help to differentiate between splenic sequestration and transient red cell aplasia (Table 52.2).
- Elevations in indirect bilirubin, alanine aminotransferase, and lactate dehydrogenase are consistent with hemolysis.
- Perform blood typing and screening if there is concern that the patient may need a transfusion.
- Patients with a fever should be evaluated for infection (Table 52.3).
- An elevated white blood cell count >20 000/microliter with an increased number of bands suggests the presence of an infection. Many patients with SCD have a baseline leukocytosis.
- Obtain cardiac biomarkers if acute coronary syndrome is suspected.
- Chest radiographs can identify the presence of a new infiltrate. The lower lobes are most commonly involved, but any lobe can be affected.
- Emergent head computed tomography (CT) should be performed in patients with suspected acute stroke.

Critical management

Vaso-occlusive crisis

- Initial management includes aggressive pain management and rehydration.
- Treatment of pain usually requires opioids. Morphine, fentanyl, and hydromorphone are all acceptable options. Meperidine should be avoided because its metabolite can cause neurotoxicity.
- In the absence of intravenous (IV) access, oral administration is preferred over the intramuscular route due to concerns for hematoma formation.
- Careful monitoring is required to prevent over-sedation and hypoventilation.
- Use acetaminophen as adjuvant analgesic pharmacotherapy.

Table 52.2. Differentiating common causes of acute anemia in sickle cell disease

Etiology	Anemia	Markers of hemolysis	Reticulocyte count
Hemolysis	Severe	Present	Increased
Splenic sequestration	Severe	Absent	Increased
Transient red cell aplasia	Severe	Absent	Decreased

Table 52.3. Diagnostic tests for patients with SCD and fever

Complete blood count
Blood cultures
Urinalysis
Urine culture
Throat culture
Chest radiography
Lumbar puncture (for toxic-appearing children)
Arthrocentesis (for acute arthritis)

- NSAIDs should be used sparingly and with caution as patients with sickle cell disease have some degree of renal dysfunction (from microinfarction and chronic anemia).
- Fluid rehydration should be performed judiciously. Use boluses of IV crystalloids if there is overt hypovolemia (sepsis, vomiting, diarrhea). Otherwise, infuse a hypotonic solution such as 5% dextrose in half-normal saline.
- IV fluid therapy should not exceed 1.5 times maintenance to avoid pulmonary edema or atelectasis, which may lead to acute chest syndrome.
- Transfusion has not been shown to be effective for routine acute VOC and should be reserved for other complications of SCD.
- Supplemental oxygen is recommended only if the patient's oxygen saturation falls below 92%.

Transient red cell aplasia
- Patients should be transfused only if they develop symptomatic anemia.
- Intravenous immunoglobulin may be administered once the diagnosis is made.
- Because parvovirus B19 is highly communicable, patients with aplastic crisis should be isolated from pregnant or immunocompromised individuals.

Priapism
- Patients with priapism for less than 2 hours duration should receive conservative treatment with IV fluids and analgesics.

- If priapism has been present for more than 2 hours, first-line therapy includes drainage of the corpus cavernosa followed by irrigation with a 1:1 000 000 solution of epinephrine in saline. If drainage and irrigation fail, consider exchange transfusion.

Infection
- Patients who are systemically ill must be treated promptly with broad-spectrum IV antibiotics. Once a causative organism is identified, therapy can be tailored according to its antibiotic sensitivity.
- Septic patients should be treated by implementation of the early goal-directed therapy protocol.

Acute chest syndrome
- Treatment of ACS parallels that of VOC, including analgesia, IV fluids, and supplemental oxygen.
- All patients with ACS should receive antibiotics to cover both typical and atypical organisms. A full course of antibiotics is recommended regardless of culture results.
- Bronchospasm may accompany ACS. Administer bronchodilators to all patients regardless of the presence or absence of audible wheezes and continue the treatment if a response is elicited.
- Transfusion therapy may be life-saving in ACS. Exchange transfusion is preferred over simple transfusion in patients with deteriorating conditions, particularly in those with relatively high hemoglobin (>9 g/dL). The goal for exchange transfusion therapy is to decrease the hemoglobin S concentration to <30%.
- Inhaled nitric oxide may reduce pulmonary pressures and improve ventilation–perfusion matching.
- Steroids are not recommended in ACS unless there is a concurrent asthma exacerbation.

Splenic sequestration
- All patients with acute splenic sequestration should immediately be transfused with packed red blood cells (PRBCs).
- Serial hemoglobin measurements should be performed to evaluate the adequacy of transfusion.

Stroke
- Exchange transfusion is the treatment of choice for children with acute ischemic stroke. Thrombolysis is contraindicated.
- Adults with SCD who present with stroke symptoms should receive conventional therapy for stroke, including thrombolysis with tissue plasminogen activator if indicated.

Eye trauma

- Patients who sustain eye trauma with or without hyphema require emergent evaluation by an ophthalmologist for evaluation of intraocular pressure.
- Treatment of hyphema includes head-of-bed elevation to 30 degrees and topical medications for lowering intraocular pressure (such as timolol).
- Mannitol and acetazolamide should be avoided because of their potential to promote sickling.
- All patients with sickle cell disease or sickle cell trait presenting with hyphema should be admitted for medical therapy and serial intraocular pressure measurements.

Sudden deterioration

Respiratory distress

- Causes of acute respiratory distress include pneumonia, pulmonary edema, pulmonary embolism, and fat embolism.
- Chest radiography should be obtained to help identify the etiology of the patient's respiratory compromise.
- A chest CT may be necessary if the chest radiograph does not provide a clear explanation for the patient's deterioration.
- Noninvasive positive-pressure ventilation improves oxygenation and ventilation in patients with pulmonary edema and decreases the need for intubation.
- Patients with impending respiratory failure should be emergently intubated.

Hypotension

- Splenic sequestration, pulmonary embolism, and septic shock can all cause a precipitous drop in blood pressure.
- Patients may require central venous access or invasive hemodynamic monitoring.
- Bedside ultrasound can be used to assess volume status (inferior vena cava collapse) and identify signs of pulmonary embolism (right heart strain).
- Inotropic support may be necessary in patients with persistent hypotension despite aggressive fluid resuscitation and PRBCs transfusion.
- Hypotension associated with sepsis should be managed according to early goal-directed therapy after the early administration of broad-spectrum antibiotics.

Altered mental status

- Patients with focal neurological deficits should undergo emergent head CT to evaluate for ischemic or hemorrhagic stroke.
- Altered mental status may be an ominous sign in patients with splenic sequestration. Emergent RBC transfusion is imperative.
- Patients with VOC may develop a depressed level of consciousness as a result of excessive opiate use. Intravenous naloxone may be used to reverse the respiratory

depression. Patients with persistent respiratory compromise will require orotracheal intubation.

Vasopressor of choice: Patients presenting with septic physiology should receive norepinephrine as first-line vasopressor.

REFERENCES

Bernard AW, Yasin Z, Venkat A. Acute chest syndrome of sickle cell disease. *Hosp Physician*. 2007; **43**: 13–18.

Gladwin M, Vichinsky E. Pulmonary complications of sickle cell disease. *N Engl J Med*. 2008; **359**: 2254–65.

Glassberg J. Current guidelines for sickle cell disease: management of acute complications. *Emerg Med Pract*. 2009; **1**: 1–9.

Glassberg J. Evidence-based management of sickle cell disease in the emergency department. *Emerg Med Pract*. 2011; **13**: 1–20.

Williams-Johnson J, Williams E. Sickle cell disease and other hereditary hemolytic anemias. In: Tintinalli J, Stapczynski J, Ma OJ, *et al.* eds. *Tintinalli's Emergency Medicine: A Comprehensive Study Guide*. 7th edn. New York: McGraw-Hill; 2011.

53

Severe sepsis and septic shock

Syed S. Ali and Laura Medford-Davis

Introduction

- **Definitions**
  - Sepsis is defined as systemic inflammatory response syndrome (SIRS) caused by an infection.
  - Severe sepsis is defined as sepsis with evidence of end-organ damage (renal failure, altered mental status, etc.).
  - Septic shock is defined as severe sepsis with cardiovascular collapse and persistent hypotension despite adequate volume resuscitation.
- **Risk factors** for sepsis include:
  - Age (very young or very old)
  - Indwelling catheters (e.g., central line, Foley catheter, etc.)
  - Immunocompromised state (HIV/AIDS, chemotherapy, etc.).
- Without rapid and aggressive intervention, sepsis has the potential to rapidly decompensate into severe sepsis, septic shock, and death.
- Early goal-directed therapy (EGDT) is a well-established and evidence-based treatment algorithm for sepsis.

Practical Emergency Resuscitation and Critical Care, ed. Kaushal Shah, Jarone Lee, Kamal Medlej, and Scott D. Weingart. Published by Cambridge University Press. © Kaushal Shah, Jarone Lee, Kamal Medlej, and Scott D. Weingart 2013.

Presentation

Classic presentation

SIRS Criteria (≥2 of the following are required)	
Fever or hypothermia	<36°C (96.8°F) or >38°C (100.4°F)
Tachycardia	HR >90 bpm
Tachypnea	RR >20 or $PaCO_2$ <32 mmHg
Leukocytosis/leukopenia	<4000/microliter, >12 000/microliter, or >10% bands

Critical presentation

- Hypotension: systolic blood pressure <90 mmHg or mean arterial pressure <65 mmHg.
  - Beware of relative hypotension in patients with chronic hypertension.
- Encephalopathy and altered mental status.
- Acute kidney injury presenting as oliguria or anuria.
- Cardiogenic shock: decreased left ventricular ejection fraction on echocardiogram, troponin leak.
- Lung injury or acute respiratory distress syndrome (ARDS).
- Disseminated intravascular coagulation (DIC).

Diagnosis and evaluation

Step 1: Confirm the diagnosis and determine the severity of illness.
- Basic metabolic panel: ↑creatinine (acute kidney injury), ↑glucose (increased insulin resistance).
- CBC with differential: WBC <4000/microliter or >12 000/microliter (SIRS), ↓platelets (DIC).
- Coagulation profile: ↑PT/INR/PTT (DIC).
- Lactate: ≥4 mmol/L (evidence of cellular anaerobic respiration and threshold to initiate EGDT).
- Arterial blood gas: ↓pH (metabolic acidosis).
- Liver function tests: ↑AST, ↑ALT, ↑bilirubin (shock liver).
- Cardiac markers: ↑troponin (cardiac injury).

Step 2: Determine the etiology.
- Chest radiograph to evaluate for pulmonary processes.
- Urine analysis to rule out a urinary tract infection.
- Lumbar puncture if symptoms are concerning for meningitis.

- Cultures:
  - Blood (two different sites + one from each chronically indwelling catheter).
  - Urine.
  - Sputum if there is a suspicion for pneumonia.
  - Cerebrospinal fluid if clinically indicated.
- Imaging as indicated by symptoms (computed tomography (CT) of the abdomen and pelvis, ultrasound, etc.).

Infectious etiologies

- Pneumonia
- Meningitis

Bloodstream infection/bacteremia
- Existing source of infection such as central line, Foley, etc.
- Endocarditis

Intra-abdominal
- Abscess
- Cholangitis
- Ruptured viscus (perforated ulcer, traumatic perforation, diverticulitis, appendicitis, etc.)
- Intestinal obstruction

Genitourinary and gynecological
- Urinary tract infection (cystitis, pyelonephritis)
- Septic abortion
- Infected intrauterine device
- Tubo-ovarian abscess

Musculoskeletal
- Necrotizing fasciitis
- Severe cellulitis
- Septic arthritis

Critical management

Early goal-directed therapy (EGDT) is the mainstay of treatment of sepsis and involves the following interventions.
- Large-volume fluid resuscitation: Bolus crystalloids (30mL/kg of normal saline (NS) or lactated Ringer's (LR) solution) *or* colloids (250–500mL albumin).
- Supplemental O_2.
- Empiric broad-spectrum intravenous (IV) antibiotics:
  - After obtaining cultures but no more than 1 hour from presentation.
  - Cover for Gram-positive and Gram-negative bacteria.
  - Coverage for viral and fungal infections should be initiated as well in the appropriate clinical setting.

- Consider the risk for healthcare-associated infections that may be multidrug resistant. Risk factors include:
  - Hospitalization within the last 90 days
  - Residence in a nursing home or long-term care facility
  - Presence of indwelling catheters
  - Intravenous therapy, wound care, or intravenous chemotherapy within the prior 30 days.
  - Attendance at a hospital or hemodialysis clinic within the prior 30 days.
- Urgent surgical consultation should be sought when indicated by the source of infection (e.g., abscess, ruptured viscus).
- Remove any indwelling catheter that is suspected of being infected.

Monitoring criteria

Criterion	Goal	Necessary lines
Mean arterial pressure (MAP)	≥65 mmHg	Arterial line
Central venous pressure (CVP)	8–12 cmH$_2$O (12–15 if mechanically ventilated)	Central line
Central venous oxygen saturation (ScvO$_2$)	≥70%	Central line
Urine output (UOP)	≥0.5 mL/kg/hour	Foley catheter
Lactate clearance	≥10%	None
Glucose	7.78–10 mmol/L (140–180 mg/dL)	None

Sudden deterioration

Patients with persistently low blood pressure despite adequate fluid administration or whose resuscitation goals are not met (ScvO$_2$ <70%, lactate clearance <10%) will require additional interventions.

- Vasopressors:
  - First line: norepinephrine (maximum dose 20 micrograms/minute).
  - Second line: vasopressin (0.03 units/minute).
  - Third line: epinephrine (1–10 micrograms/minute).
- If hypotension persists despite maximal vasopressor dose, consider administering steroids (hydrocortisone 200 mg/day).
- If ScvO$_2$ remains <70%, consider transfusing PRBCs (goal Hgb 7–9 g/dL).
- Cardiogenic shock: consider inotropes (dobutamine 2.5–20 micrograms/kg/minute).
- Respiratory failure: intubation and mechanical ventilation may need to be initiated:
  - Volume-controlled ventilation at 6 mL/kg *ideal* body weight.

- Minimize FiO_2 and increase PEEP to achieve an O_2 saturation goal of 88–95% while avoiding oxygen toxicity.
- Renal failure: emergent hemodialysis or continuous veno-venous hemodialysis (CVVHD) may be required.

REFERENCES

American College of Chest Physicians/Society of Critical Care Medicine Consensus Conference: definitions for sepsis and organ failure and guidelines for the use of innovative therapies in sepsis. *Crit Care Med.* 1992; **20**: 864–74.

Dellinger RP, Levy MM, Carlet JM, *et al.* Surviving Sepsis Campaign: international guidelines for management of severe sepsis and septic shock: 2008. *Crit Care Med.* 2008; **36**: 296–327.

Rivers E, Nguyen B, Havstad S, *et al.* Early goal-directed therapy in the treatment of severe sepsis and septic shock. *N Engl J Med.* 2001; **345**: 1368–77.

54

Pneumonia

Navdeep Sekhon and Calvin Lee

Introduction

- Pneumonia is a lung inflammation caused by a bacterial or viral infection, or irritants.
- It is the leading infectious cause of death, and the 7th overall cause of death.
- Risk factors include:
  - Patients at risk for aspiration (e.g., intoxication, seizures, stroke).
  - Endotracheal or nasotracheal intubation.
  - Smoking (damages mucociliary macrophage function).
  - Viral infections (destroy the respiratory epithelium).
  - Advanced age (the elderly exhibit decreased mucociliary clearance and elastic recoil of the lungs).
  - Immunosuppression (e.g., AIDS, asplenism, chemotherapy, transplant patients).
- Patients with pneumonia can become critically ill with respiratory distress and failure, the acute respiratory distress syndrome (ARDS), and septic shock.
- **Pneumonia classification**
  - Community-acquired pneumonia (CAP) is a pneumonia that is not acquired in a hospital or a healthcare setting (e.g., a nursing home or a dialysis unit), in an immunocompetent individual. Usual pathogens include *Streptococcus pneumoniae*, *Haemophilus pneumoniae*, *Mycoplasma pneumoniae*, *Chlamydophila pneumoniae*, and *Legionella pneumophila*.
  - Healthcare-associated pneumonia (HCAP) is a pneumonia in an individual who fulfills one of the following criteria:
    - Has been hospitalized for more than 2 days in the last 90 days.
    - Lives in a nursing home or a long-term care facility.

Practical Emergency Resuscitation and Critical Care, ed. Kaushal Shah, Jarone Lee, Kamal Medlej, and Scott D. Weingart. Published by Cambridge University Press. © Kaushal Shah, Jarone Lee, Kamal Medlej, and Scott D. Weingart 2013.

- Has received intravenous antibiotic therapy, wound care, or chemotherapy in the last 30 days.
- Attends a dialysis clinic.
- HCAP has an increased risk of multidrug-resistant organisms like methicillin-resistant *Staphylococcus aureus* (MRSA), *Pseudomonas aeruginosa*, *Klebsiella pneumoniae*, and *Acinetobacter baumannii*.

Presentation

Classic presentation

- "Typical" pneumonia presents with a sudden onset of fever and chills accompanied by productive cough with purulent sputum. It may also be accompanied by pleuritic chest pain and dyspnea. It is traditionally caused by *Streptococcus pneumoniae*, and *Haemophilus influenzae*.
- "Atypical" pneumonia presents with a subacute and nonproductive cough, fever, headache, myalgias, and malaise. It is traditionally caused by *Mycoplasma pneumoniae*, *Chlamydophila pneumoniae*, *Legionella*, and *Coxiella burnetii*.

Critical presentation

- Patients can present tachycardic, hypoxic, and in respiratory distress.
- Hypoxia can be due to lung consolidation, ARDS, or a parapneumonic effusion.
- Patients can also decompensate into septic shock.

Diagnosis and evaluation

- **History**
  - Duration and progression of symptoms.
  - Recent hospitalizations, nursing home placement, antibiotic use.
  - Assess patients' HIV risk factors.
  - Assess patients' aspiration risk.
  - Characterization of sputum:
    - Rust-colored sputum suggests *S. pneumoniae*.
    - "Currant jelly" sputum suggests *K. pneumoniae*.
- The pattern of the infiltrate on a chest radiograph can suggest an etiology (Table 54.1).
- Blood cultures should not be done in patients with uncomplicated CAP. According to the American Thoracic Society and the Infectious Diseases Society of America, blood cultures should be performed in patients going to the intensive care unit, asplenic patients, patients with cavitary lesions or pleural effusions

Table 54.1. Chest radiographic findings and their associated etiology

Chest radiographic finding	Suggested organism
Lobar consolidation	S. pneumoniae, Klebsiella pneumoniae
Patchy infiltrates	Atypical and fungal organisms
Interstitial pattern	Mycoplasma or viral organisms
Miliary pattern	Tuberculosis or fungal organisms
Apical infiltrate	Tuberculosis
Infiltrate in superior part of lower lobes or posterior part of the upper lobes	Aspiration pneumonia, anaerobic organisms
Cavitary lesion	Tuberculosis, S. aureus, anaerobic organisms, Gram-negative bacilli
Pneumothorax or pneumatocele	Pneumocystis jirovecii

on chest radiographs, patients who are leukopenic, have severe liver disease, or who severely abuse alcohol, and patients with HCAP.

- Sputum culture should be done in patients who are admitted to the ICU, those for whom outpatient antibiotic therapy has failed, those having structural lung disease, a history of severe alcohol abuse, a cavitary lesion, or pleural effusion on chest radiograph, or those with HCAP.
- For severe CAP send urine for antigen tests for *Legionella* and *S. pneumoniae*.

Critical management

- Provide supplemental oxygen to maintain a saturation higher than 90%.
- Some patients will require mechanical ventilation.
- The evidence for the use of Bi-PAP and CPAP is mixed.
- Noninvasive ventilation should be considered for preoxygenation of hypoxic patients prior to endotracheal intubation.
- Patients who are hypotensive are likely suffering from distributive shock and should be aggressively resuscitated with crystalloids.
- Place patients whose radiograph and history are suggestive of tuberculosis in respiratory isolation.
- All patients with AIDS who have pneumonia should be placed in respiratory isolation because the chest radiograph cannot discriminate between bacterial pneumonia and tuberculosis.
- Two clinical decision rules can assist the physician in deciding whether a patient needs to be admitted for inpatient management, or can be discharged home with outpatient follow-up:
  - The Pneumonia Severity Index.
  - The CURB-65 rule (Table 54.2). Two or more points warrant hospital admission. Three or more points suggests the need for an ICU admission.

Table 54.2. CURB-65 criteria for patients with a diagnosis of pneumonia

CURB-65 criterion	Points
Confusion	1
Uremia (>20 mg/dL)	1
Respiratory rate >30/minute	1
Blood pressure (systolic <90 mmHg, diastolic <60)	1
Age >65 years	1

- Initiate appropriate antibiotic therapy.
  - *CAP; outpatient therapy:*
    - No comorbidities and no antibiotic use in the past 3 months:
      - Macrolides or doxycycline.
    - Comorbidities such as diabetes mellitus, asplenism, chronic liver, lung or kidney disease, immunosuppression, alcoholism, malignancy, and patients who have received antibiotics in the last 3 months:
      - Respiratory fluoroquinolones *or* a beta-lactam and a macrolide.
  - *CAP; inpatient therapy, non-ICU:*
    - Beta-lactam (ceftriaxone, cefotaxime, ampicillin-sulbactam) *and* a macrolide or respiratory fluoroquinolone.
  - *CAP; inpatient therapy, ICU:*
    - Beta-lactam (ceftriaxone, cefotaxime, ampicillin-sulbactam) *and* a macrolide or respiratory fluoroquinolone.
  - *HCAP; inpatient therapy:*
    - Anti-pseudomonal cephalosporin or anti-pseudomonal carbapenem or piperacillin-tazobactam *and*
    - Anti-pseudomonal fluoroquinolone or aminoglycoside *and*
    - Linezolid or vancomycin to cover MRSA.
- **Special situations**
  - Aspiration pneumonia; add clindamycin or metronidazole.
  - AIDS patients with CD4 counts less than 200 cells/microliter should receive coverage for *Pneumocystis jirovecii.*
    - TMP-SMX is the first-line agent.
    - Pentamidine can be used in cases of allergy to TMP-SMX.
    - Administer steroids if the PaO_2 is <70 mmHg or the A-a gradient is >35 mmHg on arterial blood gas analysis.

Sudden deterioration

- Patients' ability to oxygenate and ventilate can decompensate rapidly. If this occurs, intubation and mechanical ventilation will be required.

- Patient can also develop hypotension secondary to septic shock. Early goal-directed therapy should be initiated with aggressive fluid resuscitation and vasopressor and/or inotrope support as needed.

Vasopressor of choice: Patients presenting with pneumonia whose blood pressure is deteriorating should be treated as septic shock. Norepinephrine is the first-line vasopressor for this condition.

REFERENCES

American Thoracic Society, Infectious Diseases Society of America. Guidelines for the management of adults with hospital-acquired, ventilator-associated, and healthcare-associated pneumonia. *Am J Respir Crit Care Med*. 2005; **171**: 388–416.

Arias E, Smith BL. Deaths: preliminary data for 2001. *Natl Vital Stat Rep*. 2003; **51**: 1–44.

Mandell LA, Bartlett JG. Update of practice guidelines for management of patients with community-acquired pneumonia. *Clin Infect Dis*. 2007; **37**: 1405–33.

55

Meningitis and encephalitis

Nathan Allen and Elizabeth Arrington

Introduction

- Meningitis is an acute inflammation of the meninges of the brain and spinal cord.
- Encephalitis is an inflammation of the brain with or without inflammation of the meninges.
- Meningitis is typically caused by bacteria or other organisms penetrating the blood–brain barrier. The immune system's response to this infection leads to vascular endothelial injury and meningeal inflammation.
- Cerebral hypoperfusion results from the associated edema and increased intracranial pressure.
- Infectious meningitis typically occurs after encapsulated organisms from the nasal or oral pharynx invade the bloodstream and then cross the blood–brain barrier into the subarachnoid space. It can also occur by direct contiguous spread or up a retrograde neuronal pathway.
- Meningitis is a life-threatening condition with up to 30% mortality and high risk of long-term neurological complications.
- Encephalitis is most commonly caused by the herpes simplex virus (HSV) but numerous other etiologies are possible.
- The differential diagnosis for meningitis and encephalitis includes subarachnoid hemorrhage, dural sinus thrombosis, metabolic encephalopathy, and other infections not involving the central nervous system (CNS).

Practical Emergency Resuscitation and Critical Care, ed. Kaushal Shah, Jarone Lee, Kamal Medlej, and Scott D. Weingart. Published by Cambridge University Press. © Kaushal Shah, Jarone Lee, Kamal Medlej, and Scott D. Weingart 2013.

Presentation

Classic presentation

- Fever, chills, headache, and nuchal rigidity.
- A prodromal upper respiratory tract infection with nausea, vomiting, and photophobia can also occur.
- A petechial or purpuric rash may be present.

Critical presentation

- Altered mental status.
- Seizures.
- Sepsis.
- Meningococcal meningitis can have a very rapid onset over hours.
- Focal neurological defects including palsy of cranial nerves III, VI, VII, and VIII can be seen.

Diagnosis and evaluation

- If bacterial meningitis is suspected, the patient should be isolated.
- Laboratory evaluations should include a complete blood count, chemistries, blood cultures, serum lactate, and a coagulation profile.
- Leukocytosis may be present but its absence does not exclude the diagnosis.
- A high index of suspicion is important for meningitis and encephalitis, and a lumbar puncture (LP) should be considered in patients with fever and altered mental status without an identified source of infection.
- Patients at risk for intracranial pathologies such as central nervous system (CNS) mass lesions or with signs of increased intracranial pressure should undergo a computed tomography (CT) scan of the head prior to lumbar puncture. The latter should be avoided in case of significant findings. Indications for performing a CT are:
  - Age older than 60 years
  - Patients who are immunocompromised
  - History of CNS lesion(s)
  - Recent seizure
  - Papilledema on retinal examination
  - Altered mental status
  - Focal neurological deficit on examination.
- Lumbar puncture with evaluation of the cerebrospinal fluid (CSF) is the diagnostic test of choice (Table 55.1).
  - CSF fluid analysis should include a Gram stain and culture, cell count and differential, and CSF glucose and protein levels. Specific antigen or PCR tests can be considered for special pathogens (HSV, *Cryptococcus*, etc.).

Table 55.1. Interpretation of lumbar puncture results.

Infection	Glucose (mg/dL)[a]	Protein (mg/dL)	Ratio CSF: blood glucose	WBC count (cells/ microliter)
No infection	45–80	15–45	>0.6	<5
Bacterial meningitis	Decreased	Elevated	<0.4	Elevated (500–5000)
Viral meningitis	Normal	Elevated	—	Elevated (10–500)

[a] Glucose: 1 mg/dL = 0.0555 mmol/L.

- CSF WBC count: Elevation of the WBC count is expected, with a typical neu-trophilic predominance in bacterial meningitis, although lymphocytes can sometimes predominate.
- CSF glucose concentration is typically decreased in bacterial meningitis.
- CSF protein concentration is typically elevated.
- Gram stain for identification of bacteria can help target antibiotic therapy.
- Encephalitis may present with nonconvulsive seizures. HSV encephalitis may have excessive red blood cells in the CSF fluid or classically frontal and/or tem-poral edema or hemorrhage on CT.

Critical management

- **Antibiotic treatment should not be delayed** for CT scan or until lumbar punc-ture results are available.
- Empiric antibiotics are based on common organisms by age:
  - 2–50 years old: *N. meningitides, S. pneumoniae.*
  - >50 years old: *S. pneumoniae, N. meningitides, L. monocytogenes.*
- A standard empiric regimen for meningitis in adults is
  - Ceftriaxone 2 g IV every 12 hours and vancomycin 30 mg/kg loading and dos-ing every 12 hours for trough concentration of 15–20 micrograms/mL.
  - Ampicillin 2 g IV every 4 hours for patients older than 50 years.
  - Acyclovir 10 mg/kg IV every 8 hours for suspected HSV encephalitis.
- Adjunctive dexamethasone is also recommended at 10 mg IV every 6 hours ini-tiated prior to or concurrent with antibiotic therapy.

Special circumstances

- Patients with a history of shunt, recent neurosurgery, or penetrating trauma should receive anti-pseudomonal coverage as well.

- Clinical findings and lumbar puncture results can be much more subtle in immunocompromised patients.

Sudden deterioration

- The most likely causes of decompensation are hemodynamic or respiratory impairment.
- Patients should be evaluated for airway protection and those who are at risk of aspiration should be endotracheally intubated.
- Patients who are hypotensive are likely septic and should be managed aggressively with fluids and pressors according to early goal-directed therapy protocols.
- Nonconvulsive or convulsive status epilepticus can occur with encephalitis and should be managed with benzodiazepines as first-line agents.

Vasopressor of choice: Hypotensive patients are likely septic and should be managed with norepinephrine as a first-line agent.

REFERENCES

Attia J, Hatala R, Cook DJ, *et al.* Does this adult patient have acute meningitis? *JAMA.* 1999; **282**: 175–81.

McIntyre PB, Berkey CS, King SM, *et al.* Dexamethasone as adjunctive therapy in bacterial meningitis: a meta-analysis of randomized clinical trials since 1988. *JAMA.* 1997; **278**: 925–31.

Straus SE, Thorpe KE, Holroyd-Leduc J, *et al.* How do I perform a lumbar puncture and analyze the results to diagnose bacterial meningitis? *JAMA.* 2006; **296**: 2012–22.

Tunkel AR, Glaser CA, Bloch KC, *et al.* The management of encephalitis: clinical practice guidelines by the Infectious Diseases Society of America. *Clin Infect Dis.* 2008; **47**: 303–27.

Tunkel AR, Hartman BJ, Kaplan SL, *et al.* Practice guidelines for the management of bacterial meningitis. *Clin Infect Dis.* 2004; **39**: 1267–84.

van de Beek D, de Gans J, Tunkel AR, *et al.* Community-acquired bacterial meningitis in adults. *N Engl J Med.* 2006; **354**: 44–53.

56

Infective endocarditis

Sandra J. Williams

Introduction

- Endocarditis refers to an inflammation of the endocardium (the inner layer of the heart) with or without heart valve involvement.
- The mitral valve is most commonly affected, except in intravenous drug abusers (IVDA), where it is the tricuspid valve that is more commonly involved.
- More than 50% of cases of endocarditis occur in patients older than 60 years.
- Risk factors include IVDA, prosthetic valve, and invasive medical procedures.
- Dental procedures and bacteremia from distant foci are the most common seeding events.
- The majority of cases are due to Gram-positive cocci (Table 56.1).
- In patients with negative blood cultures and no prior antibiotic use, the organisms often belongs to the HACEK group (*Haemophilus, Actinobacillus, Cardiobacterium, Eikenella, Kingella*).

Table 56.1. Organisms involved in infective endocarditis

History	Common causative organism
Native valve	*Streptococcus viridans, Staphylococcus aureus*
Prosthetic valve	*Staphylococcus epidermidis*
IVDA	*Staphylococcus aureus*

Practical Emergency Resuscitation and Critical Care, ed. Kaushal Shah, Jarone Lee, Kamal Medlej, and Scott D. Weingart. Published by Cambridge University Press. © Kaushal Shah, Jarone Lee, Kamal Medlej, and Scott D. Weingart 2013.

Presentation

Classic presentation

- Presentation is nonspecific and variable, but the most common symptoms are fever and malaise.
- The classic triad of fever, new heart murmur, and anemia is rare.
- Patients may present acutely with critical illness, or subacutely with low-grade fever, fatigue, weight loss, and distal emboli.

Critical presentation

- Patients may present in acute or progressive congestive heart failure with dyspnea, frothy sputum, and chest pain. This is the most common complication.
- The second most common complication is arterial embolization of valve vegetation fragments. These emboli can affect any body system:
  - Central nervous system (CNS): cerebrovascular accidents (CVA), subarachnoid hemorrhage (SAH), acute monocular blindness.
  - Renal: back pain, hematuria, renal failure.
  - Pulmonary: pneumonia, infarction, pleural effusion.
  - Gastrointestinal (GI): splenic infarction, mesenteric ischemia.
- Heart blocks and arrhythmias are also possible as the infection may extend through the septum and into the cardiac conduction system.
- Patients may present with respiratory compromise, diminished pulmonary capacity, altered mental status, or evidence of sepsis.

Diagnosis and evaluation

- Definitive diagnosis is made by positive blood culture(s), and evidence of valvular injury or vegetations on echocardiogram.
- Echocardiography should be performed as soon as possible.
- A transesophageal echocardiogram is more sensitive and should be performed in patients with a high clinical suspicion and a normal transthoracic echocardiogram.
- Nonspecific laboratory findings include leukocytosis, normocytic anemia, elevated C-reactive protein (CRP), elevated erythrocyte sedimentation rate (ESR), and hematuria.
- There are no specific findings on ECG or chest radiography.
- Other physical examination findings are due to circulating immune complexes that are embolizing (Table 56.2).
- The Duke Criteria are widely used to diagnose infective endocarditis and have a sensitivity of about 90% (Table 56.3). A positive diagnosis consists of
  - Two major criteria, *or*

Table 56.2. Physical findings in infective endocarditis

Finding	Location	Description	Frequency
Petechiae	Buccal mucosa, conjunctiva, extremities	Nonblanching erythematous pinpoint macules	20–40%
Osler's nodes	Pads of fingers and toes	Tender, small subcutaneous nodules	10–25%
Splinter hemorrhages	Under fingernails or toenails	Linear dark streaks	15%
Roth spots	Retina	Oval retinal hemorrhages with pale centers near optic disc	<10%
Janeway lesions	Palms and soles	Nontender, small hemorrhagic plaques	<10%

Table 56.3. Duke Criteria for the diagnosis of infective endocarditis

Major criteria	Minor criteria
Two separate positive blood cultures with typical endocarditis organisms: • *Staphylococcus aureus* • *Streptococcus viridans* • *Staphylococcus epidermidis* • HACEK group Evidence of echocardiographic involvement • Vegetation • Abscess • New dehiscence of prosthetic valve • New valvular regurgitation	Risk factor: IVDA or predisposing heart condition Fever >38°C Immunological phenomena: glomerulonephritis, Osler nodes, Roth spots Embolic phenomena: pulmonary infarct, arterial emboli, Janeway lesion, conjunctival hemorrhage Positive blood culture that does not meet major criteria above

- One major criterion and three minor criteria, *or*
- All five minor criteria.

Critical management

- Intravenous (IV) antibiotics should be initiated.
- Selection is based on patient history and local resistance patterns.
- Potential regimens are listed in Table 56.4.
- These patients may present with evidence of septic shock and need to be managed with early goal-directed therapy, including fluids, central line placement, measurement of central venous pressure, and use of vasopressors.

Table 56.4. Empiric therapy for suspected endocarditis

Uncomplicated history	Ceftriaxone 1–2 g IV or nafcillin 2 g IV or vancomycin 15 mg/kg IV *and* gentamicin 1–3 mg/kg IV
Prosthetic heart valve	Vancomycin 15 mg/kg IV *and* gentamicin 1–3 mg/kg IV *and* rifampin 300 mg PO
IVDA, congenital heart disease, suspected MRSA, hospital acquired or already on antibiotics	Vancomycin 15 mg/kg IV *and* gentamicin 1–3 mg/kg IV *and* nafcillin 2 g IV

- If there are signs of respiratory compromise or altered mental status, rapid sequence intubation (RSI) should be strongly considered in order to protect the airway and provide positive-pressure ventilation.

Sudden deterioration

The most likely cause for sudden deterioration in the patient with suspected infective endocarditis is acute rupture of the aortic or mitral valve.
- The placement of an intra-aortic balloon pump may be indicated for the unstable mitral valve rupture, but is contraindicated for aortic valve rupture.
- Prompt surgical evaluation is indicated.
- Rapid administration of intravenous fluid and initiation of pressor and/or inotrope may be necessary as a temporizing measure until surgical intervention can be performed.

Vasopressor of choice: Patients with infective endocarditis presenting with hypotension and evidence of hypoperfusion will usually be in septic shock. Norepinephrine is currently the pressor of choice for this condition. In patients with a suspicion of aortic or mitral valve rupture, agents with inotropic effect should be favored (i.e., norepinephrine, epinephrine, or dopamine).

REFERENCES

Marx JA, Hockberger RS, Walls RM, Adams J, Rosen P, eds. *Rosen's Emergency Medicine: Concepts and Clinical Practice*. 7th edn. Philadelphia, PA: Mosby Elsevier; 2010.

Tintinalli JE, Stapczynski JS, Cline DM, *et al.* eds. *Emergency Medicine: A Comprehensive Study Guide*. New York: McGraw-Hill Medical; 2011.

57

Necrotizing soft tissue and skin infections

Jennifer Carnell and Lindsay Oelze

Introduction

- Necrotizing soft tissue and skin infections (NSTIs) involve the deep subcutaneous tissues and adjacent fascia.
- Other names include necrotizing fasciitis, gas gangrene, and Fournier's gangrene when involving the perineum.
- They are rapidly progressive due to their spread along the fascial planes.
- The incidence of NSTI is approximately 500–1500 cases per year, and has increased in recent years secondarily to increased microbial virulence and resistance.
- Mortality is estimated to be around 24–34% and has remained largely unchanged over the past 30 years.
- NSTIs usually begin with an external trauma but can also occur spontaneously.
- Paucity of early physical examination findings can lead to a delay in diagnosis.
- Superficial findings do not occur until later in the disease course as a result of vasculitis and thrombosis of nearby vessels.
- The resultant ischemia inhibits effective antibiotic delivery to the site of infection, which is why surgical debridement should be performed as early as possible.
- Exotoxin release by clostridia, staphylococci, and streptococci can enhance virulence and cause the release of cytokines, resulting in the systemic inflammatory response syndrome (SIRS), which can then progress to sepsis and death if untreated.
- NSTIs are more common in patients with comorbidities including diabetes mellitus, chronic alcoholism, chronic renal failure, HIV, and liver failure (which is classically associated with *Vibrio vulnificus*).

Practical Emergency Resuscitation and Critical Care, ed. Kaushal Shah, Jarone Lee, Kamal Medlej, and Scott D. Weingart. Published by Cambridge University Press. © Kaushal Shah, Jarone Lee, Kamal Medlej, and Scott D. Weingart 2013.

Table 57.1. Classification of necrotizing soft tissue infections

Type	Microbial etiology
Type I	Polymicrobial (most common)
Type II	Monomicrobial (streptococci, staphylococci, clostridia)
Type III	*Vibrio vulnificus* (associated with seawater exposure)

- NSTIs can be classified based on microbial etiology, with polymicrobial etiology being the most common (Table 57.1). Staphylococcal NSTIs are increasing in prevalence due to more cases of MRSA infections in association with intravenous (IV) drug use.
- Early surgical intervention has been shown to decrease morbidity and mortality.

Presentation

Classic presentation

- NSTIs are notoriously difficult to diagnose early in the disease course, with initial signs and symptoms usually typical of cellulitis.
- Classically the pain is out of proportion to physical examination findings. As the infection rapidly spreads along the fascial planes, pain and swelling may extend beyond the areas of overlying erythema.

Critical presentation

- As an NSTI progresses, patients may present with ecchymoses, bullae, and crepitus as a result of subcutaneous emphysema. However, these occur later in the disease process (Figure 57.1).
- It is more common to see signs of systemic toxicity with NSTIs versus soft tissue infections without necrotizing component. This is due to the systemic inflammatory response from cytokine release, which can manifest as abnormal vital signs or abnormal laboratory markers.
- Type III NSTI associated with *Vibrio vulnificus* can present with cardiovascular collapse and rapid deterioration.

Diagnosis and evaluation

- NSTI is difficult to diagnose early in the disease process.
- Radiological studies can be helpful, but should not delay surgical intervention when there is a strong clinical suspicion for NSTI.

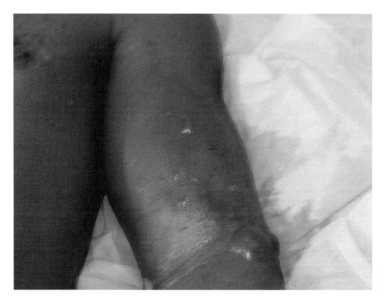

Figure 57.1. Ecchymosis and bullae of the upper extremity of a patient with an NSTI.

- Plain radiographs can demonstrate subcutaneous emphysema, but this is a late finding and should not be used to rule out NSTI (Figure 57.2).
- Advanced imaging modalities such as CT and MRI can reveal fascial thickening, edema, fluid along the fascial planes, and subcutaneous emphysema. They are not appropriate in unstable patients, or if they would result in a delay in surgical intervention.
- Emergency ultrasonography (EUS) can also aid in the diagnosis. EUS can reveal the above findings and also offers the advantage that it can be done quickly at the bedside (Figure 57.3).
- The gold standard for diagnosis remains surgical exploration for direct visualization of the deep subcutaneous tissues with histological confirmation.
- The classic intraoperative finding is "dishwater pus" and tissue necrosis.
- The Laboratory Risk Indicator for Necrotizing Fasciitis (LRINEC) score can be utilized when trying to differentiate between necrotizing and nonnecrotizing serious soft tissue infections. It includes six variables associated with NSTIs that are used to calculate a score correlating with the magnitude of the risk (Tables 57.2 and 57.3).

Critical management

- Antibiotic therapy should be initiated early with broad-spectrum coverage of Gram-positive, Gram-negative, and anaerobic organisms. Penicillin is

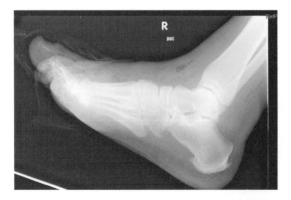

Figure 57.2. Plain radiograph of the foot demonstrating subcutaneous emphysema.

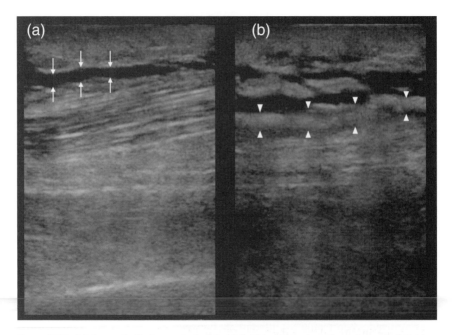

Figure 57.3. (a) Arrows indicate anechoic (black) fluid tracking along the echogenic (bright white) deep fascial plane. (b) Arrowheads delineate the thickened irregular fascia. In addition, anechoic fluid can be seen tracking along the deep fascial plane.

recommended for its coverage of streptococcal and methicillin-sensitive staph-ylococcal species.

- Clindamycin should be added to decrease exotoxin release in streptococcal and clostridial infections by inhibiting protein synthesis.

Table 57.2. LRINEC score

Laboratory parameter	LRINEC points
C-reactive protein (mg/L)	
<150	0
≥150	4
Total white blood cell count (per microliter)	
<15	0
15–25	1
>25	2
Hemoglobin (g/dL)	
>13.5	0
11–13.5	1
<11	2
Sodium (mmol/L)	
≥135	0
<135	2
Creatinine (mg/dL)	
≤1.6	0
>1.6	2
Glucose (mg/dL)	
≤180	0
>180	1

Table 57.3. LRINEC score and risk of necrotizing soft tissue infection (NSTI)

Risk category	LRINEC score	Probability of NSTI
Low	≤5	<50%
Intermediate	6–7	50–70%
High	≥8	>75%

- Vancomycin, linezolid, or daptomycin should also be included in the regimen for coverage of methicillin-resistant *Staphylococcus aureus* (MRSA).
- Early surgical consultation is imperative and should not be delayed as the mortality with antibiotics and supportive measures alone approaches 100%.
- Aggressive resuscitative measures should be initiated by placing two large-bore catheters and administering intravenous fluids if the patient is hypotensive.
- Considerations should be made for central venous access for central venous pressure and central venous oxygen saturation (ScvO$_2$) monitoring.
- Early goal-directed therapy for sepsis caused by NSTI should be implemented when indicated.

- Vasopressor support can be started as necessary for hypotension refractory to fluid resuscitation.
- Intubation for positive-pressure ventilation and 100% FiO_2 administration should be considered if the $ScvO_2$ remains <70% after appropriate fluid resuscitation and vasopressor support.
- Intravenous immunoglobulin (IVIg) and hyperbaric oxygen (HBO) are experimental treatments for necrotizing fasciitis. IVIg is postulated to bind exotoxins produced by staphylococcal and streptococcal species, potentially delaying or preventing the onset of SIRS. Consider these on a case-by-case basis and in consultation with an infectious disease specialist.

Sudden deterioration

- When a patient with NSTI deteriorates suddenly, the etiology is likely to be sepsis and septic shock. Early goal-directed therapy should be initiated immediately with additional nursing and physician staff mobilized to assist with the effort.
- While all of these interventions should ideally take place within minutes of the patient being evaluated, nothing should be prioritized over early and adequate surgical intervention.

Vasopressor of choice: Norepinephrine is the first-line vasopressor in these patients when they present in septic shock.

REFERENCES

Anaya DA, Dellinger EP. Necrotizing soft-tissue infection: diagnosis and management. *Clin Infect Dis*. 2007; **44**: 705–10.

Edlich RF, Cross CL, Dahlstrom JJ, *et al*. Modern concepts of the diagnosis and treatment of necrotizing fasciitis. *J Emerg Med*. 2010; **39**: 261–5.

Kuncir EJ, Tillou A, St. Hill CR, *et al*. Necrotizing soft-tissue infections. *Emerg Med Clin North Am*. 2003; **21**: 1075–87.

Sarani B, Strong M, Pascual J, *et al*. Necrotizing fasciitis: current concepts and review of literature. *J Am Coll Surg*. 2009; **208**: 279–88.

Wong CH, Khin LW, Heng KS, *et al*. The LRINEC (Laboratory Risk Indicator for Necrotizing Fasciitis) score: a tool for distinguishing necrotizing fasciitis from other soft tissue infection. *Crit Care Med*. 2004; **32**: 1535–41.

58

Complications of human immunodeficiency virus (HIV) and acquired immunodeficiency syndrome (AIDS)

Zubaid Rafique and Candace Pettigrew

Introduction

- HIV is more commonly seen in adult men aged 40 years or younger.
- There is a disproportionately high rate of infection among minority groups.
- Risk factors include:
  - Men who have sex with men (MSM)
  - Intravenous (IV) drug users
  - Heterosexual exposure to an infected partner
  - Vertical transmission (maternal–neonatal).
- Transmission modalities:
  - Semen
  - Vaginal secretions
  - Blood products
  - Breast milk
  - Transplacental transmission in utero.
- Acquired immunodeficiency syndrome (AIDS) is defined as evidence of human immunodeficiency virus (HIV) infection with either a CD4 count <200/microliter, or at least one AIDS-defining illness (Table 58.1).
- AIDS is a reportable disease in all 50 states of the United States. Moreover, as of 2008, all 50 states are conducting confidential name-based HIV infection reporting based on the Centers for Disease Control (CDC) recommendations.

Practical Emergency Resuscitation and Critical Care, ed. Kaushal Shah, Jarone Lee, Kamal Medlej, and Scott D. Weingart. Published by Cambridge University Press. © Kaushal Shah, Jarone Lee, Kamal Medlej, and Scott D. Weingart 2013.

Table 58.1. AIDS-defining illnesses

Pneumocystis jirovecii pneumonia (PCP)
Esophageal candidiasis
Wasting syndrome
Kaposi sarcoma
Disseminated *Mycobacterium avium* infection
Tuberculosis
Cytomegalovirus (CMV) disease
HIV-associated dementia
Recurrent bacterial pneumonia
Toxoplasmosis
Immunoblastic lymphoma
Chronic cryptosporidiosis
Burkitt lymphoma
Disseminated histoplasmosis
Invasive cervical cancer
Chronic herpes simplex

Presentation

- Primary HIV infection:
  - Acute seroconversion occurs 2–6 weeks after initial exposure.
  - Symptoms may include: fever, fatigue, lymphadenopathy, pharyngitis, diarrhea, weight loss, and rash.
- A number of complications can result from HIV and its progression to AIDS. The presentation of some of these complications is summarized in Table 58.2.

Diagnosis, evaluation, and critical management

- Enzyme-linked immunoassay (ELISA) or rapid HIV test followed by Western blot analysis for confirmation is the current gold standard for diagnosis of the condition.
- Opportunistic infections should be evaluated according to Table 58.2.

Sudden deterioration

- In the deteriorating patient with HIV/AIDS, the usual considerations of *a*irway, *b*reathing, and *c*irculation (ABC) should be made.
  - Patients with decreased level of consciousness and concern for airway compromise should be intubated.

Table 58.2. Common opportunistic infections

Opportunistic infection	CD4 count (cells/microliter)	Presentation	Diagnosis	Treatment
Cryptococcal infection	<50	Fever, malaise, headache, meningoencephalitis	CSF analysis for cryptococcal antigen, elevated CSF pressure (>20 mmH$_2$O), pleocytosis	Amphotericin B and flucytosine
Cytomegalovirus retinitis	<50	Decreased visual acuity, floaters, scotomata	Dilated fundus examination	Oral valganciclovir, or IV ganciclovir, or intraocular ganciclovir
Mycobacterium avium complex	<50	Cough, weight loss, fever, night sweats	AFB smear of blood, tissue or stool culture	Clarithromycin and ethambutol (may add rifabutin)
Toxoplasmosis	<50	Headache, confusion, weakness, fever	Ring-enhancing lesions on CT or MRI, serum anti-toxo IgG, brain biopsy	Pyrimethamine and sulfadiazine and leucovorin, or pyrimethamine and clindamycin and leucovorin
Aspergillosis	<100	Fever, cough, dyspnea, chest pain, hemoptysis, hypoxemia	Isolation from respiratory secretions, CXR or CT with suggestive findings	Voriconazole or amphotericin B
Candidal esophagitis	<100	Odynophagia, retrosternal burning pain, white plaques	Plaques visualized with upper endoscopy	Fluconazole or posaconazole
Cryptococcal diarrhea	<100	Nausea, vomiting, watery diarrhea, crampy abdominal pain	Stool studies for oocysts	Initiate ART, rehydration, electrolyte repletion. Consider nitazoxanide

Table 58.2. (*cont.*)

Opportunistic infection	CD4 count (cells/microliter)	Presentation	Diagnosis	Treatment
Microsporidial diarrhea	<100	Diarrhea, cholangitis, hepatitis, encephalitis	Light microscopy or small-bowel biopsy	Initiate ART, rehydration, electrolyte repletion. Consider albendazole or itraconazole
Bartonella	<100	Cutaneous lesions, osteomyelitis, fever, night sweats, weight loss, peliosis hepatis	Tissue biopsy: blood cultures are unreliable	Doxycycline or clarithromycin or azithromycin
Histoplasma (disseminated)	<150	Fever, fatigue, weight loss, hepatosplenomegaly, lymphadenopathy	Histoplasma antigens in blood or urine	Amphotericin B
Candida albicans (thrush)	<200	Painless white plaques	Clinical (plaques easily scrape off), light microscopy with KOH preparation	Fluconazole or posaconazole
Pneumocystis jiroveci (PCP) pneumonia	<200	Dyspnea, hypoxia, fever, nonproductive cough	CXR (diffuse interstitial infiltrates), BAL culture, low PaO_2, elevated LDH	TMP-SMX, or dapsone and TMP, or primaquine and clindamycin. Consider steroids when hypoxia is present
Varicella zoster virus	Any but more commonly <200	Typical rash (might have atypical pattern in immunocompromised patients)	Clinical diagnosis; swab open lesions for culture or PCR	Oral acyclovir or valcyclovir (outpatient); IV acyclovir (inpatient)

Organism	CD4	Clinical features	Diagnosis	Treatment
C. diff., Salmonella, Shigella, Campylobacter	Any	Watery diarrhea, crampy abdominal pain, anorexia, malaise, fever	Stool studies	Ciprofloxacin (*Salmonella, Shigella, Campylobacter*); flagyl (*C.diff.*)
Coccidioidomycosis	<250	Diffuse pneumonia or meningitis	IgG study, specimen culture	Fluconazole or itraconazole
EB virus (oral hairy leukoplakia)	Any	Painless plaques along lateral tongue borders	Unable to scrape off, biopsy	Acyclovir or valcyclovir. Initiate ART
Mycobacterium tuberculosis	Any	Cough, hemoptysis, weight loss, fever, night sweats	CXR, AFB smear	INH, RIF, PZA, EMB. Add dexamethasone for CNS infection
Streptococcal pneumonia	Any	Fever, chills, rigors, productive cough with purulent sputum, dyspnea	CXR, sputum cultures (if good sample available)	Antibiotic as for non-HIV patients; Beta-lactam and macrolide (always dual therapy)
JC virus (PML)	Any	Altered mental status, speech disturbances, visual deficits, discoordination	MRI shows hypodense white matter lesions, CSF analysis for JC virus by PCR	Initiate ART, supportive care

AFB, acid-fast bacillus; ART, antiretroviral therapy; BAL, bronchoalveolar lavage; *C.diff.*, *Clostridium difficile*; CSF, cerebrospinal fluid; CT, computed tomography; CXR, chest radiography; EBV, Epstein–Barr virus; EMB, ethambutol; TMP, trimethoprim; IgG, immunoglobulin G; INH, isoniazid; JC, John Cunningham; KOH, potassium hydroxide; LDH, lactate dehydrogenase; MRI, magnetic resonance imaging; PaO₂, partial pressure of oxygen in arterial blood; PCR, polymerase chain reaction; PML, progressive multifocal leukoencephalopathy; PZA, pyrazinamide; RIF, rifampin; SMX, sulfamethoxazole.

- Additional intravenous access should be obtained with large-bore lines in anticipation of aggressive resuscitation with fluids.
  - Broad-spectrum antibiotics should be initiated with additional coverage for suspected opportunistic infections (Table 58.2).
- Medication side effects and drug interactions can cause organ dysfunction, cardiac arrhythmias, or electrolyte abnormalities. Consider stopping the offending agent(s).
- Immune reconstitution inflammatory syndrome (IRIS) should remain a consideration.
  - IRIS is a constellation of symptoms characterized by fever and worsening of the clinical manifestations of the underlying opportunistic infection.
  - In this condition, the immune system begins to recover after the initiation of antiretroviral therapy (ART), and starts responding to the opportunistic infection with an excessive inflammatory response that worsens the initial symptoms.
  - It is typically seen within the first 4–8 weeks after initiation of ART, and most commonly with mycobacterial infections.
  - It is a clinically challenging diagnosis since its differentiation from progression of the initial opportunistic infection, the development of a new opportunistic infection, an unrelated organ dysfunction, or drug toxicity cannot be easily made.
  - Patients should receive supportive care. Systemic corticosteroids may be indicated and initiated after consultation with an infectious disease specialist.
- **Special considerations for the pregnant patient**
  - Pregnancy should not prevent diagnostic imaging that may assist in diagnosing opportunistic infections. Abdominal shielding should be considered to limit radiation exposure to the fetus.
  - Immediate initiation of ART should be considered when opportunistic infections are diagnosed in pregnant patients. This can minimize transmission of disease to the fetus.
- **System-specific complications and special considerations**
  - *Central nervous system:*
    - Reported complications: encephalitis, seizure, lymphoma, meningitis.
    - Altered mental status should be worked up with CT or MRI of the brain to evaluate for mass-occupying lesions, and lumbar puncture to evaluate for opportunistic infections.
    - Broad-spectrum antibiotics, antivirals, and antifungals should be started if there is suspicion for meningitis in the setting of a low CD4 count.
  - *Pulmonary:*
    - Reported complications: pneumonia, tuberculosis, PCP-related pneumothorax, and fungal infections.
    - A chest radiograph (CXR) may be nonspecific. A chest CT should be considered in the setting of hypoxia or dyspnea with an equivocal CXR.

- *Cardiovascular:*
  - Reported complications: pericardial effusion, dilated cardiomyopathy, myocarditis, coronary artery disease.
  - An electrocardiogram should be performed urgently if the patient presents with chest pain.
  - Consider bedside ultrasonography to evaluate for pericardial effusion and cardiac ejection fraction in the patient presenting with heart failure symptoms.
- *Gastrointestinal:*
  - Reported complications: diarrhea, esophagitis, pancreatitis, and liver failure.
  - Check for hepatitis B and C co-infections.
- *Renal:*
  - Reported complications: HIV nephropathy, and acute renal failure.
  - HIV nephropathy is an indication for the initiation of ART.
  - Stop all nephrotoxic medications and hydrate the patient.
  - Some antiretroviral drugs are associated with nephrolithiasis and should be avoided.

Vasopressor of choice: Patients with AIDS who are presenting with hypotension and evidence of shock are likely to be in septic shock. Norepinephrine is currently the initial vasopressor of choice in this situation.

REFERENCES

AIDSinfo. Guidelines for the use of antiretroviral agents in HIV-1-infected adults and adolescents [Internet]. 2011 [updated March 27, 2012]. Available from: http://aidsinfo.nih.gov/guidelines/html/1/adult-and-adolescent-arv-guidelines/21/hiv-infected-adolescents-and-young-adults/ (accessed September 22, 2012).

Centers for Disease Control and Prevention. 1993 Revised classification system for HIV infection and expanded surveillance case definition for AIDS among adolescents and adults. *JAMA.* 1993; **269**: 729–30.

Kaplan JE, Benson C, Holmes KH, *et al.* Guidelines for prevention and treatment of opportunistic infections in HIV-infected adults and adolescents: Recommendations from CDC, the National Institutes of Health, and the HIV Medicine Association of the Infectious Diseases Society of America. *MMWR Recomm Rep.* 2009; **58**(RR-4): 1–207.

Marco CA, Rothman RE. HIV infection and complications in emergency medicine. *Emerg Med Clin North Am.* 2008; **26**: 367–87.

Venkat A, Piontkowsky DM, Cooney RR, *et al.* Care of the HIV-positive patient in the emergency department in the era of highly active antiretroviral therapy. *Ann Emerg Med.* 2008; **52**: 274–85.

Endocrine emergencies

59

Diabetic ketoacidosis and hyperglycemic hyperosmolar state

Benjamin Zabar

Diabetic ketoacidosis (DKA)

Introduction

- Diabetics may enter a hyperglycemic state due to an imbalance between insulin release and glucagon production. A stressor such as infection, myocardial infarction, and stroke often precipitates this imbalance (Table 59.1).
- **Diabetic ketoacidosis (DKA)** is a critical state of hyperglycemia that results in both hyperketonemia and acidosis.
- Hyperglycemia causes glucose to spill into the urine, resulting in an osmotic diuresis that leads to dehydration and electrolyte abnormalities. In DKA the inability to use glucose leads to metabolism of fatty acids, producing ketones that cause an anion gap ketoacidosis.
- The acidosis causes K^+ to shift out of cells, leading to serum hyperkalemia. K^+ and bicarbonate are lost in the urine, depleting whole body potassium. The loss of bicarbonate further exacerbates the acidosis.
- Other causes of altered mental status, anion gap acidosis, or electrolyte abnormalities should be considered.

Practical Emergency Resuscitation and Critical Care, ed. Kaushal Shah, Jarone Lee, Kamal Medlej, and Scott D. Weingart. Published by Cambridge University Press. © Kaushal Shah, Jarone Lee, Kamal Medlej, and Scott D. Weingart 2013.

Table 59.1. Etiologies of diabetic ketoacidosis

Sepsis
Urinary tract infection
Pneumonia
Myocardial infarction
Stroke
Gastrointestinal bleeding
Medication noncompliance
Newly diagnosed diabetes

Presentation

Classic presentation
- Classic symptoms of hyperglycemia including polyuria, polydipsia, polyphagia, dizziness, and weakness.
- Abdominal pain, nausea, and vomiting.
- Altered mental status.
- Deep breathing (Kussmaul respiration) with fruity odor.
- Table 59.2 lists the differential diagnoses of patients in DKA.

Critical presentation
- Profound hypotension due to severe dehydration.
- Coma, requiring airway protection.

Table 59.2. Differential diagnosis of DKA

Ketoacidosis
- Alcoholic ketoacidosis
Anion-gap acidosis
- Salicylate toxicity
- Toxic alcohols (methanol, ethylene glycol, propylene glycol)
- Uremia
- Lactic acidosis (sepsis, shock)
Hypoglycemia
Trauma

Diagnosis and evaluation

- **Signs of dehydration**
  - Dry mucous membranes
  - Altered mental status
  - Orthostatic hypotension
  - Tachycardia.

- **Signs of hyperglycemia**
  - Kussmaul respirations
  - Fruity odor of ketones (some people cannot smell this).
- **Diagnostic tests**
  - **Glucometry** – point of care glucose level is typically greater than 250mg/dL (13.89 mmol/L) (may read "high").
  - Treatment of presumed DKA should begin with rehydration and evaluation for precipitating cause in the setting of a "high" glucometer reading. Further treatment often awaits laboratory results.
  - **Chemistry** is critical for obtaining glucose and electrolyte levels and calculating anion gap (anion gap = sodium – [chloride + bicarbonate]).
    - Serum potassium is often elevated and will correct with insulin therapy, fluid replacement, and correction of acidosis. **Remember: DKA patients are often depleted in total body potassium**.
    - Other electrolytes such as magnesium, phosphate, and calcium may also be depleted during DKA and monitoring them is important.
    - Consider checking serum lipase to exclude pancreatitis as a precipitating factor for the hyperglycemia. But keep in mind that hyperglycemia can cause pancreatitis as well.
    - Serial chemistry monitoring every 1–2 hours is recommended during treatment because of rapid fluid and electrolyte shifting.
    - Sodium should be adjusted for elevated glucose. Na^+ artificially decreases approximately 1.6 mEq/L for every 5.55 mmol/L (100 mg/dL) the glucose is above normal. For example, if the sodium is measured at 120 mEq/L, blood glucose is 400 mg/dL, the glucose is 300 units above normal ($3 \times 1.6 = 4.8$). Therefore the corrected sodium is 120 + 4.8 >124.8 mEq/L. Above glucose levels of 400 mg/dL, the correction is less reliable and a correction factor of 2.4 mEq/L appears to be more accurate.
  - **Serum acetone** measurement indicates presence of ketonemia and may correlate with the degree of dehydration and breakdown of fatty acids that occur in DKA.
  - **Blood gas** measurement is important for determining the degree of acidosis. Venous blood gas has been demonstrated to be as reliable as arterial blood gas for pH monitoring.
  - **Chest radiography** to exclude pneumonia as a precipitating cause of DKA.
  - **Urinalysis** evaluates the presence of ketonuria (commonly acetoacetate) and/ or presence of urinary tract infection.
  - *Critical pitfall: Negative urine ketone testing does not exclude the presence of DKA.*
  - **ECG** evaluates the presence of ischemia or STEMI (ST-segment elevation myocardial infarction) and provides important morphological features of electrolyte abnormalities before starting insulin and potassium therapy.

Critical management

ABCs
Aggressive fluid replacement
Insulin therapy (0.1 units/kg/hour IV drip)
Potassium repletion
Other electrolyte repletion
Treat underlying cause (e.g., infection, AMI, stroke)
Consider sodium bicarbonate for pH <7.0

- **Manage airway, breathing, and circulation**
  - Establish continuous cardiac monitoring and pulse oximetry.
  - Patients who are hypoxic should receive supplemental oxygen via a nasal cannula or nonrebreather facemask.
  - Rapid sequence intubation may be necessary for airway protection in obtunded patients or those severely hypoxic. Remember to match the ventilator respiratory rate with the patient's respiratory rate (typically tachypneic as compensation for metabolic acidosis) preintubation.
  - Start **large-bore IVs (ideally two)**, as the patient will need both IV fluids and IV insulin and electrolyte therapy.
- **Aggressive fluid replacement**
  - Patients are **often depleted 4–8 liters of total body volume**.
  - Begin with 2–4 liters of isotonic normal saline depending on the severity of the illness over the first 1–2 hours of treatment and reassess volume and electrolyte status. Children require different fluid calculations and their specific treatment regimen is beyond the scope of this chapter.
  - After initial boluses, continue either normal saline (NS) or ½NS at 250–500 mL/hour and tailor fluid replacement to the clinical status of the patient.
- **Insulin therapy**
  - Insulin therapy decreases serum glucose by shifting it into cells and signals cells to stop fatty acid breakdown and begin metabolizing existing ketones.
  - Regular insulin has a short half-life of 3–5 minutes. It will reach a steady state in five half-lives (15–25 minutes), which means that it is generally unnecessary to give a bolus dose when starting an insulin drip. Also, there is data to show potential harm when giving a bolus of insulin in DKA patients.
  - Begin an IV drip at 0.1 units/kg/hour, titrating up to 5–10 units/hour (depending on the weight of the patient), with a goal of reducing glucose 50–100 mg/dL/hour (2.77–5.55 mmol/L/hour).
  - Check blood glucose by glucometer every 30–60 minutes to prevent hypoglycemia.

Table 59.3. Potassium repletion in DKA

Measured potassium (mEq/L)	mEq of K$^+$ to give per hour
<3	40
3–4	30
4–5	20
5–6	10
>6	0

- Once serum glucose reaches 250 mg/dL (13.89 mmol/L), add dextrose to the IV fluids at a rate that allows a normal steady serum glucose level while continuing IV insulin therapy (typically D5-½NS at 100–150 mL/hour). Insulin will still be required to remove ketones despite normalization of glucose at a dose typically half the starting dose.
- Continue the insulin drip until normalization of the anion gap ("gap closure").
- One hour prior to termination of the insulin drip, administer long-acting insulin to prevent rebound hyperglycemia (i.e., insulin glargine 10–20 units subcutaneously).
- **Potassium repletion**
  - **Remember that DKA patients are often depleted in total body potassium** (Table 59.3).
  - Potassium will shift into the cells during insulin treatment and should be repleted even if slightly elevated.
  - Check potassium before starting insulin drip.
  - Resist the temptation to give further potassium-lowering agents such as Kayexalate unless the patient is exhibiting dysrhythmias as a result of hyperkalemia. Always ensure that the patient can produce urine prior to giving potassium.
- **Other electrolyte repletion**
  - Repletion of magnesium, calcium, and phosphate are often necessary, especially after the first day of treatment.
- **Sodium bicarbonate**
  - Some authors advocate administering sodium bicarbonate if pH <7.0. This is a topic of much debate because there is limited evidence to support the use of sodium bicarbonate and there is potential to worsen intracellular and cerebral acidosis.
  - Remember to continuously evaluate fluid and electrolyte status during fluid replacement and insulin therapy with repeat chemistry testing, glucose levels, anion gap assessment, potassium/magnesium levels, and physical examination.

Hyperglycemic hyperosmolar state (HHS)

Introduction

- **Hyperglycemic hyperosmolar state** (formerly hyperglycemic hyperosmolar nonketotic coma) is a critical state of hyperglycemia, hyperosmolarity, and dehydration similar to DKA but without development of ketoacidosis. As with DKA, HHS is sometimes the result of a precipitating stressor like infection, myocardial infarction, or stroke.
- In HHS it is believed that the body produces enough insulin to prevent ketoacidosis; however, the state of severe hyperglycemia continues to result in osmotic diuresis, hyperosmolar state, and electrolyte abnormalities.
- HHS occurs most frequently in elderly, confused, and bed-bound persons with underlying renal insufficiency who are unable to access enough fluids to match losses or obtain needed medications.
- The diagnosis is associated with a high mortality, up to 50% even with treatment. Note that this is much greater than in patients with DKA.
- The average fluid deficit is 9 liters.

Presentation

Classic presentation
- Altered mental status in an elderly person with multiple comorbidities.
- Polyuria, polydipsia.

Critical presentation
- Severely obtunded, comatose, lack of airway protection.
- Hypotensive.

Diagnosis and evaluation

- Same as DKA with the following differences:
  - **Glucometry** – the value is too "high" to register and presents with a glucose significantly more elevated than in DKA, at times in excess of 800–1000 mg/dL (44.40–55.50 mmol/L).
  - **Chemistry** – HHS does not primarily cause high anion gap acidosis as in DKA (there is not a primary excess of ketones); however, precipitating illnesses may lead to anion gap acidosis (i.e., renal failure, lactic acidosis). A significant osmolal gap will be present with plasma osmolality >320 mOsm/L.
  - **Blood gas** – while HHS patients are usually less acidotic than with DKA, a low pH should prompt consideration of metabolic disturbances other than HHS.
  - **Lactate** – a high lactate may indicate inadequate tissue perfusion, from dehydration or sepsis.
  - **Urinalysis** is less likely to show ketones than in DKA. Urinalysis helps evaluate the presence of urinary tract infection.

- A diagnosis of HHS must prompt the question why the patient was unable to maintain hydration. New causes of incapacity such as stroke, infection, or injury should be considered.

Critical management

- Same as for DKA with following differences:
  - **ABCs** – Due to profound mental status changes, patients with HHS more often lack airway protection than patients with DKA. Rapid sequence intubation should be performed early if coma is present.
  - **Insulin therapy** – Patients with HHS need IV fluids for profound dehydration. Although severe hyperglycemia causes osmotic diuresis, HHS occurs in individuals capable of making insulin with some degree of effectiveness. Thus, in contrast to DKA, insulin is not an urgent component of treatment. Once significant replacement of fluids occurs, electrolyte abnormalities are corrected, and adequate urine output is ensured, patients with HHS may benefit from IV insulin 0.1 U/kg/hour to slow continuing osmotic diuresis.

Sudden deterioration in DKA and HHS

- **Acute change in mental status**
  - Hypoglycemia can occur as a result of "overcorrection" of hyperglycemia with insulin drip. Immediately check bedside glucometry and if necessary stop insulin therapy and give D50W.
  - Cerebral edema may occur as a result of rapid fluid shifts, particularly in the pediatric population. If it occurs, stop fluid replacement and consider rapid sequence intubation, hyperventilation, and administration of IV mannitol.
- **Acute muscle weakness**
  - This is most often a result of an electrolyte abnormality occurring during therapy, most notably hypophosphatemia. Hold insulin and fluids and immediately obtain an ECG, chemistry panel (including calcium, magnesium, and phosphate), and whole-blood potassium. Replete the abnormal electrolyte, monitor closely, and resume therapy after improvement of weakness.
- **Acute respiratory distress**
  - Consider pulmonary vascular congestion as a result of aggressive fluid replacement. Provide additional oxygen and immediately obtain a portable chest radiograph. Avoid diuretics if the chest radiograph shows congestion as this will worsen intravascular fluid depletion and may cause a further drop in potassium. Slowing/stopping IV fluids is usually sufficient; in certain instances noninvasive positive-pressure ventilation or rapid sequence intubation are necessary.

Vasopressor of choice: norepinephrine.

REFERENCES

Cydulka RK, Gerald ME. Diabetes mellitus and disorders of glucose homeostasis. In: Marx JA, Hockberger RS, Walls RM, Adams J, Rosen P, eds. *Rosen's Emergency Medicine: Concepts and Clinical Practice*. 7th edn. Philadelphia, PA: Mosby Elsevier, 2010.

Graber MN. Diabetes and hyperglycemia. In: Adams, JG, ed. *Emergency Medicine*. Philadelphia: Elsevier Saunders, 2008.

Marino PL. *The ICU Book*. 3rd edn. Philadelphia: Lippincott Williams & Wilkins, 2007.

60

Thyroid storm

Kirill Shishlov

Introduction

- Thyrotoxicosis is a clinical state of hyperdynamic metabolism as a result of excessive circulating thyroid hormone.
- The most notable causes of thyrotoxicosis are Graves disease, Hashimoto thyroiditis, De Quervain thyroiditis, and TSH/thyroid hormone-secreting tumors.
- **Excessive circulating thyroid hormone can have critical effects on many organ systems.**
  - *Cardiovascular system:*
    - Direct positive chronotropic and inotropic effects on the heart.
    - Indirectly increases cardiac output secondary to increased peripheral tissue oxygen consumption and thermogenesis.
    - Indirectly increases cardiac output due to decreased peripheral vascular resistance and increased dilatation of arterioles.
  - *Pulmonary system:*
    - Hyperventilation secondary to increased CO_2 production resulting from elevated tissue metabolism.
    - Respiratory muscle fatigue.
  - *Renal system:*
    - Increase in blood volume and preload due to increased production of erythropoietin.
- **Thyroid storm** is a life-threatening decompensation of thyrotoxicosis, which occurs in approximately 1–2% of persons with thyrotoxicosis.
- The critical transition from thyrotoxicosis to thyroid storm is thought to be due to an acute increase in catecholamine binding sites.

Practical Emergency Resuscitation and Critical Care, ed. Kaushal Shah, Jarone Lee, Kamal Medlej, and Scott D. Weingart. Published by Cambridge University Press. © Kaushal Shah, Jarone Lee, Kamal Medlej, and Scott D. Weingart 2013.

Table 60.1. Common precipitants of thyroid storm

Infection/sepsis
Surgery
Acute coronary syndrome/myocardial infarction
Cerebral vascular accident
Trauma (especially neck trauma)
Medication noncompliance
Thyroid hormone ingestion
Iodine contrast

- Since many disease processes can increase circulating catecholamines, precipitation of thyroid storm is not simply a sudden increase in the levels of thyroid hormones but rather an exaggerated response to internal/external stressors.
- Infection is the most common precipitating factor in thyroid storm (Table 60.1).

Presentation

- The broad clinical picture is one suggestive of a hypermetabolic state with increased beta-adrenergic activity.
- Often more than one disease process may be occurring at once, which makes rapid identification of thyroid storm very difficult. The key is to have a high index of suspicion.

Classic presentation

- Marked tachycardia, often with ventricular rates exceeding 140 bpm.
- Fever, temperatures sometimes exceeding 41°C (106°F).
- Diaphoresis.
- GI symptoms, such as abdominal pain, nausea, vomiting, diarrhea.
- CNS dysfunction, agitation, confusion, delirium.

Critical presentation

- High-output cardiac failure and shock.
- Atrial fibrillation with rapid ventricular response.
- Severely obtunded state, coma, seizure.

Diagnosis and evaluation

- The diagnosis of thyroid storm is made based on clinical findings and laboratory analysis.
- **Burch and Wartofsky scoring system**
  - Given the spectrum of illness, Burch and Wartofsky developed a scoring system to help clinically distinguish uncomplicated thyrotoxicosis from impending thyroid storm and true thyroid storm (Table 60.2).
  - A score of 45 or more is highly suggestive of thyroid storm, a score of 25–44 is suggestive of impending thyroid storm, and a score below 25 makes the diagnosis of thyroid storm unlikely.

Table 60.2. Burch and Wartofsky scoring system for thyroid storm

Thermoregulatory dysfunction (°F)	
99–99.9	5
100–100.9	10
101–101.9	15
102–102.9	20
103–103.9	25
≥104	30
Tachycardia (beats/minute)	
90–109	5
110–119	10
120–129	15
130–139	20
≥140	25
CNS effects	
Mild agitation	10
Delirium/psychosis/lethargy	20
Seizure/coma	30
Heart failure	
Pedal edema	5
Bibasilar rales	10
Atrial fibrillation	10
Pulmonary edema	15
Gastrointestinal-hepatic dysfunction	
Diarrhea/nausea/vomiting/abdominal pain	10
Unexplained jaundice	20
Precipitant history	
Positive	10

- **Laboratory testing**
  - Laboratory evaluation is primarily directed at assessing the severity of the disease and searching for potential precipitants.
  - TSH, T_3, T_4, free T_4
  - CBC, basic metabolic profile, lactate, hepatic function panel, lipase.
  - Cardiac markers, brain natriuretic peptide (BNP).
  - Blood, urine and possibly CNS cultures/analysis.
  - A normal TSH virtually excludes the diagnosis of thyroid storm.
- **ECG**
  - Evaluate for the presence of atrial fibrillation, other cardiac arrhythmias, or evidence of acute myocardial ischemia.
  - The most common cardiac rhythm is sinus tachycardia.
- **Echocardiography**
  - Consider bedside echocardiography if suspecting pericardial effusion or significant cardiac dysfunction.
- **Imaging**
  - Chest radiography to rule out pneumonia and to evaluate for evidence of congestive heart failure (CHF).
  - Consider CT of the head to assess for other potential etiologies of altered mental status.

Critical management

ABC
Fluid resuscitation
Control agitation
Aggressive cooling
Treat precipitating/concomitant illness
Inhibit toxic peripheral effects of excess thyroid hormone (beta-blockade)
Inhibit further thyroid hormone synthesis (propylthiouracil [PTU]/methimazole)
Prevent peripheral conversion $T_4 \rightarrow T_3$ (dexamethasone)
Inhibit thyroid hormone release (iodine)

- **Management of ABCs and general supportive measures**
  - Insert IV line, provide supplemental O_2, and place on continuous monitoring.
  - Sit the patient upright to reduce symptomatic pulmonary congestion.
  - Consider rapid sequence intubation for respiratory distress/failure.
  - *Fluid resuscitation:*
    - Thyroid storm is a hypermetabolic state, which means patients are often severely dehydrated with depleted glycogen stores.

- Vigorous crystalloid administration is indicated unless signs of CHF are present.
- Addition of glucose containing isotonic fluid is often necessary.
- *Control hyperthermia:*
  - Antipyretics – Acetaminophen is preferred; be cautious with aspirin as it is thought to increase free T_3 and T_4 levels by affecting protein binding.
  - Consider cooling blankets, ice packs, fans, and other methods of active/passive cooling.
- *Control agitation:*
  - Benzodiazepines to control agitation and decrease sympathomimetic state.
  - Avoid agents that increase sympathomimetic tone – ketamine, amiodarone, albuterol, etc.
- **Specific therapy for thyroid storm**
  - *The order of treatment is of utmost importance in thyroid storm.* Following the ABCs, always remember to treat the life-threatening hypermetabolic state with beta-blockade first. It is also important to wait at least 1 hour from the time PTU/methimazole is given before giving iodine, or it will act as a substrate for more thyroid hormone production.
  - *Inhibit toxic effects of thyroid hormone:*
    - Initial stabilization with a short-acting IV agent such as esmolol is preferred, especially in severe disease, as it allows for rapid titration.
      - 250–500 micrograms/kg loading dose, followed by an infusion at 50–100 micrograms/kg/minute.
    - Alternatively, IV propranolol can be selected. Although more difficult to titrate, it has the physiological advantage of blocking peripheral conversion of T_4 to T_3.
      - 0.5–1 mg IV slow push, repeat every 15 minutes to effect.
  - *Inhibit thyroid hormone synthesis:*
    - Propylthiouracil (PTU) and methimazole are thioamides that block synthesis of thyroid hormone in the thyroid gland.
    - PTU is preferred for its additional advantage of blocking peripheral conversion of T_4 to T_3.
    - PTU: 600–1000 mg PO loading dose, 200–250 mg PO every 4 hours.
  - *Prevent peripheral conversion of $T_4 \rightarrow T_3$:*
    - Dexamethasone.
      - 2–4 mg IV every 6 hours.
  - *Inhibit thyroid hormone release options:*
    - Saturated solution of potassium iodide – 5 drops PO/NG/PR every 6 hours.
    - Lugol solution – 8 drops PO/NG/PR every 8 hours.
    - Sodium iodide – 500 mg IV every 12 hours.
    - If there is iodine allergy, lithium carbonate 300 mg PO/NG every 6 hours.

Sudden deterioration

- **High-output cardiac failure** can be a devastating complication in thyroid storm. It is the result of excessive tachycardia and may result in pulmonary edema despite volume depletion. This can be complicated by the development of atrial fibrillation with rapid ventricular response, further worsening hemodynamics.
- The goal is to decrease fever and heart rate and to judiciously increase intravascular volume while decreasing excessive circulating thyroid hormone.
- Avoid the use of diuretics.
- Use a titratable beta-blockade to decrease the heart rate and increase cardiac filling time.
- Consider noninvasive positive-pressure ventilation to promote pulmonary edema redistribution and reduce the work of breathing.

Vasopressor of choice: norepinephrine and milrinone.

REFERENCES

Hackstadt D, Korley F. Thyroid disorders. In: Adams JG, ed. *Emergency Medicine.* Philadelphia: Elsevier Saunders; 2008.

Mills L, Lim S. Identifying and treating thyroid storm and myxedema coma in the emergency department. *Emerg Med Pract.* EBMedicine.net, August 2009. Available at www.ebmedicine.net/ (accessed May 31, 2013).

Zull D. Thyroid and adrenal disorders. In: Marx JA, Hockberger RS, Walls RM, Adams J, Rosen P, eds. *Rosen's Emergency Medicine: Concepts and Clinical Practice.* 7th edn. Philadelphia, PA: Mosby Elsevier, 2010.

61

Adrenal crisis

Daniel Rolston

Introduction

- Adrenal insufficiency can either be primary, resulting from destruction of the adrenal gland; or secondary, resulting from a deficiency of ACTH (adrenocorticotropic hormone, corticotropin).
- Tables 61.1 and 61.2 list the causes of chronic and acute adrenal insufficiency, respectively.
- **Adrenal crisis** is either the acute development of severe adrenal insufficiency or a rapid deterioration in a patient's baseline chronic adrenal insufficiency brought on by a stressor.
- **Pathophysiology**
  - Primary adrenal insufficiency (Addison disease) occurs when the adrenal gland loses approximately 90% of its function and can no longer produce cortisol or aldosterone.
  - Secondary adrenal insufficiency occurs because of decreased production of ACTH by the pituitary gland, and therefore decreased cortisol production.
  - ACTH is released by the pituitary gland and stimulates the adrenal gland to produce and release cortisol. Additionally, the physiological stress of acute systemic illness causes the adrenal gland to secrete more cortisol.
  - Cortisol promotes gluconeogenesis/lipolysis, catecholamine synthesis, and vascular reactivity to vasoconstrictors; while inhibiting insulin secretion and inflammatory mediators.
- *The diagnosis of adrenal insufficiency is difficult to make because the most common symptoms are nonspecific, including fatigue, weight loss, GI symptoms, and depression, so a broad differential must be considered.*

Practical Emergency Resuscitation and Critical Care, ed. Kaushal Shah, Jarone Lee, Kamal Medlej, and Scott D. Weingart. Published by Cambridge University Press. © Kaushal Shah, Jarone Lee, Kamal Medlej, and Scott D. Weingart 2013.

Table 61.1. Common causes of chronic adrenal insufficiency

Chronic steroid use
HIV/AIDS
Tuberculosis
Autoimmune adrenalitis
    Congenital (congenital adrenal hyperplasia, adrenoleukodystrophy)
    Infiltrative (sarcoidosis, hemochromatosis, amyloidosis)
Cancer
Surgery/irradiation
Hepatic failure
Pancreatitis

Table 61.2. Etiologies of acute adrenal insufficiency

Drugs (steroids, etomidate, ketoconazole)
Systemic infection/sepsis
Adrenal hemorrhage (meningococcemia/Waterhouse–Friderichsen, anticoagulation,
    antiphospholipid antibody syndrome)
Pituitary hemorrhage (pituitary apoplexy)
Postpartum pituitary necrosis (Sheehan syndrome)
Trauma
Hepatic failure
Pancreatitis

Presentation

Classic presentation

- Patients with adrenal insufficiency usually present with nonspecific symptoms including weakness/fatigue, weight loss, anorexia, abdominal pain, fever, and depression.
- The classic finding in adrenal crisis is refractory hypotension.
- These patients can frequently appear to be in septic shock, and they may in fact be septic, but their body is not able to respond appropriately because of a lack of cortisol.
- A thorough history including steroid use/drug use, surgeries, history of HIV, and precipitating symptoms should be elicited.

Critical presentation

- Consider adrenal crisis in the patient who is persistently hypotensive despite multiple liters of fluid boluses and high doses of multiple vasopressors.

- Acute adrenal insufficiency can appear to be a severe gastroenteritis with fever, vomiting, and dehydration, but this can quickly progress to vascular collapse and death.

Diagnosis and evaluation

- **Vital signs** are the main identifier of illness since the symptoms are non-specific.
  - **Refractory hypotension** is the hallmark of adrenal crisis as discussed above.
  - The **lack of reflexive tachycardia** in a hypotensive state should increase concern for adrenal crisis since cortisol deficiency blunts the physiological vasoconstriction and catecholamine synthesis. However, many patients are on beta-blockers, calcium channel blockers or other antiarrhythmic drugs that can cause this discrepancy.
  - Consider adrenal crisis or neurogenic shock in a hypotensive-normocardic patient not taking heart-rate-modifying medications.
- **Physical examination** is frequently unimpressive, but a thorough examination can help determine the underlying cause.
  - First assess for signs of infection, which can precipitate a crisis:
    - Focal lung findings: crackles or rhonchi or wheezes
    - Altered mental status
    - Abdominal tenderness
    - Rashes
    - Joint swelling and erythema.
  - Dermatological examination can be especially helpful if adrenal crisis is suspected:
    - Hyperpigmentation of sun-exposed areas, axilla, palmar creases, and mucous membranes (Addison disease). The increased ACTH secreted by the pituitary stimulates melanin production.
    - Petechial rash (meningococcemia).
    - Vitiligo (white patches of amelanotic skin) can be seen in polyglandular autoimmune (PGA) syndrome type I.
- **Diagnostic tests**
  - *Laboratory tests:*
    - Hyponatremia is seen in primary adrenal insufficiency because of the aldosterone deficiency. Additionally, the lack of cortisol leads to increased antidiuretic hormone (ADH) secretion, increased free water absorption, and worsening hyponatremia.
    - The lack of aldosterone also causes hyperkalemia, with an accompanying mild hyperchloremic metabolic acidosis.
    - Hypoglycemia can be seen in both primary and secondary adrenal insufficiency because of a lack of cortisol and decreased appetite. Additionally,

in secondary adrenal insufficiency, growth hormone and ACTH deficiency contribute further to hypoglycemia.

- *Serum cortisol level:*
  - Should be elevated with acute illness because of physiological stress on the body.
  - A level <15–18 micrograms/mL is diagnostic of adrenal crisis in an acutely ill patient. A level >33 micrograms/mL excludes the diagnosis.
  - If the level is indeterminate, an ACTH (cosyntropin) stimulation test with less than a 9 micrograms/mL increase in serum cortisol is also diagnostic. Dexamethasone does not alter the cortisol assay and can be used instead of hydrocortisone if treatment is emergent and a stimulation test will be performed later.
  - Keep in mind that laboratories currently measure total cortisol only and the majority of cortisol is protein bound. As such, cortisol values might not reflect the true active cortisol level in the patient.

ABCs
Give normal saline bolus for hypotension
Rule out sepsis/other acute illness
Consider antibiotic coverage
Start inotropes/vasopressors as needed
Consider adrenal crisis in patients with hypotension refractory to vasopressors
Send serum cortisol and ACTH levels prior to steroids
Give hydrocortisone

Critical management

- **Manage ABCs**
  - Airway and breathing.
  - Place patients on cardiac monitor and pulse oximeter.
  - Hypotensive patients require 2–3 liters of normal saline fluid boluses (with D5W if the patient is hypoglycemic).
  - Vasopressors/inotropes to maintain circulation.
- **Hydrocortisone** is the initial therapy of choice once the possibility of adrenal crisis is recognized because of its glucocorticoid and mineralocorticoid effects.
  - The initial dose of hydrocortisone is 50–100 mg IV.
  - Maintenance dosing at 20 mg per hour or 50–100 mg IV every 6–8 hours. It is recommended to not give more than 300 mg per day.

Sudden deterioration

- If the patient with suspected adrenal insufficiency experiences sudden cardio-vascular collapse, adrenal hemorrhage must be considered. Hydrocortisone 100 mg IV should be started and central venous access obtained to give fluids and vasopressors for resuscitation. If the BP does not improve, fludrocortisone can be added. If the patient continues to deteriorate, another cause should be suspected.

Special circumstances

- **Steroids and sepsis**
  - The most recent meta-analysis evaluating acute management with corticoster-oids for sepsis does not demonstrate an improvement in mortality. However, subgroup analysis found improved mortality, decreased shock duration, and decreased ICU length of stay with prolonged, low-dose corticosteroids. Currently, this topic is very controversial among critical care specialists. Current guidelines recommend giving steroids only in patients with hypoten-sion not responsive to vasopressors.
- **Chronic adrenal insufficiency and sepsis**
  - Patients with known adrenal insufficiency or chronic corticosteroid use should receive hydrocortisone to generate an appropriate stress response to sepsis. If the BP is stable, 50 mg of hydrocortisone is probably appropriate.
- **Chronic adrenal insufficiency and procedures**
  - Patients with chronic adrenal insufficiency who need to have moderate seda-tion or a significant procedure in the emergency department should also receive 50–100 mg of hydrocortisone prior to the procedure.

Vasopressor of choice: norepinephrine.

REFERENCES

Annane BE. Corticosteroids in the treatment of severe sepsis and septic shock in adults: a systematic review. *JAMA*. 2009; **301**: 2362–75.

Salvatori R. Adrenal insufficiency. *JAMA*. 2005; **294**: 2481–8.

Torrey SP. Recognition and management of adrenal emergencies. *Emerg Med Clin North Am*. 2005; **23**: 687–702, viii.

Zull D. Thyroid and adrenal disorders. In: Marx JA, Hockberger RS, Walls RM, Adams J, Rosen P, eds. *Rosen's Emergency Medicine: Concepts and Clinical Practice*. 7th edn. Philadelphia, PA: Mosby Elsevier; 2010.

62

Pheochromocytoma

Jolene H. Nakao

Introduction

- Pheochromocytoma is a rare catecholamine-secreting tumor of the adrenal medulla. Chromaffin cells of the sympathetic nervous system give rise to similar extra-adrenal tumors, known as paragangliomas. Secreted catecholamines include dopamine, epinephrine, and/or norepinephrine.
- Less than 1% of cases of hypertension can be attributed to pheochromocytomas.
- It may present sporadically or as a result of genetic mutation leading to different familial syndromes that include pheochromocytomas, such as
  - Multiple endocrine neoplasia type 2 (MEN-2)
  - Neurofibromatosis type 1 (NF-1)
  - von Hippel-Lindau disease (VHL)
- In adults, approximately 10% of pheochromocytoma-like tumors are extra-adrenal (paragangliomas), 10% are bilateral, 10% are malignant, and 10% are associated with familial syndromes. In children, approximately 20% are extra-adrenal, 20% are bilateral, and 20% are malignant. Familial cases are more likely bilateral and recurrent compared to sporadic cases.
- It is known as "the great mimic" because numerous unusual presentations have been reported in the literature.
- Pheochromocytoma may be fatal if left undiagnosed, particularly in the setting of surgery or pregnancy. More than 90% of cases are curable if diagnosed early.

Practical Emergency Resuscitation and Critical Care, ed. Kaushal Shah, Jarone Lee, Kamal Medlej, and Scott D. Weingart. Published by Cambridge University Press. © Kaushal Shah, Jarone Lee, Kamal Medlej, and Scott D. Weingart 2013.

Presentation

Classic presentation

- Sustained or paroxysmal hypertension.
- Headache, palpitations, sweating, malaise, and a sensation of apprehension, anxiety, or doom.
- Less commonly: weight loss, tremulousness, flushing, nausea, constipation, and fever.
- Episodes may be related to position, meals, micturition, abdominal pressure, smoking, or physical or emotional stressors.
- Physical examination may reveal tachycardia, diaphoresis, and pallor.

Critical presentation

- The high levels of catecholamines secreted by the tumor(s) may lead to situations necessitating emergent intervention.
- Pheochromocytoma can present as a **hypertensive crisis**. This may be triggered by physiological stress including recent surgery, trauma, or pregnancy; tumor manipulation; anesthetic agents at the induction of anesthesia; or drugs including corticosteroids, antiemetics such as metoclopramide, and imipramine.
- Complications of pheochromocytoma-related hypertension result from vasoconstriction, coronary vasospasm, and hypoperfusion leading to organ ischemia (see Table 62.1).
- The most severe presentation is "**pheochromocytoma multi-system crisis (PMC).**" Manifestations include:
  - Elevated temperature >40°C
  - Encephalopathy
  - Hemodynamic instability (hypertension or hypotension)
  - Multi-system organ failure.

Diagnosis and evaluation

- **Laboratory testing**
  - Fractionated plasma and/or 24-hour urine levels of **metanephrines**, catecholamine metabolites (normetanephrine and metanephrine), have superior diagnostic sensitivity over testing for parent catecholamines.
  - 24-hour urine **catecholamine** levels may also be useful.
- **Imaging**
  - Computed tomography (CT):
    - Recommended for initial anatomical imaging.
  - Magnetic resonance imaging (MRI):
    - Recommended for initial anatomical imaging.

- ^{123}I-labeled metaiodobenzylguanidine (MIBG) scintigraphy:
  - Functional imaging – localizes adrenergic tissue.

Table 62.1. Possible manifestations of pheochromocytoma

Cardiovascular	Hypertensive crisis
	Angina
	Myocardial infarction
	Arrhythmia
	Myocarditis
	Cardiomyopathy
	Heart failure
	Cardiogenic shock
	Peripheral ischemia
Neurological	Cerebrovascular accidents
	Encephalopathy
	Generalized seizures
Pulmonary	Pulmonary edema
	Acute respiratory distress syndrome
Renal	Acute renal failure
Abdominal	Hemorrhage into the tumor
	Paralytic ileus
	Intestinal ischemia
	Colon perforation

Critical management

- Management of emergencies in patients with pheochromocytoma depends on symptoms. It should always include pharmacological treatment to block the effects of high levels of circulating catecholamines and prevent complications.
- Hypertensive crisis due to pheochromocytoma should be treated with repeated doses of **phentolamine**, a continuous infusion of phentolamine, or a continuous infusion of **sodium nitroprusside**.
- Definitive treatment for pheochromocytoma is surgery, which should be delayed until the patient is medically stable in order to improve survival.
- **Recommended preoperative pharmacological treatment options**:
  - First initiate **phenoxybenzamine**, a noncompetitive alpha-1 and alpha-2 adrenergic receptor antagonist, to reduce blood pressure fluctuation and ease vasoconstriction; side effects include orthostatic hypotension and reflex tachycardia.
  - **Metyrosine**, an inhibitor of catecholamine synthesis, may be added.
  - Selective alpha-1 receptor antagonists such as **terazosin, prazosin,** and **doxazosin** do not cause reflex tachycardia.

- **Calcium channel blockers** such as diltiazem effectively control blood pressure and prevent catecholamine-induced coronary vasospasm.
- **Beta-blockade** may be added to prevent reflex tachycardia or treat arrhythmia or angina but **should only be used in conjunction with alpha-blockade** to avoid dangerous unopposed alpha effects.
- After adequate control and stabilization of blood pressure, the tumor should be **surgically removed**.
- Patients should be **followed indefinitely**, particularly if they have familial or extra-adrenal disease.
- Inoperative disease or disease in which resection is not curative may be treated with adrenergic antagonists, chemotherapy, radiotherapy, and/or debulking.

Sudden deterioration

- Emergency surgical removal of the tumor is indicated if the patient deteriorates despite aggressive medical treatment appropriate for pheochromocytoma, even if the patient is critically ill, to increase chances of survival.

Vasopressor of choice: Vasopressors are not often indicated as patients are usually hypertensive and tachycardic, but if a patient becomes hypotensive from either over-medication or hemodynamic lability, consider norepinephrine or phenylephrine.

REFERENCES

Brouwers FM, Eisenhofer G, Lenders JW, Pacak K. Emergencies caused by pheochromocytoma, neuroblastoma, or ganglioneuroma. *Endocrinol Metab Clin North Am.* 2006; **35**: 699–724.

Chen H, Sippel RS, O'Dorisio MS, *et al.* The North American Neuroendocrine Tumor Society consensus guideline for the diagnosis and management of neuroendocrine tumors: pheochromocytoma, paraganglioma, and medullary thyroid cancer. *Pancreas.* 2010; **39**: 755–83.

Gray RO. Hypertension. In: Marx JA, Hockberger RS, Walls RM, Adams J, Rosen P, eds. *Rosen's Emergency Medicine: Concepts and Clinical Practice.* 7th edn. Philadelphia, PA: Mosby Elsevier; 2010.

Torrey SP. Recognition and management of adrenal emergencies. *Emerg Med Clin North Am.* 2005; **23**: 687–702.

Zuber SM, Kantorovich V. Hypertension in pheochromocytoma: characteristics and treatment. *Endocrinol Metab Clin North Am.* 2011; **40**: 295–311.

63

Anaphylaxis

Sebastian Siadecki

Introduction

- Anaphylaxis is a life-threatening allergic syndrome characterized by multi-organ involvement and rapid onset which can lead to life-threatening airway compromise and cardiovascular collapse.
- Anaphylaxis is an IgE-mediated (type I or immediate) hypersensitivity reaction, resulting in mast cell degranulation and release of mediators including histamine and cytokines.
- The term *anaphylactoid reaction* describes a similar clinical syndrome that is not mediated by IgE. However, the clinical presentation and treatment are identical.
- There are approximately 100 000 cases of anaphylaxis each year in the United States where the mortality is approximately 1%.
- Foods and medications are among the most common causative agents (Table 63.1); however, the offending agent is not identified in up to 1/3 of cases.
- Other etiologies may mimic the presentation of anaphylaxis (Table 63.2), although they usually lack the multi-system involvement seen in anaphylaxis.

Presentation

Classic presentation

- The severity of the presentation may vary depending on the degree of hypersensitivity, the quantity and route of exposure, and the sensitivity and responsiveness of the target organs.

Practical Emergency Resuscitation and Critical Care, ed. Kaushal Shah, Jarone Lee, Kamal Medlej, and Scott D. Weingart. Published by Cambridge University Press. © Kaushal Shah, Jarone Lee, Kamal Medlej, and Scott D. Weingart 2013.

Table 63.1. Etiologies of anaphylaxis

Foods: nuts, shellfish, eggs, cow's milk, soy, wheat
Antibiotics: penicillin, cephalosporins, sulfonamides, nitrofurantoin, tetracycline
Other therapeutics: methylparaben, rabies vaccine, egg-based vaccines
Insect stings
Latex
Heterologous and human sera
Local anesthetics (ester family)
Direct mast cell degranulation: radiocontrast media, opiates, curare, protamine
Immune complex-mediated: whole blood, immunoglobulins
Arachidonic acid metabolism: aspirin, NSAIDs, benzoates
Physical factors: exercise, temperature
Idiopathic

Table 63.2. Differential diagnoses

Flush syndromes: alcohol-induced, scombroidosis, carcinoid syndrome
Stridor: epiglottitis, retropharyngeal or peritonsillar abscess, laryngeal spasm, foreign body
Dyspnea: acute asthma, pulmonary embolism
Syncope: vasovagal, seizure, hypoglycemia, cardiac dysrhythmia, stroke, acute coronary syndrome
Shock: sepsis, spinal shock, cardiogenic, hypovolemic

- Rapid onset of symptoms (5–30 minutes) after parenteral exposure.
- Generalized warmth and tingling of the face, mouth, chest, hands, and areas of exposure.
- Pruritis.
- Generalized flushing and urticarial rash.
- Nasal congestion, sneezing, tearing.
- Crampy abdominal pain, nausea, vomiting, diarrhea, tenesmus.
- Cough, chest tightness, dyspnea, and wheezing.
- Lightheadedness or syncope.

Critical presentation

- Most fatalities occur within 30 minutes of antigen exposure.
- The rapidity of onset of symptoms after exposure is usually indicative of the severity of the reaction.
- Hoarseness, stridor, and hypersalivation may indicate oropharyngeal angio-edema or laryngeal edema.

- Cough, wheezing, ronchi, and decreased air movement indicate lower respiratory tract bronchoconstriction.
- Hypotension and tachycardia suggest circulatory collapse due to vasodilation and increased vascular permeability; dysrhythmias may also occur.
- Altered mental status or seizure may occur due to decreased cerebral perfusion.
- Fibrinolysis and disseminated intravascular coagulation, manifesting with abnormal bleeding or bruising, may develop as the reaction continues.

Diagnosis and evaluation

- **Vital signs**
  - Tachycardia and hypotension indicate impending cardiovascular collapse.
  - Hypoxia may result from upper or lower airway compromise due to edema, bronchoconstriction, and excessive secretions.
- **Physical examination**
  - Cutaneous findings: urticaria, flushing, angioedema.
  - Upper airway: rhinitis, congestion, sneezing, hoarseness, hypersalivation, stridor, oropharyngeal edema.
  - Lower airway: cough, wheezing, dyspnea, decreased air movement.
  - Eye: conjunctivitis.
  - Hematological: mucous membrane bleeding, bruising.
- **Diagnostic tests**
  - Anaphylaxis is a clinical diagnosis. However, some laboratory tests may be helpful in evaluating the severity of the reaction, guide treatment, and rule out concurrent emergencies.
  - Laboratory studies: complete blood count (CBC), metabolic panel.
  - Electrocardiogram (ECG) to rule out dysrhythmias.
  - Chest radiograph.
  - Depending on the clinical situation: cardiac enzymes, serial blood gases, cultures, computed tomography (CT) of the head, neck soft tissue radiographs, indirect or direct laryngoscopy.

Critical management

- **Initial steps**
  - Secure the airway.
  - Remove the offending agent if still present.
  - Place the patient in Trendelenburg position if hypotensive.
  - Intravenous (IV) access and crystalloid administration.
  - Cardiac monitoring, pulse oximetry.
- **Interventions**
  - Epinephrine is the primary treatment of anaphylaxis.

- The route of epinephrine administration depends on the severity of the clinical presentation.
- For typical presentations of anaphylaxis, epinephrine should be administered intrasmuscularly (IM); the adult dose is **0.3–0.5 mL** of **1:1000** concentration.
- Indications for IV epinephrine include severe upper airway obstruction, acute respiratory failure, or systolic BP <80 mmHg. Patients receiving epinephrine should be placed on cardiac monitors.
- IV epinephrine should be administered as 10 mL of a 1:100 000 dilution over 10 minutes; if there is no response, a continuous infusion of 1–10 micrograms/minute may be started.
- Much confusion exists over proper epinephrine dosing: **extreme care must be taken not to mistakenly administer the cardiac arrest dose** (1 mg of 1:10 000 concentration) in anaphylaxis, as it may lead to potentially lethal cardiac complications.
- **Antihistamines** such as diphenhydramine should also be administered.
  - H2 antagonists such as famotidine and rantidine have been shown to potentiate the effect of H1 antagonists and can be used as well.
- **Inhaled beta-agonists** may be used for bronchospasm refractory to epinephrine.
- **Systemic corticosteroids** are of limited benefit in the acute treatment of anaphylaxis as the onset of action is approximately 4–6 hours; however, they may be useful for persistent bronchospasm and to prevent delayed reactions.
- Patients on beta-blockers may be refractory to epinephrine. In these cases, glucagon may be used to counteract the beta-blockade (1–5 mg IV over 5 minutes, followed by 5–15 micrograms/minute by continuous infusion).
- **Disposition**
  - Most patients with mild to moderate anaphylaxis who respond appropriately to initial treatment may be discharged home.
  - Due to the potential for rebound reaction, patients should be observed for 2–6 hours prior to discharge, depending on the severity of the reaction.
  - Patients should be provided with oral antihistamines and corticosteroid therapy for 7–10 days.
  - Indications for admission include any hypotension, upper airway involvement or prolonged bronchospasm.

Sudden deterioration

- **Hypotension**
  - Additional crystalloid should be considered; colloid solutions such as 5% albumin may also be considered given the increased vascular permeability involved in anaphylaxis.

- If the patient remains hypotensive after fluid resuscitation, a vasopressor infusion should be initiated. Epinephrine is the first agent.
- Dobutamine may be used if myocardial depression is suspected.
- **Respiratory failure or airway obstruction**
  - Patients with anaphylactic reactions and airway compromise should be managed expeditiously in order to prevent their airway from obstructing.

Vasopressor of choice: epinephrine.

REFERENCES

Anchor J, Settipane RA. Appropriate use of epinephrine in anaphylaxis. *Am J Emerg Med.* 2004; **22**: 488–90.

Gavalas M, Sadana A, Metcalf A. Guidelines for the management of anaphylaxis in the emergency department. *J Accid Emerg Med.* 1998; **15**: 96–8.

Kanwar M, Irvin CB, Frank JJ, *et al.* Confusion about epinephrine dosing leading to iatrogenic overdose: a life-threatening problem with a potential solution. *Ann Emerg Med.* 2010; **55**: 341–4.

Marx JA, Hockberger RS, Walls RM, Adams J, Rosen P, eds. *Rosen's Emergency Medicine: Concepts and Clinical Practice.* 7th edn. Philadelphia, PA: Mosby Elsevier; 2010.

64

Hyperthermia

Amy Caggiula and Daniel Herbert-Cohen

Introduction

- Body temperature usually follows a diurnal fluctuation, going from a baseline of around 36°C in the morning, to 37.5°C in the late afternoon at rest.
- The human body has many physiological compensatory mechanisms such as shivering and sweating for maintaining a state of thermal homeostasis.
- Occasionally these mechanisms become overwhelmed resulting in a continuum of heat-related injuries and illnesses.
- Heat edema, syncope, cramps, and exhaustion comprise the milder manifestations of temperature illness. This chapter will focus on the more critical presentations of hyperthermia, including heatstroke and toxicological hyperthermia.

Heatstroke

Overview

- Two main pathophysiological mechanisms exist:
  1. *Classic heatstroke:* Occurs during heat waves and is most commonly observed in the elderly, debilitated patients, psychiatric patients, and young children. These patients may not have easy access to oral fluids, or may be taking medications that impair their body's ability to respond appropriately to increases in temperature.
     - Medications predisposing to heat illnesses include neuroleptics, sympathomimetics, diuretics, anticholinergics, and adrenergic antihypertensive agents that diminish the compensatory cardiovascular response to heat exposure.

Practical Emergency Resuscitation and Critical Care, ed. Kaushal Shah, Jarone Lee, Kamal Medlej, and Scott D. Weingart. Published by Cambridge University Press. © Kaushal Shah, Jarone Lee, Kamal Medlej, and Scott D. Weingart 2013.

2. *Exertional heatstroke:* Generally seen in athletes such as distance runners, and military personnel training in hot climates. These patients' heat-dispelling mechanisms are usually overwhelmed by endogenous heat production.

- Differential diagnosis for heatstroke
  - Sepsis
  - Meningitis/encephalitis
  - Malignant hyperthermia (MH)
  - Neuroleptic malignant syndrome (NMS)
  - Serotonin syndrome
  - Thyroid storm
  - Pheochromocytoma
  - Toxins/drugs.

Presentation

Classic presentation
- Elevated core temperature (>40.5°C).
- Central nervous system (CNS) dysfunction such as confusion, delirium, agitation, psychosis, ataxia, coma, seizures, and posturing.
- Elevated transaminases are almost universal.
- Jaundice often develops 24–72 hours after the onset of heatstroke.
- Acid–base disturbances:
  - Lactic acidosis is more frequently seen among victims of exertional heatstroke due to the increase in anaerobic metabolism occurring during strenuous physical activity.
  - Primary respiratory alkalosis with little or no metabolic acidosis is usually observed in sufferers of classic heatstroke.
- Possible electrolyte abnormalities include: hypocalcemia, hyperkalemia, hyperphosphatemia, hyponatremia, hypoglycemia.
- Impaired sweating and thus impaired evaporation contribute to the development and exacerbation of heatstroke. Medications that inhibit sweating such as anticholinergics intensify heat-related injury. However, the presence of sweating should not be used as exclusion criteria for the diagnosis of heatstroke, as anhidrosis is common but not universal in these patients.

Critical presentation
- Elevated creatine phosphokinase (CPK), rhabdomyolysis, and acute renal failure are more commonly seen in exertional heatstroke.
- Hypotension from peripheral vasodilation and dehydration can occur as well.
- Coagulopathy and disseminated intravascular coagulation (DIC) presenting as gastrointestinal bleeding, genitourinary bleeding, petechiae, purpura, epistaxis, hemoptysis, or oozing from venipuncture sites.

Diagnosis and evaluation

- A rectal temperature should be obtained on all patients with a concern for hyperthermia.
- Helpful laboratory tests include:
  - Comprehensive metabolic panel to assess electrolyte abnormalities and renal function
  - CPK to assess for rhabdomyolysis
  - Liver function tests
  - Coagulation studies including fibrinogen if there is suspicion for DIC
  - Lactic acid as a screen for sepsis but also as a marker for hypoperfusion
  - pH from arterial or venous blood gas to help determine severity of illness.
- A head CT followed by lumbar puncture should be performed in patients presenting with hyperthermia and neurological dysfunction in whom the diagnosis of heatstroke is not clearly established.

Critical management

- The goal of treatment is to decrease the core temperature quickly to less than 40°C. A urinary or rectal temperature probe should be placed for continuous monitoring of core body temperature.
- Cooling measures should be initiated even before any investigations into the etiology of the hyperthermia.
- Cooling can be initiated in the field by placing ice packs in the patient's neck, groin, and axillae until more effective cooling measures are available.
- Various methods may be utilized but evaporative cooling and ice water immersion remain the mainstays of management.
  - Evaporative cooling is quick and effective. The patient is sprayed with room temperature water and positioned under large fans to simulate the body's own response to heat.
  - Ice water immersion is also common. However, this method can induce shivering thereby increasing metabolism and core temperature. This response can be counteracted by administering benzodiazepines.
- Central cooling has been employed to some benefit. Some of these methods include cold intravenous fluids, cardiopulmonary bypass, and peritoneal, gastric, and bladder lavage. These methods are invasive and labor intensive however, and their efficacy when compared with standard measures is unknown. As such, they are often used as adjuncts to evaporative or immersion cooling.
- Cooling should be stopped when the body temperature reaches 39°C. This is done in order to avoid a hypothermic overshoot.
- Antipyretics such as acetaminophen, NSAIDs, and aspirin do not play a role in the management of heatstroke and should be avoided.

Sudden deterioration

- Airway management is the initial priority, and endotracheal intubation is often indicated in the altered or seizing patient. These patients are at high risk for aspiration, particularly if they present with persistent seizures or severe central nervous system (CNS) aberrations.
- Given the possibility of rhabdomyolysis and associated hyperkalemia in patients suffering from exertional heatstroke, a nondepolarizing muscle relaxant should be considered for rapid sequence intubation (RSI).
- Initiate fluid resuscitation with crystalloids if the patient is hypotensive or presents with signs of rhabdomyolysis. A urinary catheter should be placed to titrate fluid administration to a urine output of 1–1.5 mL/kg/hour.
- Urine alkalinization can be considered in patients with rhabdomyolysis and acidemia.
- Persistent anuria, uremia, or hyperkalemia are indications for consideration of hemodialysis.

Malignant hyperthermia

Overview

- Malignant hyperthermia (MH) is a disease state occasionally observed in patients undergoing general anesthesia.
- An inherited autosomal dominant disorder predisposes to excessive calcium release from the sarcoplasmic reticulum of skeletal muscles, resulting in hypermetabolism and hyperthermia.
- While this condition is most often seen in the operating room because of its association with inhaled anesthetic gases such as halothane, it can also be precipitated by succinylcholine which is often used in the emergency department.

Presentation

Classic/critical presentation

- MH presents during or shortly after exposure to inhaled anesthetic agents such as halothane, sevoflurane, and desflurane, or the depolarizing muscle relaxant succinylcholine.
- The hypercatabolic state results in rapid-onset, severe hyperthermia (>40.5°C), tachycardia, and tachypnea.
- Muscular rigidity, metabolic acidosis, and rising end-tidal CO_2 are also classic early findings.
- Patients can also have altered mental status, autonomic instability (including arrhythmias), rhabdomyolysis, and DIC.

Diagnosis and evaluation

- The diagnosis of MH should be suspected in the individual exposed to inhaled anesthetics or succinylcholine who develops a rising end-tidal CO_2, hyperthermia, and muscle rigidity.
- Additional investigations can help diagnose any associated complications but play no role in the diagnosis of MH and should therefore not delay essential interventions.

Critical management

- Discontinue the offending drug.
- Initiate cooling measures as described above.
- Provide sedation and muscle relaxation using benzodiazepines.
- Rising CO_2 is due to an increase in muscle metabolism as well as chest wall rigidity. Certain patients will need to be mechanically ventilated in order to assist ventilation and help overcome chest stiffness.
- Since malignant hyperthermia is due to an intrinsic problem with the muscle cells, neuromuscular blockade will provide no benefit in these patients.
- However, a nondepolarizing paralytic agent can be used to improve intubation conditions, although it is unlikely to result in complete muscle relaxation in these patients.
- Assess for rhabdomyolysis and manage electrolyte abnormalities.
- Dantrolene 2.5 mg/kg intravenously (IV) will decrease the amount of calcium released from the sarcoplasmic reticulum of muscle cells. This bolus can be repeated every 5 minutes until the signs of MH are reversed, or up to a cumulative dose of 10 mg/kg IV.

Neuroleptic malignant syndrome

Overview

- Another pathological condition in which hyperthermia is encountered is neuroleptic malignant syndrome (NMS).
- It is caused by the excessive blockage of dopaminergic receptors by some antipsychotics, as well as by withdrawal of dopaminergic drugs.

Presentation

Classic/critical presentation
- It most often presents within the first few weeks of starting antipsychotic medications.
  - It may present earlier (after as little as one dose) or later (after years on stable medication regimen).

- NMS is classically seen with "typical" neuroleptics such as haloperidol or flu-phenazine, but can also be seen with "atypical" neuroleptics such as clozapine or risperidone.
- Typical features:
  - Fever with altered mentation (e.g., agitation, delirium, catatonia)
  - Neuromuscular abnormalities often described as "lead pipe rigidity" due to increased muscle tone
    - Autonomic instability:
      - Life-threatening hyperthermia
      - Hypertension or hypotension
    - Rhabdomyolysis.
- Other possible features:
  - Arrhythmias, cardiomyopathy or myocardial infarction
  - Electrolyte abnormalities
  - Acute renal/hepatic failure
  - Hypercarbic respiratory failure from chest wall rigidity
  - Coagulopathies and DIC.

Diagnosis and evaluation

- NMS is a clinical diagnosis. Remember the **FEVER** mnemonic: **f**ever, **e**ncephalopathy, **v**ital sign instability, **e**levated enzymes (CPK), **r**igidity.
- Medication history is crucial to make the diagnosis.
- Sepsis, encephalitis, or meningitis should be in the differential diagnosis of all these patients and a sepsis workup will likely be necessary.
- Consider computed tomography (CT) of the brain as well as lumbar puncture if the diagnosis is not certain.

Critical management

- Discontinue the offending drug.
- Initiate cooling measures.
- Administer sedation and muscle relaxation using benzodiazepines.
- Neuromuscular blockade can be used for refractory hyperthermia or for airway management.
- Assess for rhabdomyolysis and manage electrolyte abnormalities.
- Bromocriptine has central dopaminergic agonist effects and can be used in patients with refractory symptoms. It is only available as an oral formulation and therefore a nasogastric tube will have to be placed for administration if the patient is intubated or at risk for aspiration. It is given in doses of 2.5–5 mg PO every 4–12 hours.

Serotonin syndrome

Overview

- Serotonin syndrome is caused by excessive stimulation of serotonin receptors.
- It is usually precipitated by medication changes such as:
  - Addition of a new serotonergic agent
  - Increase in dosage of usual medications
  - Overdose.

Presentation

Classic/critical presentation

- **Classic triad**
  - Cognitive effects: altered mental status, agitation, delirium, hallucinations
  - Autonomic effects: hyperthermia, shivering, sweating, hypertension, tachycardia, nausea, vomiting, diarrhea
  - Somatic effects: hyperreflexia, and clonus (more prominent in the lower extremities).
- **Other abnormalities**
  - Rhabdomyolysis
  - Acute renal failure
  - Seizures
  - Coagulopathies and DIC.

Diagnosis and evaluation

- The Hunter criteria (Table 64.1) can help make the diagnosis of serotonin syndrome. To meet the Hunter criteria, a patient must have recently taken a serotonergic agent and meet one of the criteria presented in the table.
- Patients usually present with clonus that is more prominent in the lower extremities. This clinical finding as well as certain historical clues can help to differentiate serotonin syndrome from neuroleptic malignant syndrome (see Table 64.2).
- Sepsis, encephalitis, or meningitis should be in the differential diagnosis of all these patients. A sepsis workup should be initiated.
- Consider computed tomography of the brain as well as lumbar puncture.

Critical management

- Discontinue the offending drug.
- Initiate cooling measures as described above.
- Patients should be supported with intravenous fluids aimed at treating dehydration and normalizing vital signs.

Table 64.1. Hunter criteria

Spontaneous clonus
Inducible clonus *plus* agitation or diaphoresis
Ocular clonus *plus* agitation or diaphoresis
Tremor *plus* hyperreflexia
Hypertonia *plus* temperature above 38°C *plus* ocular clonus or inducible clonus

Table 64.2. Serotonin syndrome (SS) vs. neuroleptic malignant syndrome (NMS)

	SS	NMS
Onset	24 hours	Days to weeks
Precipitating medications	Serotonergic agents (e.g., SSRIs, MAOIs, meperidine, linezolid, psychoactive drugs of abuse)	Antipsychotics (e.g., phenothiazines, butyrophenones, thioxanthines)
Mechanism of action	Stimulation of serotonin receptors	Dopamine blockade
Neuromuscular abnormality	Clonus	Rigidity
Specific treatment	Cyproheptadine	Bromocriptine

MAOI, monoamine oxidase inhibitor. SSRI, selective serotonin re-uptake inhibitor.

- Benzodiazepines should be administered to help decrease motor tone.
- Assess for rhabdomyolysis and managed electrolyte abnormalities.
- Neuromuscular blockade can be used for refractory hyperthermia or for airway management.
- Cyproheptadine has nonspecific serotonin antagonism effects and can be used in patients with refractory symptoms. It is only available as an oral formulation and therefore a nasogastric tube will have to be placed for administration if the patient is intubated or at risk for aspiration.

Vasopressor of choice: Patients with hypotension associated with hyperthermia can exhibit either a hypodynamic state with low cardiac index, elevated central venous pressure, and hypotension, or a hyperdynamic state with decreased peripheral vascular resistance and hypotension. A clinical assessment of the patient complemented by an evaluation of the cardiac function by ultrasound will help determine whether the patient would benefit more from additional fluids, a vasopressor, or an inotrope.

REFERENCES

Becker JA, Stewart LK. Heat-related illness. *Am Fam Physician*. 2011; **83**: 1325–30.
Boyer EW, Shannon M. The serotonin syndrome. *N Engl J Med*. 2005; **352**: 1112–20.

Glazer JL. Management of heatstroke and heat exhaustion. *Am Fam Physician*. 2005; **71**: 2133–40.

Kenny GP, Yardley J, Brown C, *et al.* Heat stress in older individuals and patients with common chronic diseases. *CMAJ*. 2010; **182**: 1053–60.

Khosla R, Guntupalli KK. Heat-related illnesses. *Crit Care Clin*. 1999; **15**: 251–63.

Marom T, Itskoviz D, Lavon H, *et al.* Acute care for exercise-induced hyperthermia to avoid adverse outcome from exertional heat stroke. *J Sport Rehabil*. 2011; **20**: 219–27.

65

Hypothermia

Viral Patel

Introduction

- Hypothermia is defined as a core temperature below 35°C.
- The body responds acutely to cold by increasing muscle tone, shivering, vaso-constriction, and behavioral changes.
- In addition, the hypothalamus increases TSH production causing an increased metabolic rate.
- In healthy patients, the body's compensatory mechanisms are overwhelmed by exposure.
- Age, health, nutrition, intoxication and medications can interfere with adequate thermoregulation.
- The human body produces approximately 250 joules (60 kcal) per m^2 of body surface area per hour.
  - Shivering, food ingestion, muscular tone, activity, fever, and acute cold exposure can increase this rate.
  - Once glycogen stores are depleted, thermoregulatory mechanisms become overwhelmed.

Presentation

Classic presentation

- Mild – from 32 to 35°C:
  - Peripheral vasoconstriction
  - Shivering

Practical Emergency Resuscitation and Critical Care, ed. Kaushal Shah, Jarone Lee, Kamal Medlej, and Scott D. Weingart. Published by Cambridge University Press. © Kaushal Shah, Jarone Lee, Kamal Medlej, and Scott D. Weingart 2013.

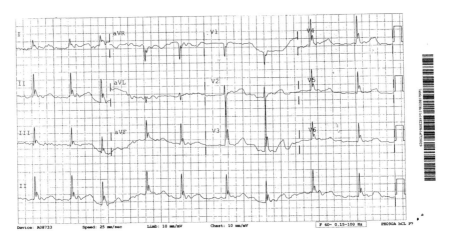

Figure 65.1. ECG of a patient with hypothermia and Osborn waves.

- Increased metabolic rate
- Normal blood pressure.

Critical presentation

- Moderate – from 28 to 32°C:
  - Stupor, apathy
  - The likelihood of dysrhythmias increases most commonly atrial fibrilation
  - The electrocardiogram (ECG) can show J-waves (Osborn waves; Figure 65.1)
  - Progressive decrease in pulse, respiration and cardiac output.
- Severe – less than 28°C:
  - Higher likelihood of ventricular fibrillation (VF)
  - Decrease in O_2 consumption, heart rate, cerebellar blood flow
  - Loss of reflexes and voluntary motion
  - Acid–base disturbances
  - Unresponsive to painful stimuli.

Diagnosis and evaluation

- Confirm hypothermia with rectal thermometer, indwelling Foley with temperature sensor, or other means of core temperature measurement.
- In general, hypothermia is a clinical diagnosis. However, laboratory tests may be helpful to look for an underlying condition that caused a patient to become hypothermic. For example, it may be the patient had a stroke or myocardial infarction and fell into a snow bank.

- Laboratory studies: complete blood count (CBC), metabolic panel, coagulation profile
- ECG
- Chest radiograph
- Depending on the clinical situation: cardiac enzymes, serial blood gases, cultures, computed tomography (CT) of the head, additional imaging.

Critical management

- **Initial management** should focus on resuscitation, rewarming, and fluid expansion
  - *Basic steps:*
    - Secure the airway.
    - Remove wet clothing.
    - Intravenous (IV) access.
    - Cardiac monitoring, temperature monitoring.
  - *Rewarming:*
    - Passive external rewarming.
    - Active internal rewarming is indicated only in severe cases:
      - Cardiovascular instability.
      - Temperature below 32.2°C.
      - Can use gastrointestinal, bladder, peritoneal, pleural, and/or mediastinal lavage in severe cases.
  - *Fluids:*
    - Start with 500 mL of D5 in 0.9% normal saline fluid challenge until laboratory results are available
- Watch for signs of **core temperature afterdrop:**
  - Thought to occur when cold blood from the extremities returns to central circulation as peripheral vessels dilate during the rewarming process.
- Correct any **unstable cardiac rhythms:**
  - Usually atrial fibrillation and atrial flutter will resolve upon rewarming.
  - Ventricular fibrillation can occur and is usually refractory until the patient is warmed, but one defibrillation attempt is recommended.
- Vasopressor support should be initiated as needed for **hypotension.**
- **Other treatments:** Cardiopulmonary bypass has been used in some cases of severe hypothermia to rewarm patients and provide circulatory support.
- **Disposition:** All patients with moderate to severe symptomatic hypothermia should be admitted to the hospital for rewarming and observation. Patients with mild hypothermia who are otherwise healthy can be rewarmed in the emergency department.

Sudden deterioration

- Hypothermic patients that are deteriorating will need to have their airway managed. There is no contraindication to performing rapid sequence induction (RSI) with the usual drug regimen in these patients.
- Patients who develop pulseless arrhythmias secondary to shockable rhythms should be managed according to advanced cardiac life support guidelines. While CPR should be initiated promptly, drug boluses should be avoided unless the patient is in asystole, and defibrillation should be attempted only once until the patient has been rewarmed to more than 30°C.

Vasopressor of choice: norepinephrine.

REFERENCES

Cline DM. *Tintinalli's Emergency Medicine Manual.* 7th edn. New York: McGraw Hill; 2012.

Marx JA, Hockberger RS, Walls RM, Adams J, Rosen P, eds. *Rosen's Emergency Medicine: Concepts and Clinical Practice.* 7th edn. Philadelphia, PA: Mosby Elsevier; 2010.

McCullough L, Arora S. Diagnosis and treatment of hypothermia. *Am Fam Physician.* 2004; **70**: 2325–32.

Mulcahy A, Watts M. Accidental hypothermia: an evidence based approach. *Emerg Med Pract.* 2009; **11**: 1.

Sawamoto K, Tanno K, Takeyama Y, Asai Y. Successful treatment of severe accidental hypothermia with cardiac arrest for a long time using cardiopulmonary bypass – report of a case. *Int J Emerg Med.* 2012; **5**: 9.

66

Overdoses

Daniel Herbert-Cohen and Daniel J. Lepp

Introduction

- Many common medications are toxic when taken at higher dosages.
- Ingestions can be accidental or a suicidal gesture.
- Patients with intentional ingestions are often unreliable historians. It is very important to get additional history from family, friends, or emergency medical services personnel with regard to observed and reported behavior, medication history, or empty pill bottles found at the scene.
- History and physical examination are crucial to establish a diagnosis and to guide treatment.
- Co-ingestions are common in intentional overdoses.
- Urine toxicology screens do not pick up the drugs most commonly used in the setting of overdose, are notoriously inaccurate, and do not add much to the toxicological workup of a patient.
- Patients may become critically ill if not promptly assessed, and the appropriate antidote given.
- This chapter will cover a selection of drug overdoses such as acetaminophen, aspirin, tricyclic antidepressants, beta-blockers, calcium channel blockers, and digoxin.

Acetaminophen

Overview

- Acetaminophen (APAP) is the most common medication overdose reported to poison control centers in the United States.

Practical Emergency Resuscitation and Critical Care, ed. Kaushal Shah, Jarone Lee, Kamal Medlej, and Scott D. Weingart. Published by Cambridge University Press. © Kaushal Shah, Jarone Lee, Kamal Medlej, and Scott D. Weingart 2013.

- It is responsible for the highest number of toxicological fatalities every year, and the leading cause of acute liver failure in the United States.
- APAP is a common co-ingestant.
- It is rapidly absorbed, but large overdoses may delay absorption.
- The peak plasma concentration is usually detected within 4 hours of ingestion.
- The majority is metabolized by the liver into harmless conjugates that are excreted in the urine.
- A small percentage is metabolized by cytochrome P450 into a highly toxic metabolite called NAPQI (N-acetyl-p-benzoquinone imin), which is then reduced to nontoxic conjugates by glutathione.
- In overdose, normal metabolic pathways are saturated and glutathione is depleted, resulting in NAPQI accumulation and subsequent hepatocellular damage.

Presentation

Classic presentation
- During phase 1 (0–24 hours from ingestion), patients can be asymptomatic, or present with mild gastrointestinal upset (nausea, vomiting, and anorexia) or general malaise.
- During phase 2 (24–72 hours after ingestion), patients usually develop right upper quadrant (RUQ) abdominal pain. Serum transaminase levels are continuously rising at this point, and tachycardia and hypotension can be present as well.

Critical presentation
- Critical symptoms generally appear during phase 3 (72–96 hours after ingestion).
- Hepatic necrosis and failure can lead to a number of clinical manifestations:
  - Jaundice
  - Encephalopathy
  - Coagulopathy and hemorrhage
  - Hypoglycemia
  - Acute renal failure
  - Metabolic acidosis
  - Multi-organ failure
  - Sepsis
  - Acute respiratory distress syndrome (ARDS)
  - Cerebral edema.

Diagnosis and evaluation

- A thorough history is imperative. The time of ingestion and amount of drugs taken is critically important.

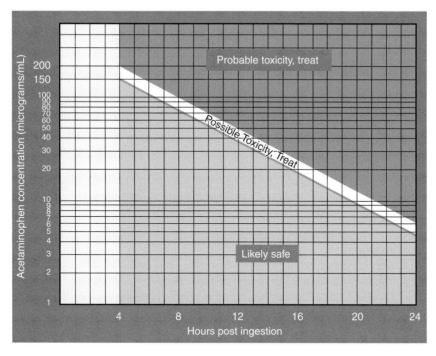

Figure 66.1. Rumack–Matthew nomogram. (Courtesy of Graham Walker, MD.)

- Examination findings such as RUQ tenderness, jaundice, altered mental status or unstable vital signs suggest a late presentation.
- Acetaminophen level:
  - Plot on the Rumack–Matthew nomogram (Figure 66.1).
  - 150 mg/kg is considered a toxic dose.
- Liver enzymes (ALT, AST), bilirubin, and prothrombin time (PT):
  - Should initially be normal but will rise over time as liver injury develops.
- Imaging has a limited role:
  - Chest radiography if ARDS or other pulmonary process is suspected.
  - It is possible to see some radiopaque co-ingestants on plain abdominal films, but this is nonspecific.
  - If the patient is demonstrating signs of encephalopathy, consider a computed tomography (CT) head scan.
- The electrocardiogram (ECG) is expected to be normal but remains an important screening tool.
- Pregnancy status must be established as acetaminophen freely crosses the placenta.

Critical management

- Activated charcoal can be given as a gastric decontaminant:
  - It is most effective if given in the first hour.
  - It can absorb co-ingestants as well.
  - It is harmful if aspirated. The patient must be alert and cooperative.
- Gastric lavage is rarely indicated.
  - It can be considered in cases of recent highly toxic co-ingestions.
- N-Acetylcysteine (NAC) is life saving if given early enough.
  - Draw an acetaminophen level and plot it on the nomogram if the time of ingestion is known.
    - Note that the nomogram starts at 4 hours post ingestion. Levels drawn earlier than this will generally not be helpful to guide treatment.
  - Begin treatment if the level is above the treatment line on the nomogram.
  - Preparing the appropriate NAC infusion should be done after discussion with a pharmacist.
  - N-Acetylcysteine has been shown to completely reverse the effect of an acetaminophen overdose if administered within 8 hours after the ingestion. It still offers protective effects up to 24 hours after ingestion although the success rate decreases proportionally to the delay.
  - If a patient presents at 8 hours or later after a toxic ingestion, do not delay treatment while waiting for an acetaminophen level.
  - NAC can be given orally or intravenously (IV).
    - Oral NAC can cause nausea and vomiting, making its administration sometimes difficult.
    - IV NAC can rarely cause anaphylactoid reactions.
    - The intravenous route has not been shown to be superior to the oral regimen, but intravenous treatment is usually preferred.
  - Therapy is discontinued once acetaminophen metabolism is complete (level <10 micrograms/mL) and liver injury is resolving (normal or near normal enzymes, absence of encephalopathy or coagulopathy).
- Some patients with severe overdoses and meeting certain criteria may be candidates for liver transplantation. Various scoring systems exist to help decide which patients should be referred to a liver transplantation center:
  - King's College Criteria (Table 66.1)
  - Lactic acidosis >3.5 mg/dL after early fluid resuscitation
  - Phosphorus >3.75 mg/dL at 48 hours
  - Apache II score >15.

Sudden deterioration

- These patients can develop sepsis with multi-organ failure.
  - Initiate hemodynamic support with intravenous fluids and vasopressors or inotropes as per the early goal-directed therapy protocol.

Table 66.1. King's College Criteria

pH <7.30 *or all three* of the following:
  INR >6.5 (PTT >100 seconds)
  Creatinine >3.4 mg/dL
  Grade 3 or 4 hepatic encephalopathy

- Respiratory support with oxygen, noninvasive ventilation, or intubation may be required.
- ARDS should be managed by endotracheal intubation and ventilator settings in accordance with the ARDSNet guidelines.
- Patients with evidence of renal failure should have their electrolytes checked and corrected. Hemodialysis may have to be initiated after consultation with a nephrologist.
- Cerebral edema and herniation are very difficult to treat successfully. Mannitol, hypertonic saline, or cranial decompression can be attempted in the rapidly decompensating patient.

Aspirin

Overview

- Aspirin (acetylsalicylic acid, ASA) is a weak acid that is widely used and is present in many mixed preparations.
- It is rapidly absorbed in its uncharged, nonionized form, in the acidic environment of the stomach.
- In nontoxic ingestions, the majority of the salicylate is protein-bound and free salicylate is mostly ionized.
- In overdose, albumin becomes saturated and free salicylate concentration increases:
  - As acidosis worsens, more salicylate exists in nonionized form.
  - This crosses into tissues and exerts toxicity, especially in the central nervous system (CNS).
- Aspirin is normally metabolized by the liver through conjugation.
  - In overdose, enzymes become saturated and renal elimination becomes important.

Presentation

Classic presentation
- May be asymptomatic
- Tinnitus or impaired hearing

- Hyperventilation
- Nausea and vomiting
- Hyperthermia
- Dehydration
- Mixed acid–base disturbance:
  - Respiratory alkalosis from direct stimulation of the medulla
  - Anion gap metabolic acidosis from uncoupling of oxidative phosphorylation.

Critical presentation
- Cerebral edema resulting in altered mental status, coma, convulsions
- Pulmonary edema
- Coagulopathy
- Acute renal failure
- Gastrointestinal (GI) hemorrhage
- Severe acid–base imbalance.

Diagnosis and evaluation

- A good history is critical, including the amount of drug taken and the time of ingestion.
- Early signs usually include tinnitus, nausea, and vomiting.
- On examination the patient may be hyperthermic, tachycardic, hyperpneic, diaphoretic, and confused.
- A salicylate level should be ordered even though it does not always correlate with toxicity.
- Electrolytes should be checked specifically for renal function and potassium level:
  - Renal failure will prevent elimination of salicylates.
  - Hypokalemia will hinder urinary alkalinization.
- Arterial or venous blood gas to monitor pH.
- Lactic acid concentration.
- Always check an acetaminophen level in any suspected toxic overdose as co-ingestion is common.

Critical management

- Activated charcoal should be given as gastric decontaminant.
  - It can absorb co-ingestants as well.
  - It is harmful if aspirated. The patient should be alert and cooperative.
- Gastric emptying with lavage can be considered in early presentations of massive overdoses.

- Aggressive fluid resuscitation is indicated as most patients are hypovolemic due to vomiting, tachypnea, and hyperthermia.
- Airway management:
  - Although endotracheal intubation may be necessary for airway protection, attempt to avoid intubation if possible as it is difficult for the ventilator to maintain as high a minute ventilation as a tachypneic person.
  - The patient may not tolerate even a brief episode of apnea if severely acidemic.
  - Consider awake intubation.
  - If awake intubation is not possible, consider a sodium bicarbonate bolus with 100 mEq of sodium bicarbonate prior to the initiation of rapid sequence intubation.
- Ventilator settings:
  - These patients are usually acidemic and will require a high minute ventilation to compensate for the metabolic acidosis.
  - An arterial or venous blood gas should be drawn 10–15 minutes after intubation and the tidal volume and respiratory rates should be adjusted to achieve a $PaCO_2$ of 35–40 mmHg.
- Urinary alkalinization is the mainstay of therapy.
  - It is achieved by administering a sodium bicarbonate bolus followed by a drip:
    - Bolus 1–2 mEq/kg IV.
    - Prepare a drip by mixing three ampules (50 mEq each) of sodium bicarbonate in 1 liter of D5W. Run at twice the maintenance rate.
    - Titrate to a urine pH >7.5.
    - Consider adding 40 mEq of potassium chloride to fluids.
    - Do not mix the sodium bicarbonate into normal saline or the solution will be hypertonic.
  - Alkaline urine will trap salicylate ions and allow for excretion.
  - Alkalinization of serum relative to CSF will prevent transfer of salicylate into the brain.
  - Maintain normal potassium levels by repleting if necessary as hypokalemia will prevent the excretion of acid into the urine.
- Serial salicylate levels should be checked to monitor therapy effects.
  - Continue therapy until the levels are at or below 30 mg/dL.
  - Concretions of aspirin may exist in the GI tract and cause a delayed peak of salicylate level.
- Hemodialysis is the definitive treatment:
  - Treats acid–base disturbances and removes salicylate from blood.

- Indications for hemodialysis in aspirin overdose

  - End-organ damage such as altered mental status, acute lung injury, or coagulopathy
  - Renal failure resulting in the inability to eliminate the drug
  - Inability to tolerate the necessary fluid load for alkalinization
  - Refractory acidemia
  - Absolute serum concentrations >100 mg/dL in acute ingestions, or 60 mg/dL in chronic ingestions
  - Clinical deterioration despite alkalinization and other supportive management

Sudden deterioration

- Decline in mental status, coma, or seizure can be caused by cerebral edema.
  - Any alteration in mental status should lead to consideration for hemodialysis.
- Fluid overload can result in pulmonary edema and respiratory failure.
  - Dialysis should be initiated in patients that are not able to tolerate the fluid load necessary for urine alkalinization.
  - Intubation may be necessary and should be done early before the development of severe acidemia.
- Patients with salicylate overdose are also at risk of life-threatening GI bleeding and administration of blood product should be initiated in those patients.

Tricyclic antidepressants

Overview

- Tricyclic antidepressants (TCAs) are mostly used for the treatment of neuropathic and chronic pain.
- TCAs are rapidly absorbed in the GI tract.
- They have multiple physiological effects.
  - Sodium channel blockade:
    - Type Ia (quinidine-like) dysrhythmic effect: blocks fast inward sodium channels at phase 0 of myocyte depolarization.
    - Decreases conduction with QRS prolongation.
    - Negative inotropy.
  - Anticholinergic effect: mental status changes, seizures, coma.
  - Alpha-1 adrenergic blockade: vasodilation, hypotension.
  - Antihistamine effect: sedation.
  - Serotonin, norepinephrine, and dopamine reuptake inhibition:
    - Antidepressant effect at therapeutic doses.
    - In overdose, transient hypertension is followed by hypotension and bradycardia as catecholamines are depleted.

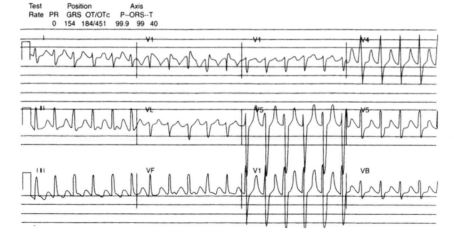

Test	Position	Axis
Rate PR	GRS OT/OTc	P--ORS--T
0 154	184/451	99.9 99 40

Figure 66.2. Classic ECG changes after TCA overdose: sinus tachycardia, QRS duration >100 milliseconds, right axis deviation, terminal R wave in aVR (or S wave in I or aVL).

- Also contributes to agitation and seizures.
- Death is most often due to refractory hypotension and cardiovascular collapse.

Presentation

Classic/critical presentation
- Anticholinergic effects initially predominate:
  - Sinus tachycardia, hypertension, agitation, pupillary dilation, dry and flushed skin, hyperthermia.
- QRS complex widening on ECG with terminal R wave in lead aVR.
- Rapid deterioration usually occurs within 30–60 minutes of presentation.
- Altered mental status, coma, seizures.
- Ventricular dysrhythmias.
- Hypotension.

Diagnosis and evaluation

- The diagnosis is made based on history, clinical presentation and ECG findings (Figure 66.2).
- A dose of >10 mg/kg of most TCAs is considered life-threatening.
- ECG findings:
  - The most common findings are sinus tachycardia and a right axis deviation.
  - QRS prolongation (>100 milliseconds):
    - <100 milliseconds: no significant toxicity.
    - >100 milliseconds: 30% will have seizures.

- >160 milliseconds: 60% will have ventricular dysrhythmias.
- Rightward deviation of the terminal 40 milliseconds of QRS.
  - Lead aVR: large (>3 mm) terminal R wave or R/S ratio >0.7.
- Quantitative and qualitative tests for TCAs are not helpful in the acute management.

Critical management

- Airway management: early intubation for depressed consciousness and airway protection.
- GI decontamination:
  - Orogastric lavage, preferably if ingestion occurred less than 1 hour prior to presentation.
  - Activated charcoal can be used as well within the first hour.
- Sodium bicarbonate: if QRS >100 milliseconds.
  - Provides sodium load and serum alkalinization leading to improved myocyte conduction.
  - 1–2 mEq/kg boluses until QRS narrows or arterial pH is 7.50–7.55.
  - Once QRS narrows, start a drip at 2–3 times maintenance (by adding three ampules of 50 mEq/ampule sodium bicarbonate to 1 liter of D5W).
  - If QRS fails to narrow with bicarbonate or pH >7.55, consider hyperventilation and hypertonic saline.
- Management of seizures:
  - Intravenous lorazepam or diazepam are first-line agents for seizures and agitation.
  - Phenobarbital and diprivan can be used for refractory seizures.
  - Avoid phenytoin due to sodium channel blockade and increased risk of ventricular dysrhythmias.
- Management of hypotension:
  - Intravenous crystalloids.
  - Sodium bicarbonate increases inotropy and intravascular volume.
  - Norepinephrine for refractory hypotension.
  - Physostigmine is contraindicated due to increased risk of bradycardia and asystole.
- Management of arrhythmias:
  - Class IA (quinidine, procainamide, disopyramide, and moricizine) and class IC (flecainide, propafenone) antiarrhythmics are contraindicated as they have a similar mode of action as TCAs.
  - Lidocaine is most commonly advocated for the treatment of dysrhythmias refractory to treatment with sodium bicarbonate.
- Disposition:
  - Intensive care unit (ICU) admission with at least 12 hours of bicarbonate therapy for any patient with:

- QRS >100 milliseconds
- Altered mental status
- Respiratory depression
- Seizure
- Dysrhythmia
- Hypotension.
- Patients who have had GI decontamination and remain asymptomatic with stable vital signs and normal ECGs may be medically cleared after 6 hours of monitoring.

Beta-blockers

Overview

- Beta-blockers are used as antihypertensives, antidysrhythmics, glaucoma agents, and for migraine prophylaxis.
- They are available as oral, intravenous, and ophthalmic preparations.
- They are rapidly absorbed and have rapid onset of action.
- Specific drugs vary in degree of selectivity for different β receptors:
  - Selective = β only.
  - Nonselective = β1 and β2.
- Some agents (e.g., labetalol, carvedilol) also have some alpha-adrenergic blockade.
- Effects of stimulation at beta-adrenergic receptors:
  - β1: increased heart rate, cardiac conduction, and contractility; increased renin release from kidneys; increased aqueous humor production.
  - β2: relaxation of smooth muscle (bronchi, blood vessels, GI tract, uterus); increased heart rate; increased glucose release (gluconeogenesis and glycogenolysis).
- In overdose, selectivity for beta receptors is lost and β1 and β2 effects are seen.
- Toxicity of various beta-blockers depends on:
  - *Cardioselectivity:* nonselective beta-blockers (e.g., propranolol) are associated with higher mortality than selective beta-blockers (e.g., metoprolol).
  - *Lipid solubility:* highly lipid-soluble beta-blockers (e.g., propranolol) are more toxic due to larger volumes of distribution and CNS permeability.
  - *Intrinsic sympathomimetic ability:* certain beta-blockers (e.g., pindolol, oxprenolol) have partial beta-agonist effect. At high doses, tachycardia and hypertension are more common and are relatively safe.
  - *Membrane stabilizing effect:* certain agents (e.g., propranolol, oxprenolol, acebutolol) have type Ia sodium channel blockade effect with resultant bradydysrhythmias and ventricular dysrhythmias.
- Propranolol accounts for the most fatalities of any beta-blocker.

Presentation (Table 66.2)

Table 66.2. Most common symptoms of beta-blocker overdose in order of frequency

Bradycardia
Hypotension
Unresponsiveness
Respiratory depression
Hypoglycemia
Seizures (with lipid-soluble agents)

Classic presentation
- May be mild or even asymptomatic, especially in young healthy patients.
- Bradycardia due to SA and AV nodal blockade.
- Hypoglycemia (more common in children).

Critical presentation
- Symptomatic bradycardia: hypotension, cardiogenic shock.
- Respiratory depression (bronchospasm is less common).
- Seizures, coma.

Diagnosis and evaluation

- Known access to these agents in the appropriate clinical setting should raise suspicion for beta-blocker overdose.
- An ECG should be performed to assess for bradydysrhythmias.
- Bedside blood sugar testing will rule out hypoglycemia.
- Laboratory studies are generally unhelpful.

Critical management

- ABCs:
  - Supplemental oxygen can be provided. Intubation may be needed for airway protection or respiratory depression.
  - 20–30 mL/kg of intravenous crystalloids should be administered if the patient is hypotensive.
- GI decontamination:
  - Activated charcoal: preferably given in the first hour but can be given later if the patient is not at risk for aspiration.
  - Whole-bowel irrigation (with polyethylene glycol): consider for all ingestions of sustained-release preparations.
- Glucagon:
  - Activates adenyl cyclase downstream from the beta receptor.

- Has chronotropic and inotropic effects.
- Can cause nausea and vomiting.
- Usually given as 3–5 mg IV push.
- Effect should be seen within minutes, but is usually inadequate on its own.
- Higher doses up to 10 mg IV can be given if no response is noted.
- An infusion can be started at the dose per hour at which the response was observed.
- In patients with high suspicion for beta-blocker overdose who do not respond to glucagon boluses, it is still recommended to initiate an infusion at 10 mg/hour.
- Atropine:
  - Given as 0.5 mg IV pushes.
  - May help with bradycardia but not hypotension.
- Calcium:
  - Administration of calcium can help improve the hypotension but will not have any effect on the bradycardia according to animal models.
  - 13–25 mEq of calcium gluconate or calcium chloride can be administered as slow boluses every 15–20 minutes up to 4 doses.
- High-dose insulin:
  - Beta-blocker toxicity shifts myocardial metabolism from free fatty acids to carbohydrates.
  - Insulin increases myocardial carbohydrate uptake.
  - Insulin also has inotropic and chronotropic effects.
  - *Dose:* begin with regular insulin 0.5–1 unit/kg and 0.25–0.5 g/kg dextrose IV push, followed by insulin 0.5–1 units/kg/hour with dextrose 0.5 g/kg/hour. Titrate to serum glucose of 5.55 mmol/L (100 mg/dL).
- Catecholamines:
  - They are reserved for patients not responding to other therapies.
  - Isoproterenol, epinephrine, norepinephrine, and dopamine can be used.
- Cardiac pacing:
  - Transcutaneous and transvenous pacing can be initiated but are often ineffective secondary to failure to capture.
- Phosphodiesterase inhibitors (e.g., amrinone, milrinone):
  - Inhibit cyclic AMP breakdown leading to increased inotropy and chronotropy.
  - They have undesired effect of causing smooth muscle relaxation and peripheral vasodilation.
- Lipid emulsion therapy:
  - May act as "lipid sink" aiding in the elimination of lipophilic drugs.
  - Provides a source of fatty acids to the myocardium and may therefore have an inotropic effect.
  - It consists of 20% soybean oil in water given as 1.5 mL/kg bolus followed by 15 mL/kg/hour infusion.
  - Dosing is not standardized and based on animal studies and case reports.

- Hemodialysis:
  - May be beneficial for beta-blockers with lower volumes of distribution and high hydrophilicity (e.g., atenolol, sotalol, nadolol, timolol).
- Sodium bicarbonate:
  - Can be used if signs of sodium channel blockade exist (e.g., QRS widening).
- Disposition:
  - Symptomatic patients should be admitted to the ICU.
  - Patients with ingestions of sustained-release preparations should be admitted for 24 hours to a monitored setting.
  - Patients with ingestions of regular-release preparations who received adequate GI decontamination and remain asymptomatic can be medically cleared after 6 hours.
    - Sotalol is an exception as it may cause serious prolonged toxicity.

Calcium channel blockers

Overview

- Calcium channel blockers inhibit calcium channels in:
  - The myocardium: decreased contractility, decreased SA node activity, decreased AV node conduction
  - Vascular smooth muscle: coronary and peripheral vasodilation.
- Dihydropyridine (e.g., amlodopine, nicardipine).
  - More specific to smooth muscle calcium channels.
- Nondihydropyridine (e.g., verapamil, diltiazem).
  - More specific to myocardial calcium channels.
- As with beta-blockers, selectivity is lost in overdose.
- Verapamil is the most toxic in overdose and accounts for most fatalities.

Presentation

Classic presentation
- Rapid onset of symptoms due to rapid GI absorption.
- Bradycardia.
- Reflex tachycardia may occur in dihydropyridine overdose.
- Hyperglycemia.

Critical presentation
- Symptomatic bradycardia, hypotension, and tissue ischemia.
- Cardiogenic shock.

Diagnosis and evaluation

- Mainly based on history and clinical presentation.
- ECG with normal intervals (except bepridil which prolongs QT interval).
- May be indistinguishable from beta-blocker overdose.
- Bedside blood sugar testing may show hyperglycemia.

Critical management

- ABCs:
  - Supplemental oxygen can be provided. Intubation may be needed for airway protection or respiratory depression.
  - 20–30 mL/kg of intravenous crystalloids should be administered if the patient is hypotensive.
- GI decontamination:
  - Activated charcoal: preferably in the first hour, but can be given later if the patient is not at risk for aspiration.
  - Whole-bowel irrigation (with polyethylene glycol): consider for all ingestions of sustained-release preparations.
- Glucagon:
  - Less effective than in beta-blocker overdose because the effect on cAMP is upstream from the calcium channel blockade.
- Atropine:
  - Given as 0.5 mg IV pushes.
- Calcium:
  - Increases intracellular calcium influx.
  - Dose depends on type of calcium preparation used.
    - *Calcium chloride:*
      - 1 g contains 13.4 mEq calcium.
      - Initial dose is 10–20 mL of 10% solution (1–2 ampules).
      - Avoid in children and in peripheral IVs due to sclerosis of vessels.
    - *Calcium gluconate:*
      - 1 g contains 4.3 mEq calcium.
      - Initial dose is 30–60 mL of 10% solution (3–6 ampules).
  - Effect is often transient, which requires re-dosing.
    - Repeat boluses every 15 minutes to a maximum of 5 g before rechecking serum electrolytes.
  - Raise serum calcium levels to no higher than 14 mg/dL.
- High-dose insulin:
  - Calcium channel blocker toxicity shifts myocardial metabolism from free fatty acids to carbohydrates.
  - Insulin increases myocardial carbohydrate uptake.
  - Insulin also has inotropic and chronotropic effects.

- *Dose:* begin with regular insulin 0.5–1 unit/kg and 0.25–0.5 g/kg dextrose IV push, followed by insulin 0.5–1 units/kg/hour with dextrose 0.5 g/kg/hour. Titrate to serum glucose of 5.55 mmol/L 100 mg/dL.
- Catecholamines:
  - They are likely to be more effective with lower dose requirements than in beta-blocker overdose because adrenergic receptors are not blocked.
- Cardiac pacing:
  - Transcutaneous and transvenous pacing can be initiated but are often ineffective secondary to failure to capture.
- Phosphodiesterase inhibitors (e.g., amrinone, milrinone):
  - Inhibit cyclic AMP breakdown, leading to increased inotropy and chronotropy.
  - They have the undesired effect of causing smooth muscle relaxation and peripheral vasodilation.
- Lipid emulsion therapy:
  - May act as "lipid sink" aiding in the elimination of lipophilic drugs.
  - Provides a source of fatty acids to the myocardium and may therefore have an inotropic effect.
  - It consists of 20% soybean oil in water given as 1.5 mL/kg bolus followed by 15 mL/kg/hour infusion.
  - Dosing is not standardized and is based on animal studies and case reports.
- Disposition:
  - Symptomatic patients should be admitted to the ICU.
  - Patients with ingestions of sustained-release preparations should be admitted for 24 hours to a monitored setting.
  - Patients with ingestions of regular-release preparations who have received adequate GI decontamination and remain asymptomatic can be medically cleared after 6 hours.

Digoxin

Overview

- Digoxin is derived from the foxglove plant (*Digitalis purpurea*).
- Indications for use include congestive heart failure, and rate control in atrial fibrillation.
- Mechanism of action:
  - Increases vagal tone.
    - Leads to decreased SA node and AV node activity.
    - At toxic levels can lead to bradydysrhythmias.
  - Blocks sodium–potassium ATPase.
    - Ultimately leads to increased intracellular calcium in myocardium and increased contractility.

Table 66.3. Comparison of acute versus chronic digoxin overdose.

Acute	Chronic
Lower mortality	Higher mortality
Bradydysrhythmias more common	Ventricular dysrhythmias more common
Younger patients	Older patients
Serum potassium high or normal	Serum potassium low or normal

- At toxic levels enhances automaticity and may cause tachydysrhythmias.
- It has a relatively slow onset (1.5–6 hours) and long elimination half-life (30 hours).
- It can cause acute and chronic intoxication (Table 66.3).
- Mortality in chronic intoxication may be related to higher incidences of underlying heart disease.
- Digoxin toxicity is potentiated by:
  - Renal insufficiency
  - Underlying cardiac disease
  - Electrolyte abnormalities (e.g., hypokalemia, hypomagnesemia, hypercalcemia)
  - Other cardioactive medications (e.g., beta-blockers, calcium channel blockers)
  - Drugs that slow digoxin clearance (e.g., quinidine, quinine, macrolides).

Presentation

Classic presentation
- Gastrointestinal symptoms are most common, especially nausea and vomiting. Abdominal pain and diarrhea may also occur.
- CNS effects include headache, weakness, and lethargy.
- Yellow-green chromatopsia (objects appearing yellow and green) is classic, but photophobia, blurry vision, and other nonspecific visual disturbances are common as well.
- Hyperkalemia may occur due to sodium–potassium ATPase blockade.
- Digoxin can cause almost any arrhythmia but most commonly causes premature ventricular contractions (PVCs).

Critical presentation
- Digoxin toxicity can cause lethal ventricular dysrhythmias including ventricular tachycardia, torsades de pointes, and ventricular fibrillation.
- Bidirectional ventricular tachycardia is pathognomonic for digoxin toxicity.
- Hypokalemia, which may be seen in patients with chronic overdoses, predisposes to ventricular dysrhythmias.
- Delirium, hallucinations, and seizures may occur.

Diagnosis and evaluation

- Usually based on history of digoxin use or abuse with clinical symptomatology.
- The differential diagnosis is broad as many signs and symptoms are nonspecific.
- The ECG may show the classic "digitalis effect," comprising scooped, down-sloping ST depressions ("Salvador Dali mustache"). However, this effect is not a sign of toxicity.
- Serum digoxin levels can help confirm the diagnosis but are not entirely sensitive or specific for toxicity.
  - Patients may be toxic at therapeutic levels (especially in hypokalemia).
  - Patients may be asymptomatic at supratherapeutic levels.

Critical management

- Digoxin Immune Fab is the definitive antidotal therapy.
- Other treatments are either temporizing or for patients who do not meet indications for antidotal therapy.
- GI decontamination:
  - Activated charcoal binds digoxin well and should be used ideally within 1 hour of presentation.
  - Orogastric lavage is generally not recommended as it stimulates vagal tone and can worsen bradydysrhythmias.
- Electrolyte abnormalities:
  - *Hyperkalemia:*
    - Usually not clinically significant but is a predictor of mortality.
    - If severe, treat with insulin, glucose, sodium bicarbonate, sodium polystyrene.
    - Avoid calcium therapy until the antidote is given.
    - Calcium supplementation has traditionally been contraindicated in these patients because of fear of the development of life-threatening dysrhythmias. While recent studies have challenged this belief, the administration of calcium should still be performed cautiously and as a slow infusion over 30 minutes.
  - *Hypokalemia:*
    - In chronic intoxication, hypokalemia increases myocardial sensitivity to digoxin.
    - Replete the potassium to 3.5–4 mEq/L as it may help to treat tachydysrhythmias.
- Dysrhythmias:
  - *Bradydysrhythmias:*
    - Atropine can be used for severe bradycardia or high-degree AV block.

- Cardiac pacing:
  - Transcutaneous pacing is generally safe but its efficacy varies.
  - Transvenous pacing can trigger ventricular arrhythmias and should be avoided.
- *Tachydysrhythmias:*
  - Magnesium therapy:
    - May be effective even if serum magnesium levels are normal.
    - It is contraindicated in bradycardia or AV blocks.
  - Antidysrhythmics:
    - Amiodarone, phenytoin, and lidocaine can be used.
    - Avoid AV nodal blocking agents.
  - Electrical cardioversion:
    - Should be performed for ventricular fibrillation (VF) or pulseless ventricular tachycardia (VT).
    - Avoid in other tachydysrhythmias as it can precipitate VT, VF, or asystole.
- Digoxin-specific Fab fragments:
  - The mainstay of treatment as it is safe and highly effective.
  - Derived from sheep immunized with digoxin.
  - Bind intravascular digoxin and prevent it from binding to its sites of action on target cells.
    - Free digoxin levels drop rapidly upon administration.
    - Most laboratory assays measure both bound and free digoxin; thus, levels may stay elevated for up to a week despite adequate treatment.
  - Fab therapy is generally reserved for serious cardiotoxicity rather than routine treatment of elevated serum levels.
  - *Indications for use:*
    - Ventricular dysrhythmias.
    - Bradydysrhythmias not responding to atropine.
    - Serum potassium >5 mEq/L.
    - Acute ingestion of >10 mg in adults and >4 mg in children.
    - Acute ingestion with steady state digoxin level >10 ng/mL.
    - Co-ingestion of other cardiotoxic medications.
  - *Dosing:*
    - One vial contains enough Fab fragments to bind 0.5 mg of digoxin.
    - Empiric dosing:
      - 10 vials for acute ingestion.
      - 20 vials in cardiac arrest.
    - If the dose ingested is known:
      - Numbers of vials = (mg digoxin ingested × 0.8)/0.5.
    - If the steady-state serum digoxin concentration (ng/mL) is known:
      - Numbers of vials = (digoxin concentration × patient weight in kg)/100
- Disposition:
  - Symptomatic patients should be admitted for cardiac monitoring.

- Patients with arrhythmias and patients treated with Fab therapy should be admitted to the ICU.
- Patients with suspected toxicity who remain asymptomatic after 6 hours of monitoring and whose repeat digoxin levels are not trending upward may be medically cleared.

REFERENCES

Boehnert MT, Lovejoy FH. Value of the QRS duration versus the serum drug level in predicting seizures and ventricular dysrhythmias after an acute overdose of tricyclic antidepressants. *N Engl J Med.* 1985; **313**: 474–9.

Levine M, Nikkanen H, Pallin DJ. The effects of intravenous calcium in patients with digoxin toxicity. *J Emerg Med.* 2011; **40**: 41–6.

Marx JA, Hockberger RS, Walls RM, Adams J, Rosen P, eds. *Rosen's Emergency Medicine: Concepts and Clinical Practice.* 7th edn. Philadelphia, PA: Mosby Elsevier; 2010.

Nelson L, Lewin NA, Howland MA, Hoffman RS, Goldfrank LR, Flomenbaum NE, eds. *Goldfrank's Toxicologic Emergencies.* New York: McGraw-Hill Medical; 2010.

Rumack BH, Matthew H. Acetaminophen poisoning and toxicity. *Pediatrics.* 1975; **55**: 871–6.

Smilkstein MJ, Knapp GL, Kulig KW, *et al.* Efficacy of oral N-acetylcysteine in the treatment of acetaminophen overdose. Analysis of the national multicenter study (1976 to 1985). *N Engl J Med.* 1988; **319**: 1557–62.

Tintinalli JE, Stapczynski JS, Cline DM, *et al.* eds. *Emergency Medicine: A Comprehensive Study Guide.* New York: McGraw-Hill Medical; 2011.

67

Care of the dying patient

Ashley Shreves

Introduction

- Palliative medicine focuses on maximizing the quality of life of patients with serious illnesses.
- For many patients in the critical care setting, the best medical treatments and technologies are unable to reverse advanced disease processes, as evidenced by the fact that 20% of Americans died in or after ICU care.
- Even when treatments can prolong life, they may not ultimately allow patients to achieve a quality of life acceptable to them. Functional and cognitive independence are highly valued by patients and yet most chronically, critically ill patients never live independently again.
- Honest, transparent, empathetic communication is the cornerstone of determining how to deliver effective, patient-centered medical care in this setting.
- When critical care interventions are no longer able to achieve the stated goals of the patient and family, transitioning away from life-prolonging care often makes the most sense, especially because these treatments can be burdensome and contribute to patient suffering.
- The "withdrawal" of life-sustaining treatments like ventilatory support and hemodialysis often signify to the medical staff and family that the patient has entered the dying process.
- Care of the dying patient is complex as patients and families have intense emotional, spiritual, psychosocial, and medical needs.

Practical Emergency Resuscitation and Critical Care, ed. Kaushal Shah, Jarone Lee, Kamal Medlej, and Scott D. Weingart. Published by Cambridge University Press. © Kaushal Shah, Jarone Lee, Kamal Medlej, and Scott D. Weingart 2013.

- While optimizing comfort through effective symptom-based therapies is essential, high-quality end-of-life care typically extends beyond these measures, involving an interdisciplinary team to tend to a wide range of needs that patients and families manifest.

Presentation

Classic presentation

- At the end-of-life, there are two classically described trajectories of dying:
  - *Easy road:* Decreased functionality marked by increasing time spent in bed and sleeping, with the patient eventually becoming comatose, followed by death.
  - *Difficult road:* Functional loss occurs but end-of-life symptoms are also pronounced, particularly terminal delirium, dyspnea, and pain.

Critical presentation

- Dying in the critical care setting most often follows the withholding or withdrawal of life-sustaining treatments and therefore has its own unique trajectory.
- Symptom burden and the dying trajectory vary widely depending on a multitude of factors such the underlying disease process, the severity of illness, and types of life-sustaining intervention being withdrawn.
- While the prevalence of distressing symptoms such as pain, discomfort, thirst, anxiety, and dyspnea are high in critically ill patients, high rates of comfort have been reported in those undergoing withdrawal of life-sustaining therapies.

Diagnosis and evaluation

- When critical care is no longer achieving patient-centered goals and/or the patient is dying despite aggressive use of life-sustaining therapy, a meeting should be held to determine the "goals of care."
- Many dying patients are sedated, comatose, or delirious and can no longer participate in medical decision-making; therefore, legally appropriate surrogate decision-makers should be identified.
- Previously completed advance directives, including the designation of a health care proxy, should be reviewed.
- Efforts should be made to gather all the important decision-makers in the patient's family and hold a meeting with the treatment team, ideally with members of the palliative care service present.

Table 67.1. The goal-setting conference

Ten-step guide	Tips/examples
Establish a proper setting	Quiet, appropriate parties invited, pagers turned off.
Introductions	"Can you tell me something about your mom?"
Assess patient/family understanding	"What have the doctors told you about your mom's condition?"
Medical review/summary	Start with a warning shot. Give small pieces of information. Avoid jargon. "I'm afraid I have some bad news. Your mom is dying."
Silence/reactions	"I wish we had better treatments for her disease." "I can only imagine how disappointed you must be." "You've been so devoted and loving to your mom."
Discuss prognosis	Assess the amount of information desired. Present prognostic data using ranges.
Assess goals	Not prolonging the dying process, a peaceful death, being surrounded by family? "If your mom could talk to us right now, what would she tell us is most important to her?"
Present broad options	"Based on what we've discussed and what you've told me about your mom, *I recommend* that we refocus our efforts on maximizing her comfort and not prolong her dying process."
Translate goals into care plan	"Maintaining your mom on life support does not seem consistent with what her wishes would be, therefore I'm recommending that we liberate her from the machine and allow her to have a natural death."
Document	Write DNR orders, discontinue and add appropriate therapies, give a new care plan.

Source: Adapted from Weissman DE. "The Family Goal Setting Conference" and "Communication Phrases Near the End of Life" pocket cards from Medical College of Wisconsin.

- Clear, compassionate, culturally sensitive language should be used to communicate the patient's overall prognosis and elicit previously expressed values, goals, and preferences.
- Many departments have protocolized this "goal-setting conference" (Table 67.1).
- If all agree that life-sustaining treatment is no longer able to achieve the patient's goals, an ideal plan often includes a transition to care that maximizes comfort and dignity while not prolonging the patient's dying process.

Critical management

- **Withdrawal of ventilator support** or "liberation from the ventilator": a common step preceding death in the ICU.
  - *Preparation:*
    - Ensure that "Do not resuscitate" (DNR)/"Do not intubate" (DNI) orders and paperwork are completed.
    - Ensure that the spiritual needs of patient and family are met, which may include completion of important religious rituals.
    - Chaplaincy or even physician instruction regarding end-of-life communication that expresses gratitude and forgiveness can be a helpful tool in allowing patients and families to achieve peace and closure (Table 67.2).
    - Discontinue unnecessary laboratory testing and therapies that are not supporting goals, such as artificial nutrition and hydration, vasopressors, and antibiotics.
  - *Premedication:*
    - Glycopyrrolate 0.2 mg every 6 hours to minimize respiratory secretions.
  - *Procedure:*
    - Turn off monitors as alarms will be distracting and the patient's visible signs of discomfort, rather than vital signs, should guide management.
    - The ETT can be easily removed after cuff deflation.
    - Adequate analgesia and sedative medications should be available, either through continuous drips that can be titrated for symptom control or in prefilled syringes that be delivered as IV pushes at the bedside.
    - *Dosing instructions:* for patients already on opiate and benzodiazepine infusions, bolus doses used for dyspnea should be approximately double the hourly infusion rate (i.e., if fentanyl is infusing at 100 micrograms/hour, the patient should receive 200-microgram boluses every 10–15 minutes until comfort is achieved).
    - Oxygen does not need to be administered as it might prolong the patient's dying process, and opiates can adequately palliate dyspnea.
    - *Goal:* no signs of respiratory distress and/or dyspnea, which would include gasping, accessory muscle use, or labored breathing.
  - *Prognosis:*
    - If desired, families should be informed regarding the estimated survival time once ventilator support is discontinued, as this allows for adequate preparation and planning. Prognostic estimates should be communicated as time frames: minutes to hours, hours to days, or days to weeks.
    - Once ventilator support is removed, the median time to survival is just under an hour, though some patients may survive for days. Predictors of shorter survival include such variables as multi-organ failure, use of vasopressors, and brain death.

Table 67.2. Six things to say before you die

1. I love you
2. Thank you
3. Please forgive me
4. I forgive you
5. Good-bye
6. I'm going to be okay

- **Other symptom considerations**
  - *Terminal delirium:*
    - This is common and easily treatable with antipsychotics.
    - Haldol 0.5–2 mg IV every 6 hours is an adequate dosing regimen for most patients.
  - *Pain:*
    - Pain is common in critically ill patients.
    - Dying patients are often sedated and/or unable to communicate, so nonverbal cues such as grimacing, moaning, and restlessness should be used.
    - Opiates are the mainstay treatment. Dilaudid is preferred over morphine in patients with renal or liver failure.
- **Other considerations**
  - *Transferring patients to the palliative care unit or inpatient hospice:*
    - Hospitals are increasingly incorporating palliative care and hospice units into their institutions. These can be ideal settings for transitions from LST to comfort-focused care.
  - *Improving the family's experience:*
    - Families rate factors such as "preparation for death"; timely, compassionate communication; care maintaining comfort, dignity, and personhood; open access and proximity of the family to the patient; interdisciplinary care; and bereavement support as highly important in the setting of a dying patient.
    - Surprisingly, families of patients who have died rather than survived in the ICU show higher satisfaction with the care delivered.

Special circumstances

- **Young children**
  - Family members of dying patients may include young children. Depending on their age and maturity, children will have varying abilities to process death and dying. Child life specialists and social workers can be incredibly valuable resources in facilitating communication and coping in this group.

- **Organ donation**
  - The local organ donor network should be contacted early and often for patients in whom the withdrawal of life-sustaining treatments is planned. Assumptions should never be made regarding the patient's suitability as a donor and/or the family's preferences regarding this option.

A helpful resource

The Center to Advance Palliative Care has created a website called **IPAL-ICU** (www.capc.org/ipal-icu) that is an invaluable resource for clinicians hoping to improve the practice of palliative care within the ICU setting.

REFERENCES

Angus DC, Barnato AE, *et al.* Use of intensive care at the end of life in the United States: an epidemiologic study. *Crit Care Med.* 2004; **32**: 638–43.

Camhi SL, Mercado AF, *et al.* Deciding in the dark: advance directives and continuation of treatment in chronic critical illness. *Crit Care Med.* 2009; **37**: 919–25.

Cooke CR, Hotchkin DL, *et al.* Predictors of time to death after terminal withdrawal of mechanical ventilation in the ICU. *Chest.* 2010; **138**: 289–97.

Kompanje EJ, van der Hoven B, *et al.* Anticipation of distress after discontinuation of mechanical ventilation in the ICU at the end of life. *Intensive Care Med.* 2008; **34**: 1593–9.

Mularski RA, Heine CE, *et al.* Quality of dying in the ICU: ratings by family members. *Chest.* 2005; **128**: 280–2.

Nelson JE, Puntillo KA, *et al.* In their own words: patients and families define high-quality palliative care in the intensive care unit. *Crit Care Med.* 2010; **38**: 808–18.

Prendergast TJ, Claessens MT, *et al.* A national survey of end-of-life care for critically ill patients. *Am J Respir Crit Care Med.* 1998; **158**: 1163–7.

Rocker GM, Heyland DK, *et al.* Most critically ill patients are perceived to die in comfort during withdrawal of life support: a Canadian multicentre study. *Can J Anaesth.* 2004; **51**: 623–30.

Wall RJ, Curtis JR, *et al.* Family satisfaction in the ICU: differences between families of survivors and nonsurvivors. *Chest.* 2007; **132**: 1425–33.

Index

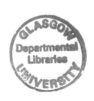